Being a Nursing Aide

second edition

Hospital Research
and
Educational Trust

Chicago, Illinois

ACKNOWLEDGMENTS

This edition of *Being a Nursing Aide* was prepared by **Rose Schniedman,** R.N., B.S., M.S. Ed., and **Susan Lambert,** M.A. Ed. For more than fifteen years, Mrs. Schniedman has directed the training of nursing aides for community hospitals in the Miami, Florida area; Mrs. Lambert is an education consultant currently specializing in adult and vocational education. The Trust gratefully acknowledges their wisdom, their perseverance and, above all, their dedication in completing this revision.

Deeply appreciated also are the contributions of the many reviewers and consultants in the fields of nursing service and education who gave so generously of their knowledge and experience to ensure the accuracy and quality of this book.

Special mention also must be made of the hundreds of instructors of nursing aide students who took the time to complete and return evaluation questionnaires in which they reported their experiences in using the first edition. Their comments and suggestions aided greatly in determining the form and content of this second edition.

PUBLISHED FOR HRET BY THE ROBERT J. BRADY CO. BOWIE, MARYLAND 20715.

Library of Congress Cataloging in Publication Data

Hospital Research and Educational Trust.
Being a Nursing Aide.

1. Nurses' aides.   2.   Care of the sick.
I. Title.
RT84. H67   1978   610.73   78-13512
ISBN 0-87914-050-X

Prentice-Hall International, Inc., London
Prentice-Hall of Australia, Pty., Ltd., Sydney
Prentice-Hall of India Private Limited, New Delhi
Prentice-Hall of Japan, Inc., Tokyo
Prentice-Hall of Southeast Asia (Pte.) Ltd., Singapore
Whitehall Books, Limited, Wellington, New Zealand
Printed in the United States of America

79 80 81 82   10 9 8 7 6 5 4 3

CONTENTS

LIST OF PROCEDURES   vii

INTRODUCTION   xi

1   ORIENTATION TO HEALTH CARE INSTITUTIONS   1

SECTION 1: THE HEALTH CARE INSTITUTION   1
Nursing Personnel   2
SECTION 2: YOUR JOB AS A NURSING AIDE   5
The Nursing Aide: An Important Person   8
Being a Successful Nursing Aide   13
Incidents   14

2   INTRODUCTION TO THE PATIENT   17

SECTION 1: THE PATIENTS YOU WILL CARE FOR   17
SECTION 2: COMMUNICATION   23
SECTION 3: OBSERVING THE PATIENT   31

3   INFECTION CONTROL IN THE HEALTH CARE INSTITUTION   39

SECTION 1: MEDICAL ASEPSIS   39
SECTION 2: THE PATIENT IN ISOLATION   50
Isolation Gowns   55
Personal Care of the Patient in Isolation   59

4   YOUR WORKING ENVIRONMENT   63

SECTION 1: THE PATIENT'S UNIT AND EQUIPMENT   63
SECTION 2: BEDMAKING   70
The Closed Bed   73
The Open Bed, Fan-Folded Bed, Empty Bed   80
The Operating Room Bed   82
The Occupied Bed   84
SECTION 3: SAFETY AND FIRE PREVENTION   89

5   LIFTING, MOVING, AND TRANSPORTING PATIENTS   95

SECTION 1: BODY MECHANICS   95
Lifting and Moving Patients   97
SECTION 2: TRANSPORTING A PATIENT   110
Transporting a Patient by Wheelchair   111
Using A Stretcher   119

6   PERSONAL CARE OF THE PATIENT   123

SECTION 1: DAILY CARE OF THE PATIENT   123
Schedule of Daily Care   123

Oral Hygiene   **124**

Helping the Patient To Bathe   **130**

Changing the Patient's Gown   **143**

Shampooing the Patient's Hair   **145**

Combing the Patient's Hair   **148**

Shaving the Patient's Face   **149**

Giving the Bedpan or Urinal   **151**

SECTION   2:   PREVENTING DECUBITUS ULCERS
                (BEDSORES)   **158**

7   FOOD SERVICE   **163**

SECTION   1:   THERAPEUTIC DIETS   **163**

Regular and Special Diets   **165**

SECTION   2:   NUTRITION FOR THE PATIENT   **165**

Preparing the Patient and Serving a Meal   **167**

Feeding the Helpless Patient   **170**

Between-Meal Nourishments   **174**

Passing Drinking Water   **175**

8   INTAKE AND OUTPUT   **178**

SECTION   1:   FLUID BALANCE   **177**

SECTION   2:   FLUID INTAKE   **179**

Measuring Fluid Intake   **182**

SECTION   3:   FORCING AND RESTRICTING FLUIDS   **183**

Force Fluids   **183**

Restrict Fluids   **184**

Nothing by Mouth   **185**

SECTION   4:   FLUID OUTPUT   **186**

Measuring Fluid Output   **186**

Plastic Urine Container   **187**

9   SPECIMEN COLLECTION   **189**

Asepsis in Specimen Collection   **191**

Routine Urine Specimen   **191**

Midstream Clean-Catch Urine Specimen   **193**

24-Hour Urine Specimen   **195**

Sputum Specimen   **197**

Stool Specimen   **199**

Straining the Urine   **200**

Testing for Sugar and Acetone   **202**

10   SPECIAL TREATMENTS   **209**

Rectal Treatments   **209**

The Oil Retention Enema   **216**

The Harris Flush (Return-Flow Enema)   **218**

Perineal Care   **225**

Daily Catheter Care   **226**

Care of the Patient's Artificial Eye   **227**

11   OBSERVING AND RECORDING VITAL SIGNS   **231**

SECTION 1:   VITAL SIGNS   **231**

SECTION 2:   MEASURING THE PATIENT'S
TEMPERATURE   **232**

Body Temperature   **233**

Taking a Rectal Temperature   **241**

SECTION 3:   TAKING A PULSE   **249**

The Apical Pulse and Pulse Deficit   **252**

SECTION 4:   COUNTING RESPIRATIONS   **253**

SECTION 5:   TAKING BLOOD PRESSURES   **255**

12   PATIENT ADMISSION, TRANSFER, AND
DISCHARGE   **263**

SECTION 1:   ADMITTING THE PATIENT   **263**

SECTION 2:   TRANSFERRING THE PATIENT   **268**

SECTION 3:   DISCHARGING THE PATIENT   **271**

13   PHYSICAL EXAMINATIONS, BODY POSITIONS, TUBES
AND TUBING   **275**

SECTION 1:   YOUR ROLE IN THE PHYSICAL
EXAMINATION   **275**

SECTION 2:   DRAPING AND POSITIONING THE PATIENT   **278**

SECTION 3:   CATHETERS, TUBES, AND TUBING   **283**

Intravenous (IV) Equipment   **284**

Nasogastric Tubes   **286**

Suction   **287**

Urinary Catheters   **289**

14   WARM AND COLD APPLICATIONS   **293**

Reasons for Warm and Cold Applications   **293**

Localized and Generalized Applications   **296**

The Alcohol Sponge Bath   **318**

15   PREOPERATIVE AND POSTOPERATIVE NURSING
CARE   **323**

SECTION 1:   PREOPERATIVE NURSING CARE   **323**

SECTION 2:   POSTOPERATIVE NURSING CARE   **333**

Deep-Breathing Exercises   **337**

SECTION 3:   BINDERS AND ELASTIC BANDAGES   **340**

16   CARE OF THE DYING PATIENT   **347**

SECTION 1:   CARE OF THE DYING PATIENT   **347**

SECTION 2:   POSTMORTEM CARE (PMC)   **352**

17   HUMAN ANATOMY AND PHYSIOLOGY   **357**

MEDICAL TERMINOLOGY: CONTINUING TO
LEARN   **397**

SECTION 1:   MEDICAL TERMINOLOGY-ABBREVIATIONS   **397**
  Abbreviations and Their Meanings   **397**
  Guide to Pronunciation   **401**
  Formulating Medical Terms   **413**
  Diseases and Diagnoses   **416**
  Surgical Procedures   **419**
  Medical Specialties   **420**
SECTION 2:   CONTINUING TO LEARN   **422**

WORDS TO REMEMBER   **425**
INDEX   **439**

LIST OF PROCEDURES

3 INFECTION CONTROL IN THE HEALTH CARE INSTITUTION

Handwashing   *49*

Mask Technique   *56*

Putting on an Isolation Gown in the Hall   *57*

Removing an Isolation Gown   *58*

4 YOUR WORKING ENVIRONMENT

Making the Closed Bed   *74*

Making the Open Fan-Folded Empty Bed   *81*

Making the OR Bed or Stretcher Bed   *82*

Making the Occupied Bed   *84*

5 LIFTING, MOVING AND TRANSPORTING PATIENTS

Locking Arms with the Patient To Raise His Head and Shoulders   *98*

Helping the Patient to Stand from a Sitting Position   *99*

Moving the Helpless Patient Up in Bed   *101*

Moving a Patient to the Head of the Bed with His Help   *103*

Moving the Mattress to the Head of the Bed with Patient's Help   *103*

Rolling the Patient Like a Log (Log Rolling)   *104*

Moving a Helpless Patient to One Side of the Bed on His Back   *106*

Turning a Patient onto His Right Side Toward You   *107*

Turning a Patient onto His Left Side Away from You   *109*

Helping a Patient Who Can Stand into a Chair or a Wheelchair   *112*

Moving the Helpless Patient into a Wheelchair   *114*

Helping a Patient Back into Bed from a Chair or Wheelchair   *115*

Using a Portable Mechanical Patient Lift to Move the Helpless Patient   *116*

Moving a Patient from the Bed to a Stretcher   *119*

Moving a Patient from a Stretcher to the Bed   *121*

6 PERSONAL CARE OF THE PATIENT

Giving Oral Hygiene to the Conscious Patient   *126*

Cleaning Dentures (False Teeth)   *126*

Giving Oral Hygiene to the Unconscious Patient   *128*

Giving the Complete Bed Bath   *131*

Giving the Partial Bed Bath   *137*

Giving the Tub Bath   *139*

Helping the Patient Take a Shower   *141*

Giving the Patient a Back Rub   *142*

Changing the Patient's Gown   *144*

Shampooing the Patient's Hair   *146*

Combing the Patient's Hair   *149*

Shaving the Patient's Face   *150*

Giving the Bedpan   *152*

Giving the Urinal   *155*

Using the Portable Bedside Commode   156

Preventing Decubitus Ulcers (Bedsores) in the Incontinent Patient   161

7 FOOD SERVICE
Preparing the Patient for a Meal   167
Serving the Food   168
Feeding the Helpless Patient   171
Serving Between-Meal Nourishments   174
Passing Drinking Water   175

8 INTAKE AND OUTPUT
Determining the Amounts Consumed   183
Measuring Urinary Output   186
Emptying a Plastic Urine Container   187

9 SPECIMEN COLLECTION
Collecting a Routine Urine Specimen   192
Collecting a Midstream Clean-Catch Urine Specimen   193
Collecting a 24-Hour Urine Specimen   196
Collecting a Sputum Specimen   197
Collecting a Stool Specimen   199
Straining the Urine   200
Collecting a Fresh Fractional Urine (FrU) Specimen   203
The Clinitest
  (2-Drop Method and 5-Drop Method)   204
The Clinistix Test   205
Testing Urine for Acetone: the Acetest   206
The Ketostix Reagent Strip Test   206
Collecting a Routine Urine Specimen from an Infant   207

10 SPECIAL TREATMENTS
Giving the Cleansing Enema   210
Giving the Ready-To-Use Cleansing Enema   214
Giving the Ready-To-Use Oil Retention Enema   217
Giving the Harris Flush (Return-Flow Enema)   219
Using the Disposable Rectal Tube with Connected Flatus Bag   222
Caring for an Old Colostomy   224
Giving Perineal Care   225
Giving Daily Catheter Care   226
Caring for the Artificial Eye   228

11 OBSERVING AND RECORDING VITAL SIGNS
Shaking Down the Thermometer   234
Reading a Fahrenheit Thermometer   234
Reading a Centigrade (Celsius) Thermometer   235
Taking an Oral Temperature   239
Taking a Rectal Temperature   241
Taking an Axillary Temperature   244
Using a Battery-Operated Electronic Oral Thermometer   245

Using a Battery-Operated Electronic Rectal Thermometer 247
Using a Battery-Operated Electronic Oral Thermometer
   to Take an Axillary Temperature 248
Taking a Radial Pulse 250
Taking an Apical Pulse 252
Measuring the Apical Pulse Deficit 253
Counting Respirations 255
Taking Blood Pressure 258

12 PATIENT ADMISSION, TRANSFER, AND DISCHARGE
Admitting the Patient 263
Weighing and Measuring the Patient 267
Transferring the Patient 268
Discharging the Patient 272

13 PHYSICAL EXAMINATIONS, BODY POSITIONS, TUBES AND TUBING
Preparing the Patient for a Physical Examination 276

14 WARM AND COLD APPLICATIONS
Applying the Warm Compress (Moist Heat Application) 300
Applying the Cold Compress (Moist Cold Application) 302
Applying the Cold Soak (Moist Cold Application) 304
Applying the Warm Soak (Moist Warm Application) 305
Applying the Warm Water Bottle (Dry Heat Application) 307
*Applying the Ice Bag, Ice Cap and Ice Collar
   (Dry Cold Application)* 308
*Applying the Commercial Unit Cold Pack
   (Dry Cold Application)* 310
*Applying the Commercial Unit Heat Pack
   (Moist Warm Application)* 311
Applying a Heat Lamp (Dry Warm Application) 312
Applying the Aquamatic K-Pad (Dry Heat Application) 313
Applying the Cool Wet Pack (Moist Cold Application) 314
Applying the Disposable Sitz Bath (Moist Warm Application) 315
*Using the Portable Chair-Type or Built-In Sitz Bath
   (Moist Warm Application)* 317
Giving the Alchohol Sponge Bath (Moist Cold Application) 319

15 PREOPERATIVE AND POSTOPERATIVE NURSING CARE
Shaving a Patient in Preparation for Surgery 326
Helping with Deep-Breathing Exercises 337
Applying Elastic Bandages 345

16 CARE OF THE DYING PATIENT
Giving Postmortem Care 353

Introduction

HOW TO USE THIS MANUAL

Welcome to being a nursing aide. You are or will be working in a health care institution. Such institutions are hospitals, nursing homes, clinics, and other places where sick and injured people are treated and cared for.

You will be working with nurses, doctors, technicians, and other health care personnel.

Working in a health care institution is a very special job. You can take pride in your work. You are helping people and making your community a better place to live in.

The most important person in the health care institution is the patient. Everyone is there to meet the needs of the patient.

This book has been written to help you do well in your job. The first step is to learn how to use the book efficiently so you will be able to get the most out of it.

This manual is designed to guide you in your training. It is a learning tool, a reference book, like a dictionary. Use it in class for taking notes. Look at it whenever you have a chance. Use this book at home for study and reading before class. Use it on the hospital floor, during your work, to review the procedures you may not be sure of. Check the pictures. They will help to make things clear. Keep working on your vocabulary.

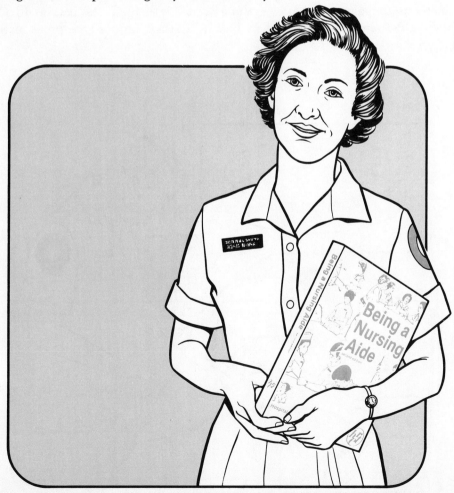

TABLE OF CONTENTS

All of the nursing tasks described in this manual are listed in the table of contents. Use the table of contents to find the page number of any procedure you might want to review.

SECTIONS

Most chapters are divided into sections. This is to make it easier for you to study, to understand the lesson, and to learn the many nursing tasks that make up your job.

OBJECTIVES: WHAT YOU WILL LEARN

The objectives should serve as realistic goals for you to reach as you go through each section. Objectives tell what a successful learner is able to do at the end of the course. For example, you will be able to make an occupied bed. Objectives are your destination, all the things you can expect to accomplish.

KEY IDEAS

Under the heading of *Key Ideas* you will find the reasons behind each procedure you will be doing. Knowing why you are doing something will help you to prepare for and carry out the procedures in the best possible way.

Often there are basic principles, ideas, and methods that must be remembered for the overall care of a patient. As an example, you will always treat the patient with courtesy, kindness, and sympathy. Such a principle or rule does not make up a full procedure. In some situations the order in which the tasks are done doesn't matter. For example, you will check the patient unit (the room) to make sure that everything needed is there. Tasks like this do not follow a definite numerical order. Therefore, they are not true procedures. They are called *Rules To Follow*.

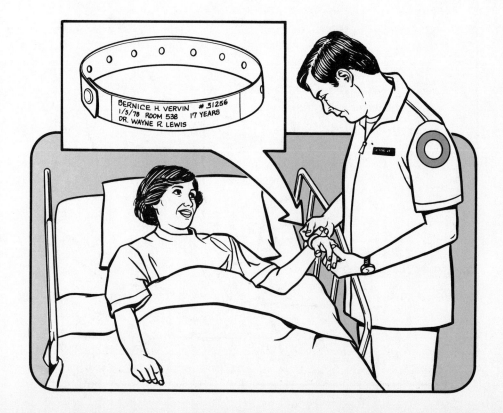

PROCEDURES

A task is an assigned duty, something you are expected to do. In this manual, each nursing task has been divided into a logical, orderly series (sequence) of actions or steps. The full set of steps is a procedure. In health care institutions, procedures are done according to a set method. Nursing procedures will be somewhat different in different hospitals. The underlying principles or ideas are always the same. But the wording, sequence, or style for a task may be different. Be sure you know the methods, the policies, and the style of the institution where you are working. Usually, however, the way things are done will be very similar to the series of steps given in this manual for a procedure.

Sample Procedure

1. Assemble all necessary equipment.

2. Wash your hands before and after each procedure.

3. Check the identification bracelet or band to make sure the procedure is done with the right patient.

4. Ask all visitors to step out of the room. The patient should have privacy.

5. Tell the patient what you are going to do. For example, "I'm going to take your temperature." Explain that you are doing this procedure according to the instructions of your head nurse or team leader.

6. Pull the curtain around the unit.

7. Do the procedure at the correct time, as instructed.

8. Get rid of all disposable equipment and supplies as soon as the procedure is completed. Put the material in the proper containers.

9. Clean the standard equipment and put it in its proper place, or return the equipment to the central supply room (CSR) as soon as you have finished the procedure.

10. Report what you did to your head nurse or team leader:
    a. The name of the procedure
    b. When it was done
    c. How long it took (for example, 3 minutes)
    d. Area (of the patient's body) where you did the procedure
    e. Your observations of anything unusual

THINGS TO REMEMBER

- We will use the term *health care institution* to mean hospital, nursing home, or clinic.

- You will be working under the supervision of the head nurse or team leader. They are not necessarily the same person, although they might be. We will use the term *head nurse* to refer to the person who supervises you and keeps track of your performance.

- If you don't know how to do a procedure, ask your head nurse for help. If you are not sure of yourself, tell her. It is better to get help than to do something wrong.

- Use this book. Read through the procedures until you remember every step. Check the *Words to Remember* in the back for the meanings of words you don't know.

WHAT YOU HAVE LEARNED

Each chapter has a summary at the end. Reading this should remind you of what you have learned. You can quickly review the chapter's main ideas and how they affect your job as a nursing aide .

NOTES COLUMN

Use the blank space on each page to make notes. Or underline the important information on each page. Writing things down helps you to remember them. Keep a pencil in hand as you study. Jot down key words and "thought clues." They will come back to you later when you need them. As your instructor goes over each procedure with you, he or she will explain things that are done differently in your hospital. Taking notes is a good way to record those differences.

WORDS TO REMEMBER

New words are tools for communication. In your work, you will be introduced to medical terminology. You should increase your vocabulary as much as you can so you always understand what the head nurse or team leader tells you. Besides, it is a personal achievement. Learning new words can help to make you more self-confident.

When you are reporting to your supervisors, you must make yourself clearly understood. It is important that you accurately communicate information about the patient and his or her situation or condition. Chapter 18 and the *Words to Remember* will help you understand the meaning of many words used in the hospital. Use the list throughout this course and on the job.

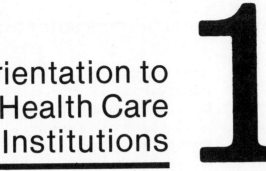

Orientation to Health Care Institutions

Section 1: The Health Care Institution

OBJECTIVES: WHAT YOU WILL LEARN

When you have completed this section, you should be able:

- To explain the purpose and organization of health care institutions
- To describe the organization of the nursing division of a hospital
- To identify the nursing team
- To explain the difference between the registered nurse (RN) and the licensed practical nurse (LPN)

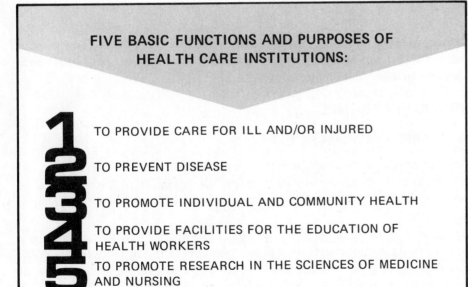

FIVE BASIC FUNCTIONS AND PURPOSES OF HEALTH CARE INSTITUTIONS:

1 TO PROVIDE CARE FOR ILL AND/OR INJURED

2 TO PREVENT DISEASE

3 TO PROMOTE INDIVIDUAL AND COMMUNITY HEALTH

4 TO PROVIDE FACILITIES FOR THE EDUCATION OF HEALTH WORKERS

5 TO PROMOTE RESEARCH IN THE SCIENCES OF MEDICINE AND NURSING

KEY IDEAS

During the orientation period your instructor will give you the names and correct titles of the personnel in key positions in your nursing service department. Your instructor will also tell you about the policies in effect in

ORGANIZATION OF HEALTH CARE INSTITUTIONS

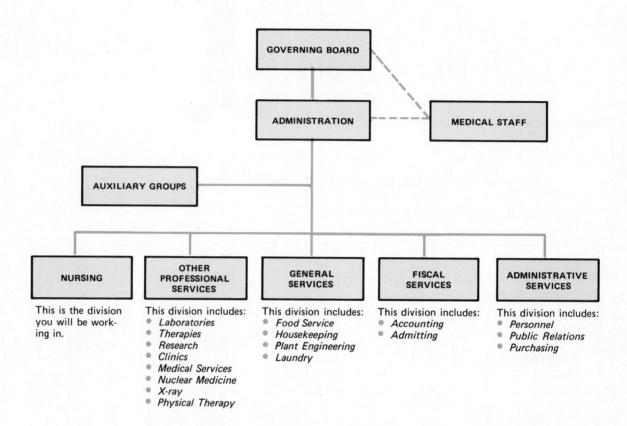

your hospital. For example, you will carry out all orders given to you by your head nurse or team leader. Finally, your instructor will explain what is expected of you as a nursing aide.

NURSING PERSONNEL

The Nursing Aide: Part of a Team

As a nursing aide, you are a member of a health care team. Everyone on the team must understand teamwork. Teamwork means that everyone knows what he is supposed to do and does it to the best of his ability with a spirit of cooperation.

You will be working under the supervision of a professional nurse. Also, you will be working cooperatively with other members of the nursing service staff. Remember that the nurse recognizes the nursing aide as a valuable worker, as a member of the team. Look to your head nurse or team leader as a friend who will help you to learn and understand your job.

Nursing care in your hospital may be organized in one of several ways:

- *Direct assignment.* The head nurse assigns and directs all patient-care responsibilities for the nursing staff.

- *Team nursing.* The head nurse is sometimes called the resource nurse. She divides her staff into teams. Each team has a leader. The head nurse assigns a group of patients to each team. The leader then makes out

ORGANIZATION OF NURSING DIVISION

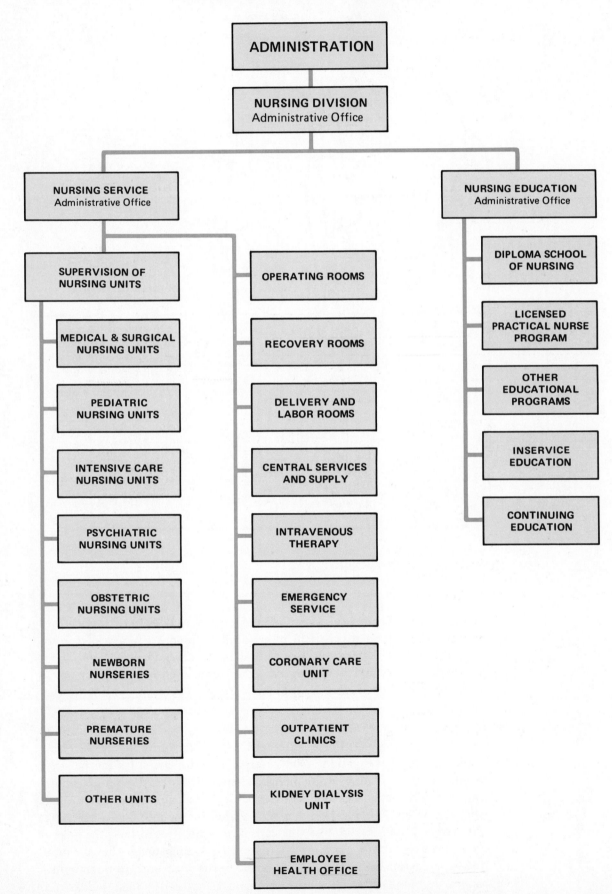

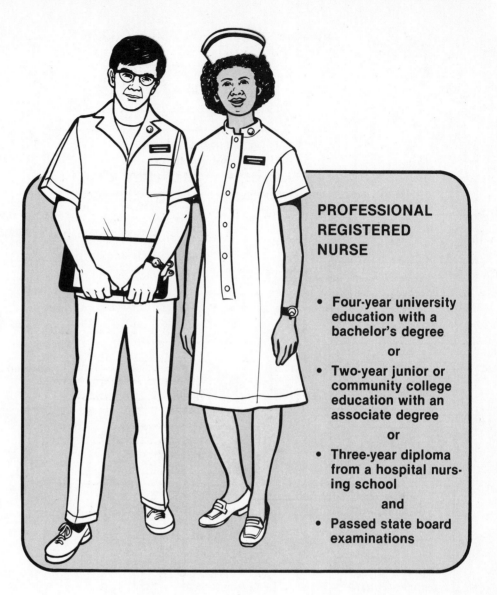

PROFESSIONAL REGISTERED NURSE

- **Four-year university education with a bachelor's degree**

    or

- **Two-year junior or community college education with an associate degree**

    or

- **Three-year diploma from a hospital nursing school**

    and

- **Passed state board examinations**

patient care assignments for members of her team. They may be registered nurses (RN), licensed practical nurses (LPN), or nursing aides. It is the responsibility of the team leader to make sure everything is done. She is teacher, adviser, and helper to all of her team members. This system is *task oriented*. This means that nursing care is arranged according to what must be done.

- *Primary nursing*. Primary nursing is a method of patient care delivery in which the professional nurse is responsible and accountable for the entire nursing care of the patient. She is responsible for assessing the patient's needs and for planning, implementing, and evaluating the patient's nursing care. The purpose is to ensure that the professional nurse work directly with the patient. In addition, her responsibilities include family teaching, discharge planning, and involving community agencies to assist the patient after discharge. This system is *patient oriented*. This means that the nursing care is arranged according to the total needs of the individual patient.

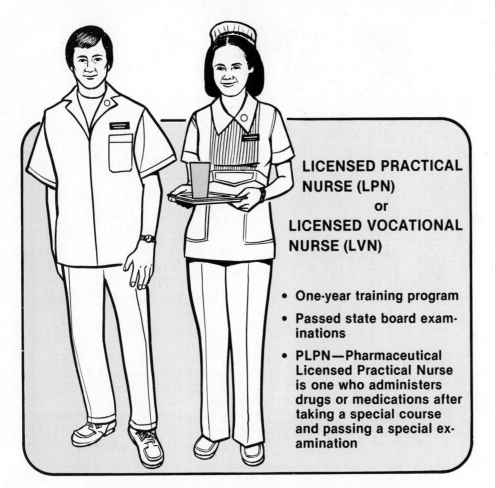

LICENSED PRACTICAL NURSE (LPN)
or
LICENSED VOCATIONAL NURSE (LVN)

- **One-year training program**
- **Passed state board examinations**
- **PLPN—Pharmaceutical Licensed Practical Nurse is one who administers drugs or medications after taking a special course and passing a special examination**

Section 2: Your Job as a Nursing Aide

OBJECTIVES: WHAT YOU WILL LEARN

When you have completed this section, you should be able:
- To list the nursing tasks you will be doing on the job
- To display qualities that are desirable for good nursing aides to have

KEY IDEAS

The nursing tasks and procedures you will learn to do in your work are listed here. Some may be added or taken out, according to your hospital's policy. But this list is your basic "job description." When you have finished your training, you will be able:
- To answer the patient's signal light
- To report useful information
- To assist in admission, transfer, and discharge of patients
- To dress and undress patients
- To weigh patients
- To feed patients
- To bathe patients
- To measure and record intake and output

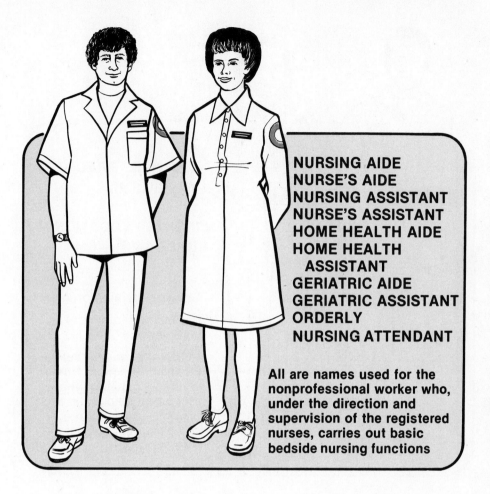

**NURSING AIDE
NURSE'S AIDE
NURSING ASSISTANT
NURSE'S ASSISTANT
HOME HEALTH AIDE
HOME HEALTH
  ASSISTANT
GERIATRIC AIDE
GERIATRIC ASSISTANT
ORDERLY
NURSING ATTENDANT**

All are names used for the nonprofessional worker who, under the direction and supervision of the registered nurses, carries out basic bedside nursing functions

- To collect specimens
- To test patients' urine for sugar and acetone
- To make patients' beds
- To lift and move patients
- To observe and record information about patients objectively
- To take vital signs
- To use the proper techniques of good medical asepsis
- To use bedside rails correctly
- To maintain a safe environment
- To shave male patients' faces
- To take care of the colostomy patient
- To take care of the obstetrical patient
- To care for the psychiatric patient
- To offer bedpans and urinals
- To apply binders and ace bandages
- To straighten up the utility room
- To apply warm or cold applications

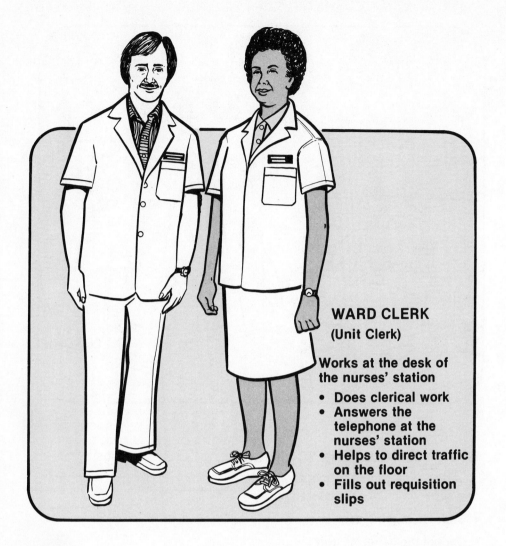

WARD CLERK
(Unit Clerk)

Works at the desk of the nurses' station

- Does clerical work
- Answers the telephone at the nurses' station
- Helps to direct traffic on the floor
- Fills out requisition slips

- To deliver drinking water
- To give preoperative and postoperative care
- To change the patient's position
- To care for equipment
- To give enemas
- To care for the patient's skin
- To give back rubs
- To care for the diabetic patient
- To care for the cardiac patient
- To care for the pediatric patient
- To care for the patient with tumors
- To give oral hygiene
- To care for the patient in isolation
- To care for the geriatric patient
- To care for the dying patient
- To take care of the patient's body after death

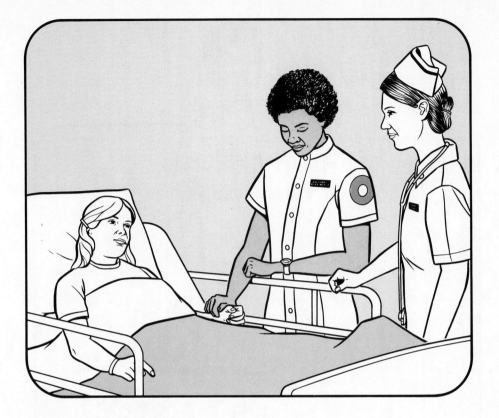

WHAT YOU WILL DO IN YOUR JOB

**Everything you will do will be under
the supervision of a registered nurse**

- **Bedside nursing care**
- **Care of the patient's unit**
- **Food service**
- **Handling equipment and supplies**

THE NURSING AIDE: AN IMPORTANT PERSON

Being a nursing aide is not just another job. There are so many things to learn, so many things to do. Yours is a serious occupation. Making mistakes can cause extra pain and suffering for patients, even death. Doing a good job is something to be proud of. You will be helping sick people and making their stay in the hospital easier to bear.

During your training and while you are at work, always think about the patient as a person. Try to imagine what it's like to have his or her problems. The main point is: As much as possible, try to develop a *feeling* for the patients, a sensitivity to their needs. Sympathy and understanding by those caring for a patient are part of the treatment. Sometimes these are as important as medicine in helping the patient to get well.

Good Qualities To Have

You have decided that you want to be the best nursing aide you can be. You want to do the best possible job. What kind of person makes a good nursing aide? Certain traits, attitudes, and habits are often seen regularly in people

PATIENT CARE RESPONSIBILITIES

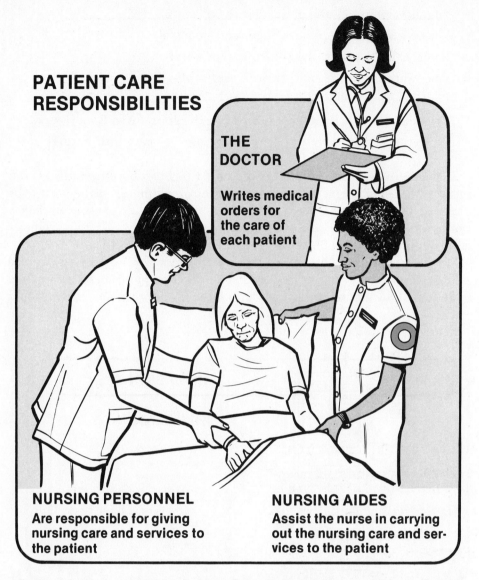

THE DOCTOR

Writes medical orders for the care of each patient

NURSING PERSONNEL

Are responsible for giving nursing care and services to the patient

NURSING AIDES

Assist the nurse in carrying out the nursing care and services to the patient

who have been successful in their work in the hospital, especially on the nursing team. Some of these traits are built into one's personality—you have had them all along. Others can be learned through practice and become part of one's changed (improved) personality.

Run through this list and see where you stand. Review those qualities you already have. Then check out those you think you could learn and actually make a part of yourself. You are an excellent nursing aide if:

- You are a person who can be trusted and depended on.
- You relate easily to new people.
- You make friends quickly.
- You enjoy working with people.
- You get along well with others.
- You are sensitive to the feelings of others.
- You want to help people when they are in pain.
- You are considerate and tactful.
- You try to be gracious and polite at all times.
- You get satisfaction out of being of service to others.

- You show sympathy and patience with others.
- You try always to keep your temper under control.
- You believe that you are doing important work.
- You want to improve your performance.
- You like to learn new things.
- You never (or only rarely) let your private life interfere with your work.
- When the work is heavy and everyone is tense, you try a little harder.

Dependability. Your hospital is organized to function efficiently when a certain number of people are on the job. If you aren't there, a patient could be deprived of the care he needs. Also, your absence may cause your fellow workers to have an overload of work. It is essential that you arrive promptly every day unless you are ill. If you are sick, call the nursing office.

Moreover, dependability means more than coming to work every day and coming in on time. It means that the head nurse or team leader who asks you to do something can rely on you to do it at the proper time and in the proper way.

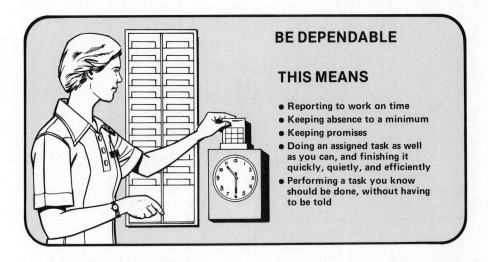

BE DEPENDABLE

THIS MEANS

- Reporting to work on time
- Keeping absence to a minimum
- Keeping promises
- Doing an assigned task as well as you can, and finishing it quickly, quietly, and efficiently
- Performing a task you know should be done, without having to be told

Accuracy. Accuracy is part of being dependable. In a hospital you are concerned with human lives. What might appear to you to be a tiny mistake or oversight could delay the recovery of a patient.

Be accurate when you are recording a temperature. Be careful in making a bed. Stay alert when you answer the patient's call light. It is vitally important for you to follow your head nurse's or team leader's instructions exactly. If you make a mistake, report it. If you do not understand something, ask again. Always remember: There is a reason for every step in the routine of the hospital.

Following Rules and Instructions

Everybody follows instructions and goes by rules. Otherwise, the job would never get done. Even the top people in the hospital have to follow rules.

Here are some good rules to remember in your work. These can help to make you a better nursing aide.

- Be accurate to the best of your ability.

- Follow carefully the instructions of your head nurse or team leader.

- If you do not understand something, ask your supervisor.

- There are good reasons for every rule and every procedure in the hospital. Be aware of them all.

- Report accidents or errors immediately to the head nurse or team leader.

- Keep confidences to yourself, except when it might be dangerous to a patient. For example, a patient tells you she isn't taking her medicine. Report this to your head nurse or team leader.

- Don't waste supplies and equipment.

- Be ready to adjust quickly to new situations, say, a medical crisis.

- Try to get things done on time. Use a systematic work schedule.

- Remember that you are helping those who are unable to help themselves. Your head, your heart, and your hands should be strong, willing, and capable.

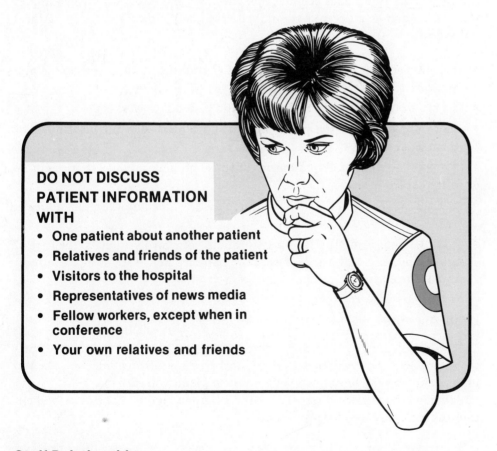

DO NOT DISCUSS PATIENT INFORMATION WITH

- One patient about another patient
- Relatives and friends of the patient
- Visitors to the hospital
- Representatives of news media
- Fellow workers, except when in conference
- Your own relatives and friends

Staff Relationships

You will find your fellow workers and other hospital personnel more agreeable and helpful if you treat them right. Some good practices are:

- Report to the head nurse or team leader whenever you leave the unit for any purpose and at the end of your shift. Report to her again when you return.

- Take all questions you may have about patients and their care to your head nurse or team leader.
- Tell your head nurse or team leader about important personal problems that you feel might be interfering with your work.
- Don't talk about your personal problems with other staff members.
- Don't discuss your personal problems with patients.
- Follow all instructions given to you by your head nurse or team leader. If you are confused about any of your assignments, discuss this with the head nurse or team leader.
- Report all complaints from patients and visitors to the head nurse or team leader. Never ignore complaints, no matter how silly or unreasonable they may seem to you.
- Perform all of your duties in a spirit of cooperation and follow orders willingly.

Ethical Behavior

Ethical behavior means keeping your promises and doing what you ought to do. As a nursing aide, you should observe the following code for ethical behavior:

- Be conscientious in the performance of your duties. This means do the best you can.
- Be generous in helping your patients and your fellow workers.
- Faithfully carry out the instructions you are given by your head nurse or team leader.
- Respect the right of all patients to have beliefs and opinions that might be different from yours.
- Let the patient know that it is your pleasure, not just your job, to assist him.
- Try to demonstrate that you are sincere in your involvement in the care of a human being. Always show that the patient's well-being is of the utmost importance to you.

Legal Aspects

Laws concerning patients and workers in health care institutions were written to protect both the patient and the worker. As a nursing aide, you need to understand how the law affects you and the patients you care for.

Patients are entitled to respect for their human rights. They must be kept safe and must be cared for properly.

Negligence. The words *negligence* and *malpractice* are often used interchangeably, as if they were the same thing. Officially, "Negligence is the commission of an act or failure to perform an act where the respective performance or nonperformance would deviate from that act which should have been done by a reasonably prudent person under the same or similar conditions. Malpractice is negligence when applied to the performance of a professional." Examples are:

- If the nursing aide fails to fasten the safety strap over a patient on a stretcher and as a result the patient falls, the aide has been negligent.

- When a nursing aide performs procedures not included in her job description or for which she has not been trained, or performs any procedure incorrectly, she is guilty of negligence.

- When a nursing aide serves a regular diet to a diabetic patient, she is guilty of negligence.

- Any nursing aide who neglects to wash her hands after contact with a patient is guilty of negligence.

BEING A SUCCESSFUL NURSING AIDE

All members of the nursing team are *teachers* by the example they set. They influence each other to become better in their jobs. The practice of good personal hygiene as used in a hospital environment becomes a teaching tool. Here are things to learn and remember about care of your person—your body—and your appearance. Most of these apply to both male and female nursing aides. Some are obviously for women.

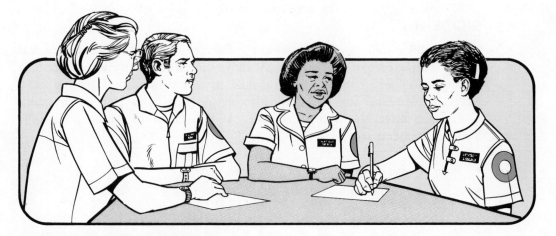

DEVELOP THESE QUALITIES

- Dress properly and neatly.
- Use good personal hygiene.
- Bathe daily.
- Use an unscented deodorant.
- Keep your mouth and teeth clean.
- Keep your hair clean, neat, and off the collar.
- Keep your nails short and clean.
- Wear conservative makeup.
- Try to be completely free of odor. Don't use perfume or scented sprays.

- Wear clean clothes every day.
- Wear comfortable low-heeled shoes with nonskid soles and heels.
- Polish your shoes every day. Be sure the laces are clean.
- Repair rips and hems, and replace missing buttons right away.
- Never wear jewelry—earrings, bracelets, pendants.
- Wear a white sweater if you are cold.
- Wear pantsuits only if approved.
- Always wear your name pin.
- Always wear a wristwatch with a second hand.
- Always carry a pen or pencil and paper.

Stay Healthy. When patients see that you take good care of yourself, they are more likely to trust you to take good care of them.

- Have a physical checkup every year.
- Eat a well-balanced diet every day.
- Eat a good meal before coming on duty.
- Get plenty of sleep. Be alert when you come to work.
- Take some time for recreation. It's good for you.
- Do your exercises. Keep your body fit. You'll feel better.
- Protect yourself from infection. Wash your hands properly and thoroughly before and after each contact with a patient.

INCIDENTS

An incident is an event that does not fit the routine operation of the hospital or the routine care of the patients. It may be an accident or something that might cause one. For example, a staff person runs into a patient in a wheelchair, because someone spilled liquid and failed to wipe it up. Such incidents can affect the patients, visitors, and members of the hospital staff. Types of incidents are:

- Patient, visitor, or employee accidents
- Thefts from patients, visitors, or employees
- Thefts of hospital property
- Accidents occurring on outlying hospital property, such as sidewalks, parking lots, or entrances

Whenever an incident occurs, a report must be made out. Report any incident you observe. Also report any bad conditions you think might lead to an incident. Reporting is very important to the safety program of the hospital and for the protection of all health care workers. For the hospital to be prepared for possible liability suits or damage claims, all the facts related to such incidents must be known.

WHAT YOU HAVE LEARNED

You are now a part of the nursing team. As much as you can, be sympathetic and understanding toward the patients. Remember that the hospital exists only for the care and the treatment of the patient. His or her welfare

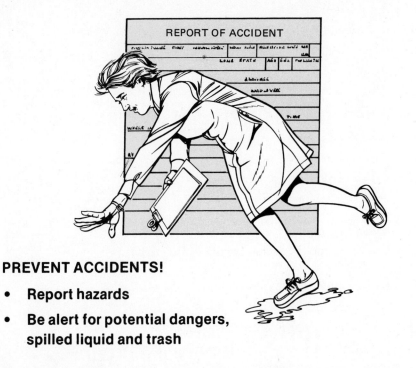

PREVENT ACCIDENTS!

- **Report hazards**
- **Be alert for potential dangers, spilled liquid and trash**

comes first. Keep this in mind as you do your work with dependability and accuracy.

Remember who you are. You are in a serious learning process. As you develop skills, as you grow in experience, you will have more and more self-confidence. As you become more sure of yourself, the work will get easier. Soon you will be enjoying your work. Then you can look for advancement. Then you can begin to see this job as the start of a career.

Introduction to the Patient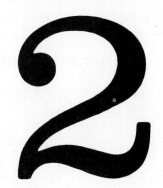

Section 1: The Patients You Will Care For

OBJECTIVES: WHAT YOU WILL LEARN

When you have completed this section, you should be able:

- To describe the five main kinds of patients
    a.   The medical-surgical patient
    b.   The obstetrical patient
    c.   The pediatric patient
    d.   The geriatric patient
    e.   The psychiatric patient
- To describe the patient care departments in the hospital

THE PATIENTS YOU WILL CARE FOR

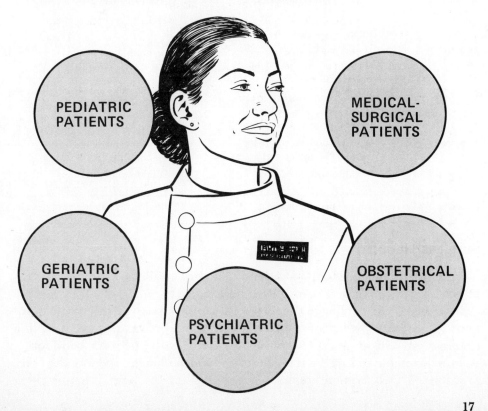

KEY IDEAS

As a nursing aide, you must consider each patient as a person with emotional as well as physical needs. In this chapter you will be introduced to the five major groups of patients in most hospitals.

Medical-Surgical Patients

Medical-surgical patients are those who have an acute or chronic illness that is treated with medication or surgery.

Acute illness: Comes on suddenly and runs its course within a few days. Examples are appendicitis and pneumonia.

Chronic illness: Continues over years or a lifetime. Examples are leukemia and diabetes.

Classification of Disease. Diseases, conditions, infections, and illnesses can all be chronic or acute. These categories often overlap. They are based on the cause of the disease, the body system that has been affected, or the way the disease has been acquired.

Types of Disease Classified by Cause

Type (cause)	Meaning	Disease (examples)
Aging	Degeneration of all the body systems	Hardening of the arteries
Chemical	Foreign substance interfering with normal processes	Alcoholic cirrhosis of the liver
Congenital (or birth injury)	Occurring during pregnancy (or at birth)	Cleft palate (congenital) Cerebral palsy (birth injury)
Deficiency	Lacking the right foods or nutrients	Scurvy (lack of vitamin C)
Hereditary	Passed on through genes	Sickle-cell anemia
Infectious	Communicable—caused by microorganisms	Measles, chickenpox, mumps
Mechanical blocks	Formation of an obstruction of body wastes, fluids, or natural chemicals	Gallstones, kidney stones, blood clots
Metabolic	Failing to produce or break down substances needed for normal processes	Diabetes (lack of insulin)
Neoplastic	Abnormal growth of tissue—tumors (benign or malignant)	Fibroids (benign) Cancer (malignant)
Occupational	Peculiar to a job	Lead poisoning (painter) Black lung disease (miner)
Trauma	Injury, usually physical	Fracture, broken bone

Surgical Patients

Surgical patients need an operation because of an illness or injury. It may be necessary to repair or remove a part of the body.

Some surgery may change the form of a person's body or the way it functions. For example, when amputation is necessary a body part is taken off (for example, an arm or leg). Of course this changes the person's body form. Another example of surgery is a colostomy, which changes the way the body functions. This operation creates a new outlet for the large intestine. It is

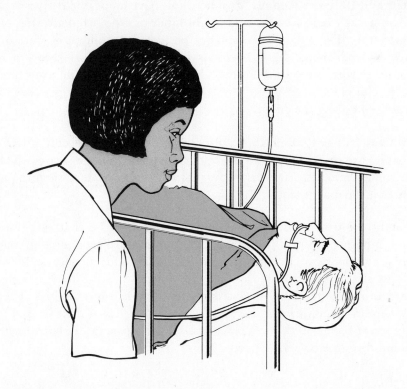

made in the wall of the abdomen. The person's feces are discharged through this outlet instead of through the rectum and anus.

A surgical patient usually has to get used to (or adapt to) changes in the form of his or her body or in the way the body functions.

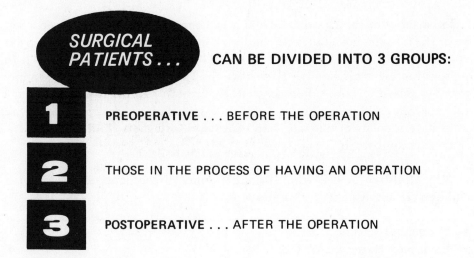

SURGICAL PATIENTS . . . CAN BE DIVIDED INTO 3 GROUPS:

1 PREOPERATIVE . . . BEFORE THE OPERATION

2 THOSE IN THE PROCESS OF HAVING AN OPERATION

3 POSTOPERATIVE . . . AFTER THE OPERATION

Obstetrical Patients

Obstetrical patients are women having babies. These women are different from all other kinds of patients. This is because pregnancy without complications is a normal, natural event. Sometimes obstetrical patients do have complications. These happen either because of the pregnancy itself or because of a disease that is not related to the pregnancy. For example, complications can affect a pregnant women who has diabetes.

Labor and Delivery Rooms. Most hospitals have labor and delivery rooms. These are areas where women who are in labor or who are delivering babies are cared for. The labor and delivery patient care unit is a part of the obstetrical department. Most hospitals have an obstetrical recovery room where women who have just delivered a baby will stay for awhile. New mothers need a special place to rest until they recover from any anesthesia they might have received during the delivery.

Newborn Nursery. A newborn nursery is a patient care unit where full-term babies are cared for. *Full term* means that the mother carried the baby for the full normal nine months of pregnancy. Newborn nurseries are part of the obstetrical department.

Premature Nursery. Babies are sometimes born early, that is, before the full nine months are over. They are called premature babies. A premature nursery is a patient care unit for premature babies. This nursery is also a part of the obstetrical department.

Premature babies are almost always smaller than full-term babies. They are usually kept in incubators for the first few days or weeks of their lives. The incubator is a special crib that makes it possible for a premature baby to get the extra humidity and oxygen he needs.

Pediatric Patients

Pediatric patients are children. In most hospitals, anyone under age 16 is called a pediatric patient. These patients may be grouped in several ways. For example, pediatric patients are sometimes grouped according to age. That is because children of different ages need different kinds and amounts of care. Children may also be grouped according to the medical condition they have.

Importance of the Family. A child is still a member of a family, even when he or she is in the hospital. The child may have only one parent, but there is always someone (or several persons) to care for the child in his home. These persons represent his family. The small child's mother is usually the family member closest to him. Often the mother, or both parents, will want to stay with the sick child in the hospital. Many hospitals and pediatric patient care units have a policy of allowing parents to stay with their child and even encourage them to do so.

Why Children Are in the Hospital. Some of the conditions for which children are admitted to the hospital are:

- Congenital defects
  Examples: Harelip, club foot
- Accidents
  Examples: Falls, poisoning
- Tumors
  Examples: Cysts, cancerous growths
- Long-term or chronic conditions
  Examples: Diabetes, rheumatic heart disease

- Infectious diseases
  Examples: Pneumonia, meningitis
- Emotional disturbances
  Examples: Severe depression, acute anxiety
- Nutritional disorders
  Examples: Rickets, iron-deficiency anemia

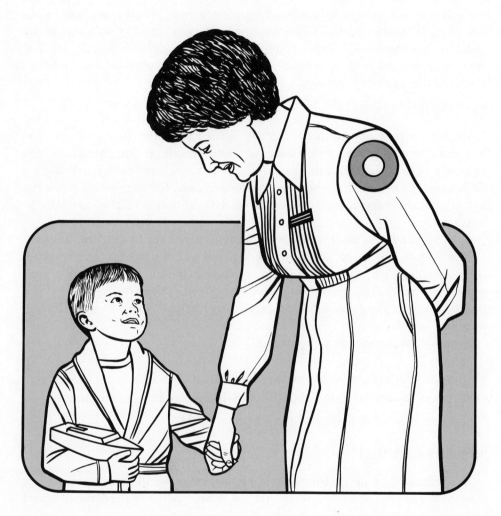

- Babies who are born three weeks or more before full term, or who weigh less than 5½ pounds at birth, are known as *premature* babies.
- Full-term babies from birth until the age of 1 month are known as *newborn* babies (*neonates*).
- Babies from 1-month to 1-year old are known as *infants*.
- Children from 1 to 3 years old are known as *toddlers*.
- Children from 3 to 5 years of age are known as *preschoolers*.
- Children from 6 to 12 years of age are known as *school-age* children.
- Children 12 to 18 are known as *teenagers*.

Geriatric Patients

A geriatric patient is usually defined as a patient over 65 years old. This is the age at which many employees retire. It is also the age at which the federal Medicare benefits go into effect.

However, people don't suddenly grow old on their 65th birthday. Aging is a gradual process. It takes place all during life. One person at 65 may be "old" and ready to retire. Another person of the same age is neither "old" nor ready to retire.

Each person develops, matures, and deteriorates at his own rate, not by the calendar. It is not unusual to see an elderly person who has an alert, active mind but who has some condition that prevents his body from functioning as it once did. An example is the person who likes to read a lot but now has cataracts that restrict his vision.

Psychiatric Patients

Psychiatric patients are those who have a mental illness, which means there is a disturbance in the person's feelings and emotions. Mental illness may cause changes in the way a person talks and acts. Sometimes mentally ill people change so much that they can no longer care for themselves properly. Sometimes they are dangerous to themselves and others and need to be restrained.

Until recent years, most psychiatric patients were kept in separate hospitals built especially for them. However, today, more and more general hospitals have special patient care units for psychiatric patients. In these units most psychiatric patients are in bed only when they sleep. They are up, around, and dressed all day. They are not handicapped by physical illness or the effects of surgery.

Examples of psychiatric patients are:

- Persons who are very depressed or agitated
- Persons who are confused about people, events, and their surroundings
- Persons who think that everyone is against them

Intensive Care Unit

An intensive care unit is for patients who are critically ill. These patients are always in bed. Nurses are always present. These patients need much closer observation and more nursing care than ordinary patients.

Coronary Care Unit

A coronary care unit is for patients who have had a severe heart attack. In some hospitals the coronary care unit is part of the intensive care unit.

Postoperative Recovery Room

A postoperative recovery room is where patients who have had surgery are cared for until they recover from anesthesia. Lifesaving equipment is kept ready at all times in the surgical recovery room.

Emergency Department

An emergency patient care unit is a place for people who need emergency treatment. A *crisis intervention center* is usually part of the emergency department. Emergency patients are those who have suddenly become ill. Others have had an accident. Others think they need medical attention and cannot reach their own doctor.

Section 2: Communication

OBJECTIVES: WHAT YOU WILL LEARN

On completing this section, you should be able:

- To maintain a courteous and professional manner toward patients, visitors, and co-workers
- To keep your emotions under control while on the job
- To deal with patients and visitors in a sympathetic and tactful manner
- To show interest and concern about the patient's welfare
- To answer the patient's signal promptly
- To use communication skills effectively

KEY IDEAS

Developing the habit of getting along with people—parents, visitors, fellow workers—is a very important part of your job. Keep cool under pressure. Don't let your feelings get out of control. Being courteous and sympathetic to others is at least as necessary to your success as job skills. The key to getting along with people is being able to *communicate* well with them.

Relating to People

Relating to people is a way of saying how you get along with them. In your work, always try to relate well to people, even when they are unhappy, angry, or afraid.

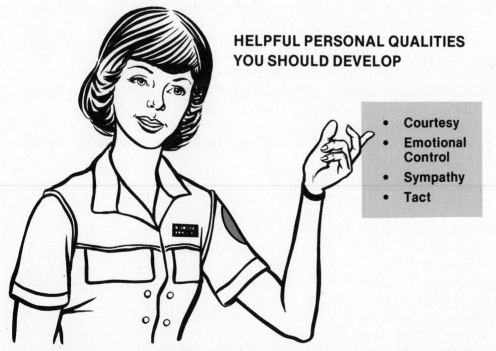

HELPFUL PERSONAL QUALITIES YOU SHOULD DEVELOP

- **Courtesy**
- **Emotional Control**
- **Sympathy**
- **Tact**

Courtesy. Courtesy means being polite and considerate and cooperating with others. You should be courteous all the time. Never be critical or impolite in your contacts with patients. Imagine yourself in their place. Be cheerful. Don't complain about how busy you are. Avoid judging others. Think about how you would feel if you were in the patient's shoes.

Courtesy is very important in your relationships with your fellow workers. Your supervisor and instructors will be giving you advice and directions. Show them you are willing and eager to learn. Convince them that you want to do a good job.

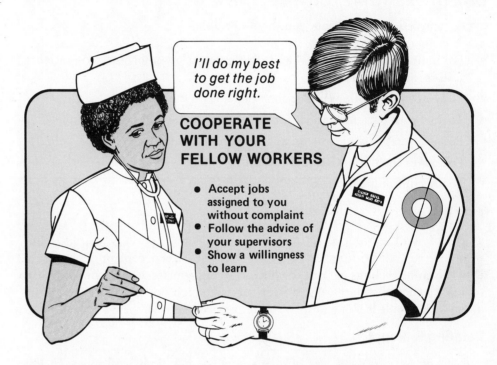

Emotional Control. Sometimes a patient, another staff member, or a visitor can upset you so much you get angry. You feel like making a rude or nasty remark. Don't do it. Remember that a patient is probably worried about himself, his illness, his family, or his job.

Learn to take criticism and accept suggestions without feeling you're being attacked. Try to avoid becoming defensive. Your supervisor may criticize you or tell you to do something. You may feel like saying "That isn't my job" or "Why do you pick on me?" Stop, think, and examine your attitude. Calm down and go ahead and do the right thing.

Children's crying is the normal, natural way for them to express their feelings. Or to tell you that something is wrong. Try to understand why a child is crying. Don't let it irritate you.

Sympathy and Tact. A sick patient's problems are all-important to him. Try to be understanding. Be a good listener, even when you would rather leave.

Patients and visitors often relieve their feelings of helplessness and hopelessness through words. They may try to take it out on you. Bear with them as much as possible. Also, remember that the patient may be suffering emotionally as well as physically.

Try to be as tactful as you can. *Tact* means doing and saying the right things at the right time. When a patient begins to recover from being in pain or uncomfortable, tell him that you can see improvement. He seems to move more easily. He appears to be standing straighter. He seems to be moving his arm or leg better. Remarks like these often lift the patient's spirits.

Always listen when a patient makes a complaint or brings up a problem. The patient may ask you questions about his doctor or when he will be discharged. Refer such questions to the head nurse or team leader.

Sometimes a child cries when his visiting parents are getting ready to leave the hospital. You can show sympathy to both the child and his parents by making the separation easier for all of them. Pick up the child (if permitted), pat him, and soothe him. Turn his attention to something other than the pain of being left in the hospital by his parents.

Never tell a child that you are going to *take* his temperature or blood pressure. He may think you are going to take something away from him. Say you are going to *measure* his temperature or blood pressure instead.

**WHAT
A PATIENT
WORRIES
ABOUT . . .**

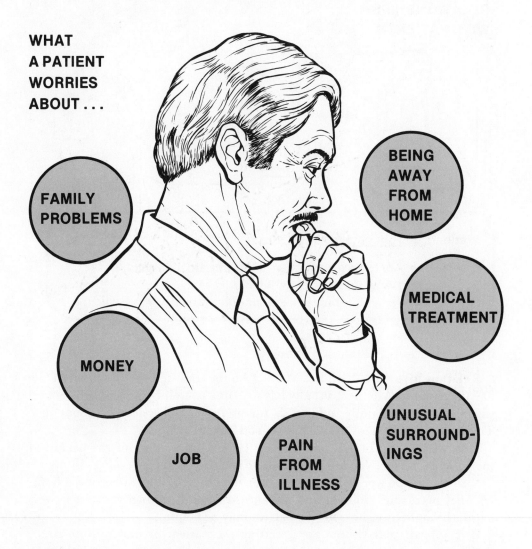

FAMILY PROBLEMS

BEING AWAY FROM HOME

MEDICAL TREATMENT

MONEY

UNUSUAL SURROUND-INGS

JOB

PAIN FROM ILLNESS

Relationships with Patients. Many things make a difference in a patient's behavior and attitude during an illness. The patient may be frightened, angry, or sad. Some factors or influences are the diagnosis, seriousness of the illness, age, previous illnesses and experience in hospitals, and mental condition. Other things that can make a difference are the patient's personality and disposition and perhaps his financial condition.

Each patient is different in his reaction to pain, treatment, annoyances, and even kindness. Always treat each patient as an individual, a person who needs your help. Practice the kind of special consideration that all patients need on an individual basis.

Never talk to anyone except your supervisor about a patient's condition. Never discuss one patient's medical condition with another patient. That would be an invasion of privacy.

Always try to give the patient confidence in the hospital, the doctors, and the nursing staff. Never criticize any of your fellow staff members in front of a patient.

Also, remember that the patient's behavior is the result of things that worry or bother him. He may be hostile or mean and nasty. And you may simply be the nearest person to talk to.

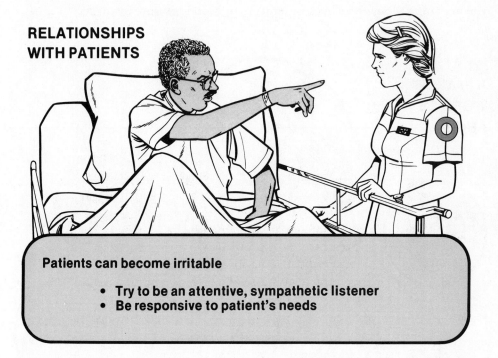

RELATIONSHIPS WITH PATIENTS

Patients can become irritable

- **Try to be an attentive, sympathetic listener**
- **Be responsive to patient's needs**

Relationships with Visitors. Visiting hours are often the highlight of the day for patients. A patient usually has a feeling of well-being and satisfaction when he knows his family and friends are interested and concerned about him. This feeling can do a lot to give him a good mental attitude.

Most visitors realize that hospital regulations are written for the benefit of the patients. Be sure you know the rules in your hospital concerning visitors.

Visitors may be worried and upset over the illness of a member of the family. They need your kindness and patience. Pleasant comments about flowers or gifts brought by visitors for the patient may be helpful.

If it appears that visitors are upsetting the patient or making him tired, notify the head nurse or team leader. She can caution visitors or ask them to leave.

If the patient is seriously ill or is an obstetrical patient, visiting hours may be different. Your instructor will tell you about the visiting hours and any rules for visitors in your hospital. These rules, of course, must be followed.

Three main rules usually apply to visitors in all hospitals:

- Visitors are not allowed to take hospital property away with them.
- Visitors are not allowed to give nursing or medical care to a patient.
- Visitors can't bring food or drink to the patient unless permission has been given by the head nurse or team leader.

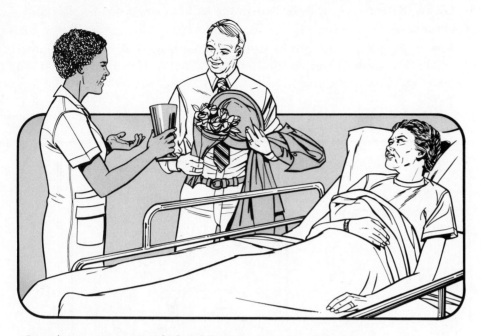

Certain ways to act are helpful in your contacts with visitors:

- Listen to the family member. Whether it is a suggestion, a complaint, or "passing the time of day," listen to the person. Some suggestions by visitors can be very helpful. Some complaints may be valid, others not. When a complaint is first presented, you probably need to get more information. You might ask, "Where did this happen?" or "What did you do?" Say to the person, "I will tell the head nurse about this," and then report it to the head nurse or team leader.

- Don't get involved in the family's private affairs and feelings. Never take sides in family quarrels. Never give information or opinions to someone about other family members.

- Be prepared to give information to visitors. Tell them under what circumstances family members are allowed to eat in the employee cafeteria. Mention where the coffee shop is and what hours it is open. Tell them where a public telephone is. Direct them to other places in the hospital, for example, the business office or the gift shop.

When the Patient Is a Child. Several important things need to be considered and remembered with the pediatric patient:

- Parents need to be with their children, and children need their parents.
- Parents are normally concerned and often are worried, frightened people.
- Most children first learn about the world from their parents.
- The younger the child, the more he needs his parents.

Things you can do to help:

- Do the best possible job of caring for the child. This is usually reassuring to the parents.

- Show interest and concern about the parents' welfare. Ask, "Is there something we can do?"

- Don't make judgments about the parents' attitudes or behavior, even if they seem strange to you.

- Let the parents help to take part in the child's care, when possible and if permitted.
- Sometimes parents seem to be worried about something concerning their child in the hospital and are afraid to talk about it. If you see this, tell your team leader or head nurse.

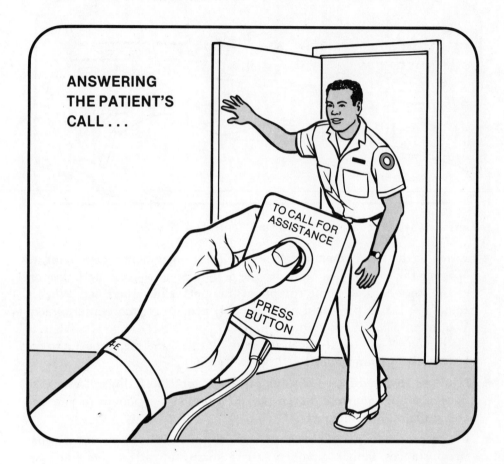

ANSWERING THE PATIENT'S CALL . . .

TO CALL FOR ASSISTANCE

PRESS BUTTON

Answering the Patient Call Signal

Every patient has a way of sending a signal to the nursing staff when he wants something. One thing you will do often in a hospital is answer the patient's call for service or help without delay.

All patients have a signal cord. When the patient presses a button on the end of the cord, a light flashes in the head nurse's station and over the patient's door. This device may be called a *signal cord* or *call bell.* You should always keep alert for such signals. Answer the signal as soon as it flashes. Every minute seems forever to the patient who is waiting.

When the patient signals:

- Go to the patient at once, quietly and in a friendly way.
- Turn off the call signal, and address the patient by name.
- Say, "Mr. Jones, what can I do for you?"
- Do whatever the patient asks, but be sure it is correct and safe for this patient. If you are in doubt, ask the head nurse or team leader. Tell her what the patient wants and then follow her directions.

- When necessary, use the emergency signal to get qualified personnel to assist you.

- Replace the signal cord where the patient can reach it easily.

- *Caution:* A young child or a helpless adult may not be able to use the signal cord. Listen for calls for help from these patients and go quickly to see what they need. Check these patient's rooms often to see if they need something.

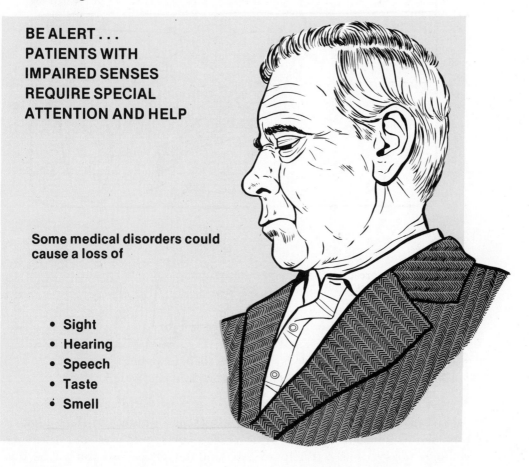

BE ALERT...
PATIENTS WITH
IMPAIRED SENSES
REQUIRE SPECIAL
ATTENTION AND HELP

Some medical disorders could cause a loss of

- **Sight**
- **Hearing**
- **Speech**
- **Taste**
- **Smell**

When the Patient Is Handicapped. For patients who have serious hearing and seeing losses, the signal cord is used differently. Blind or visually handicapped patients must be shown how to use the signal. Have them feel around for the cord and practice using it while you are there.

If the signal is the kind that you push to turn on, you can call it a "push" button. If it works like a light switch, you can compare it to that. When working with patients who have serious visual losses, you should not expect them to turn off the signal. You can do that routinely when you respond to the signal.

Patients with serious hearing losses can easily learn how to pull or push the signal cord on if you show them how to do it. Show them, don't tell them. Remember: they can't hear you.

Communicating with Patients and Other People

Being successful as a nursing aide depends partly on understanding the various responsibilities of the job.

Patients must have help to recover. You are the person who provides most of the personal bedside assistance. Every time you bathe or turn a patient in his bed, you are helping him get better.

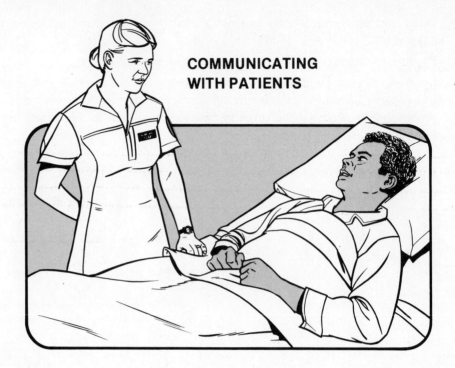

COMMUNICATING WITH PATIENTS

- Show an interest in what the patient is saying.
- Let your face show that you are interested.
- Use good manners.
- Speak clearly and slowly. Speak in a pleasant tone.
- Use normal words.
- Respect the patient's moods sometimes silence can help.
- Make your body movements look pleasing and energetic.

When someone in need asks you for assistance—whether to clean him, or turn him, or for something out of his reach—you should give your assistance willingly and graciously. It helps to have kind thoughts. Then you will be able to handle a situation with kindness.

Spoken and written words are used for most communication. But there are other ways—sometimes better ways—to get a message across. Hand movements (gestures), expressions on your face, and body movements may tell the story better than words.

As a nursing aide, you are close to the patient during his stay in the hospital. Often he tells you about his wants, his pains, and his worries. As you listen, you are both in close communication.

Every time you touch a person's body, whether you speak any words or not, you are saying something to him. You are communicating. How you assist him in any action that involves touching his body tells him something. If you are careful, firm, and gentle, it tells him something far different than if you are rough and jerking him around.

Pay attention to your posture. The way you move when you enter a patient's room or how you stand by his bed are ways of communicating through body language. Try to make these movements communicate energy, a sense of interest, and a willingness to help. A frown or an impatient body movement, a shrug, may give the patient the message, "Don't bother me." Also, a certain way of standing or walking may send the message, "I'm lazy."

Look at the patient when you speak to him. This tells him that he has your attention. If you are looking away as you talk with him, he gets the impression that your attention is elsewhere. Speak clearly and distinctly. This is especially necessary when you are talking with older people. Some of them, as part of the aging process, may have a hearing loss. Talk *with* the patient, not just to or at him. Ask him what he likes and dislikes. Ask what he thinks or what he wants. Listen to his responses in an interested manner.

Slang or coarse or vulgar words are not appropriate or necessary. Also, don't use medical terms or abbreviations when talking to patients and their visitors. If you do use medical language, you might give the impression that you are showing off, or you might give the patient the wrong idea about what is happening to him.

Keep your voice pleasant, not too loud or too high pitched. Speak clearly and slowly enough to be easily understood. Never whisper or mumble, even when you think the patient is asleep or cannot hear you. This is annoying to the patient. Besides, he may hear more than you think.

Remember that, although some patients seem to be unconscious, they may be fully aware of what is happening around them. Therefore, always speak and behave as if the patient can hear every word.

Be sensitive to those times when the patient doesn't want to talk. Respect his moods. At times saying nothing may have more meaning than any words or facial expressions on your part. Sometimes a pat on the shoulder or hand means more to a patient than anything you might say. Simply being by the stretcher or bed at the moment of trouble may be the most comforting message of all.

Using the Telephone. When you use the telephone or an intercommunication device (intercom), speak clearly and slowly. When you answer the telephone, for example, say, "Third floor west. Mrs. Brown, nursing aide, speaking." When you take a message for someone else, write it down immediately. Then, if possible, repeat it to the person calling to make sure it is correct. Ask the caller how to spell his name so you are sure you have it right. Record the following:

- The person being called
- The time the call was received
- The caller's name
- The message
- Your name

Section 3: Observing the Patient

OBJECTIVES: WHAT YOU WILL LEARN

When you have completed this section, you should be able:

- To use your senses of sight, touch, hearing, and smell to observe the patients you care for
- To notice changes in patients' appearance or behavior
- To describe the difference between *objective* and *subjective* reporting
- To report your observations promptly, accurately, and objectively

KEY IDEAS

Get into the habit of observing the patient during all your contacts with him. These contacts include the bed bath, bed making, meal times, visiting hours, and any other time you are with him. Observation of the patient is a continuous process. Observing begins the first time you see a patient and ends when he is discharged from the hospital.

Observation means more than just careful watching. It includes listening to the patient, talking to him, and asking questions. Be extra alert to anything unusual whenever you are with a patient. Notice any changes in the patient's condition or appearance that may be important. Watch also for changes in the patient's attitude, his moods, his emotional condition. Pay attention to any complaints. For example, report to the head nurse or team leader if:

- A patient who had an abdominal operation two or three days ago says, "The calf of my leg is sore."

- A patient who is being given a blood transfusion says, "I feel itchy."

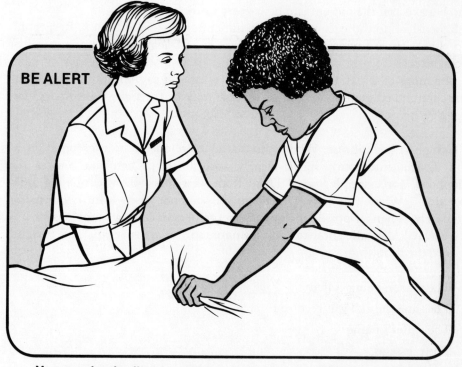

You may be the first to notice a change in the patient's condition, attitude, or emotional behavior

Methods of Observation

Use all of your senses when making observations:

- You can *see* some signs of change in a patient's condition. By using your eyes, you can observe a skin rash (breaking out), reddened areas, or swelling (edema).

- You can *feel* some signs with your fingers—a change in the patient's pulse rate, puffiness in the skin, dampness (lots of perspiration).

- You can *hear* some signs, such as a cough or wheezing sounds, when the patient breathes.

- You can *smell* some signs, such as an odor on the patient's breath.
- Listen to the patient talking, for other changes in his condition. Some can be felt and described only by the patient himself. Examples are pain, nausea, dizziness, a ringing in the ears, or headache.

Making useful observations is one of the most important things you will do in your work. Learning how to make useful observations will give you satisfaction, a feeling of achievement. The process never ends. You learn by doing it. Doctors and nurses never stop learning more about observing a patient. This is because observations are so important in the total medical care of the patient.

Things To Observe in a Patient

- *General appearance.* Has this changed? If so, in what way? Is there a noticeable odor (smell)?
- *Mental condition or mood.* Does the patient talk a lot? Very little? Does he talk about the future or the past? Does he talk about where he hurts? Is the patient anxious and worried? Is he very calm? Or is he very excited? Is he talking sensibly? Or not making sense? Is he speaking rapidly? Slowly? Is he cooperative? Uncooperative?
- *Position.* Does the patient lie still? Or does he toss around? Does he like to lie in one position better than others? Does he prefer being on his back? Or on his side? Is he able to move easily?
- *Eating and drinking habits.* Does he complain that he has no appetite? Does he dislike his diet? How much does he eat? Does he eat some of each kind of food? Is he always thirsty? Or does he very seldom drink water? Does he eat all of the food on his tray? Does he eat half the food on his tray? Does he refuse to eat?
- *Sleeping habits.* Is he able to sleep? Is he restless? Does he complain about not being able to sleep? Do these complaints agree with your observations? Does he sleep more than is normal? Is he constantly asleep?
- *Skin.* Is the patient's skin unusually pale (pallor)? Is it flushed (red)? Is the skin dry or moist? Are his lips and fingernails turning blue (cyanotic)? Is there any swelling (edema) noticeable? Are there reddened areas? Are these at the end of the spine, or on the heels, or at other pressure points? Is the skin shiny? Is there any puffiness? Is there puffiness in the legs and feet? Is his skin cold or clammy? Is it hot?
- *Eyes, ears, nose, and mouth.* Does the patient complain that he sees spots or flashes before his eyes? Does bright light bother him? Are his eyes inflamed? Is it hard for him to breathe through his nose? Does he seem to have a lot of mucous discharge from the nose? Does he say that he has a bad taste in his mouth? Is there an odor on his breath? Is the patient able to hear you?
- *Breathing.* Does the patient wheeze? Does he make other noises when he breathes? Does he cough? Does he cough up sputum? Lots of it? What is the color? Is it bloody? Does he have difficulty breathing (dyspnea)?
- *Abdomen, bowels, and bladder.* Does the patient's stomach appear to be puffed up? Does he complain of gassiness, belching, or nausea? Is he vomiting (having emesis)? Is he constipated? How often does he have a bowel movement? What is the color and consistency (hard or soft) of feces (stool)? Does the stool look like black tar or coffee grounds? Is the amount large or small? Is there any blood, or clumps of mucus, or pieces of white

material in the feces? How often does the patient void (urinate)? How much does he void each time? Does he say that he has pain during urination? That it is hard to start? Is there sediment (cloudiness) or blood in the urine? Does the urine have a peculiar odor or color? Is the patient unable to control his bowels or urine (incontinent)?

- *Pain.* Where is the pain? How long does the patient say he has had it? How does he describe the pain? Is it constant? Or does it come and go? Does he say that it is sharp, dull, aching, or knifelike? Has he had medicine for the pain? Does the patient say that the medicine relieved the pain?

- *Daily activities.* Did he dress himself? Did he walk without help? Did he walk with help? Did he avoid walking altogether?

- *Personal care.* Without help, did the patient brush his teeth? Comb his hair? Go to the bathroom? Wash his face? Did he need assistance?

- *Movements.* Is he shaking (having tremors or spasms)? Is he limp? Are his movements jerky, shaky, or jumpy?

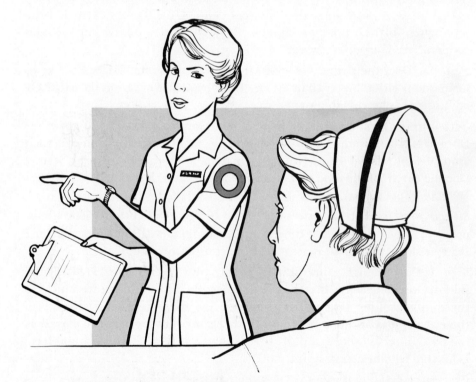

RULES TO FOLLOW WHEN REPORTING YOUR OBSERVATIONS

Write down patient's name, room number, and bed number

Write or report your observations to the head nurse or team leader as soon as possible

Report the time you made the observation

Report the location of the abnormal or unusual sign

Report exactly, but report only what you observe, that is, report objectively

Reporting

Objective and Subjective Reporting. It is very important for you to understand the difference between *objective* reporting and *subjective* reporting.

Objective reporting means reporting exactly what you observe—that is, reporting what you see, hear, feel, or smell. The nursing assistant must always use objective reporting.

Subjective reporting means giving your *opinion* about something, or what you think might be the case. One might report, for example, what he or she thinks is the cause of a change in a patient's condition or what might be the proper treatment. The nursing aide should never use subjective reporting.

Objective Reports. Here are some examples of objective reports of observations:

1. Mrs. Smith (404-B bed) is breathing rapidly and the breaths appear to be shallow.
2. Mr. Williams's (204-C bed) urine looks as if there is blood in it.
3. Cindy Jones (107-A bed) says that she has pain in her right upper abdomen.
4. Mr. Jones (101-A bed) picked up his selective menu but could not read it. He asked me to read it for him.
5. For Mr. Brown (104-B bed) to hear me, I had to speak louder than normal.
6. Mrs. Adams (119-C bed) said she didn't want to get out of bed.
7. Mr. Cass (103-D bed) can't hold a glass without spilling its contents.

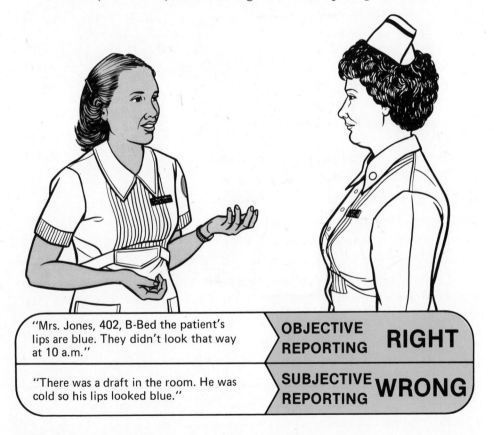

"Mrs. Jones, 402, B-Bed the patient's lips are blue. They didn't look that way at 10 a.m." | **OBJECTIVE REPORTING RIGHT**

"There was a draft in the room. He was cold so his lips looked blue." | **SUBJECTIVE REPORTING WRONG**

Observation of an Infant or Child. Observing an infant or a child means looking at his appearance and physical condition, his bodily functions and secretions, his movements, and his behavior. When you observe changes in any of these, it is very important that you report them to the head nurse or team leader right away. Report things that can be measured, such as a high temperature. Also report the things you see in a *pattern* of change, such as the child's behavior. Your careful observation and quick reporting could save a baby's life. The following are things to report when you observe them in infants or children:

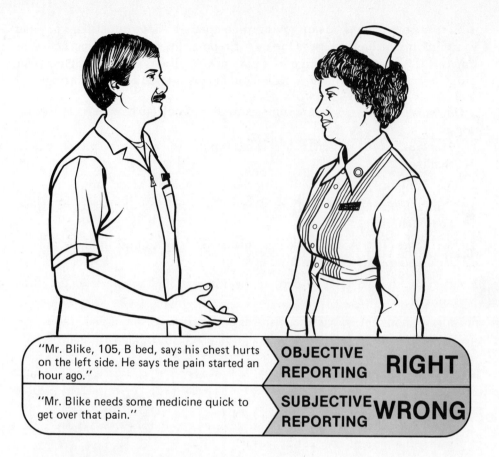

"Mr. Blike, 105, B bed, says his chest hurts on the left side. He says the pain started an hour ago." | OBJECTIVE REPORTING **RIGHT**

"Mr. Blike needs some medicine quick to get over that pain." | SUBJECTIVE REPORTING **WRONG**

Appearance and Physical Condition

- The child's temperature is high or very low.
- The pulse is unusually fast, slow, or irregular.
- The child is breathing rapidly or is having trouble breathing.
- The abdomen seems to be swollen.
- The child's skin does not look right. It may be yellow, or show purplish patches, or appear unusually pale, or have a blue cast. There may be blueness (cyanosis) in the fingernails or lips.
- There are secretions, bleeding, or odor coming from the baby's navel (umbilicus).

Bodily Functions and Secretions

- The child has not urinated during your hours of work or has voided very little.
- The child has diarrhea.
- There is a large amount of mucus being secreted in the mouth or nose.
- The child is producing a large amount of saliva.
- The child is having trouble swallowing.
- The child is coughing or choking.
- The child is vomiting.

Movement and Behavior

- The child is lying in an abnormal position.
- The muscles are twitching.
- There is no movement in the legs or arms.
- The child is lying very quietly or seems unusually still.
- The child is crying or is very irritable.

WHAT YOU HAVE LEARNED

Patients who have the same illness or medical condition often show the same behavior and have similar needs. Knowing what certain patients look like, how they act, and what their problems are likely to be will help you in your work. You will be better able to meet each patient's needs. You will be a more effective nursing aide and will give better care.

Your attitude is very important in your relationships with patients and visitors. A good attitude by everyone makes good relationships. The result is a pleasant working environment. The work in the unit goes more smoothly. In this pleasant atmosphere, patients and visitors have more confidence. Everyone feels better and the patients get the benefit.

Your attitude toward visitors should be just as courteous and friendly as it is toward patients and other staff members. Try always to be sympathetic and a good listener.

Be sure every patient knows how to use the signal cord. Always leave the cord where the patient can reach it easily.

Keep improving your skills in communication. The better you can communicate with everyone—patients, visitors, other staff members—the better you will feel about your work and the more self-confidence you will have.

You are in the best position to spot changes in the patient's condition and report them. Being with the patient so much of the time gives you many opportunities to learn and practice making observations.

Your head nurse or team leader depends on you to make good objective observations. She expects you to be prompt and accurate in reporting them.

The alert nursing aide is often the first person to see a major change in a patient's condition. Reporting it can be very important to the head nurse and especially to the patient.

Infection Control in the Health Care Institution

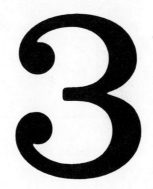

Section 1: Medical Asepsis

OBJECTIVES: WHAT YOU WILL LEARN

When you have completed this section, you should be able:

- To define medical asepsis
- To explain how microorganisms are destroyed
- To demonstrate the procedure for handwashing

KEY IDEAS

People who work in health care institutions soon learn the importance of cleanliness. Everyone tries constantly in many ways to achieve ideal sanitary conditions. You, too, take part in this team effort to keep everything absolutely clean. Why? Because cleanliness is a part of the hospital's effort to control disease and keep communicable diseases from spreading.

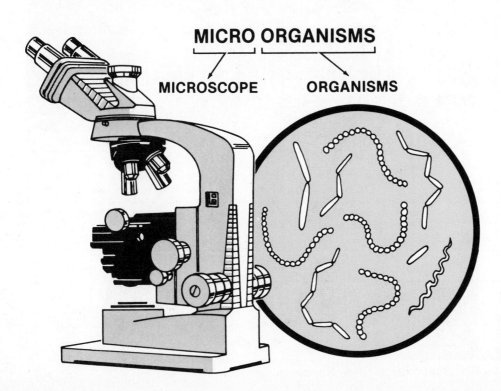

MICRO ORGANISMS

MICROSCOPE   ORGANISMS

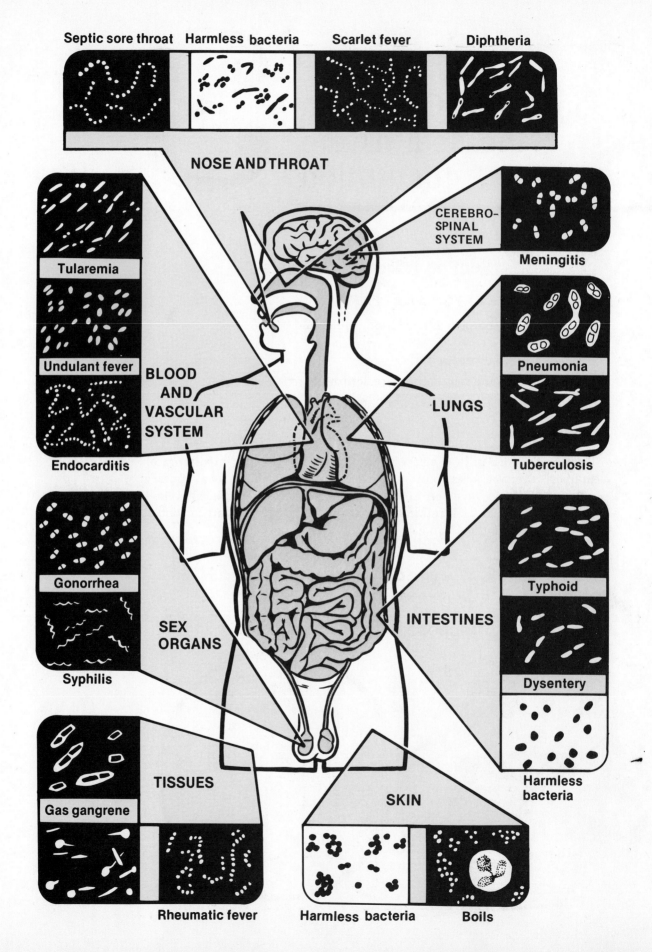

Septic sore throat   Harmless bacteria   Scarlet fever   Diphtheria

NOSE AND THROAT

CEREBRO-SPINAL SYSTEM

Meningitis

Tularemia

Undulant fever

BLOOD AND VASCULAR SYSTEM

Pneumonia

LUNGS

Endocarditis

Tuberculosis

Gonorrhea

Typhoid

Syphilis

SEX ORGANS

INTESTINES

Dysentery

Gas gangrene

TISSUES

SKIN

Harmless bacteria

Rheumatic fever   Harmless bacteria   Boils

You will understand the importance of cleanliness in the hospital if you know something about germs—the microorganisms that cause diseases. It may help to know what they are, how they spread, and how they can be destroyed.

The Cause of Disease

People once believed that sickness was caused by evil spirits. About 500 years ago scientists began to suspect that some diseases were caused by very small living things they called germs.

Germs are a kind of *microorganism*. *Micro* means very small. Germs can be seen only under a microscope. And *organism* means a living thing. Different kinds of microorganisms (also called microbes) are:

- Protozoa (microscopic animals)
- Fungi, including molds and yeasts
- Bacteria (microscopic plants)
- Rickettsiae
- Viruses

The Nature of Microorganisms

Most microorganisms are helpful to people. For example, certain microbes cause a chemical change in food called *fermentation*. Fermentation is the change that produces cottage cheese from milk, beer from grains, cider from apples, and sauerkraut from cabbage. Other microorganisms in the human digestive system break down the foods not used by the body and turn them into waste products (feces).

There are other kinds of microorganisms, however, that are harmful to man. These are the microbes that cause disease and infection. Disease- producing microorganisms are called *pathogens*. They grow best at body temperature, 98.6° F (37° C). Pathogens destroy human tissue by using it as

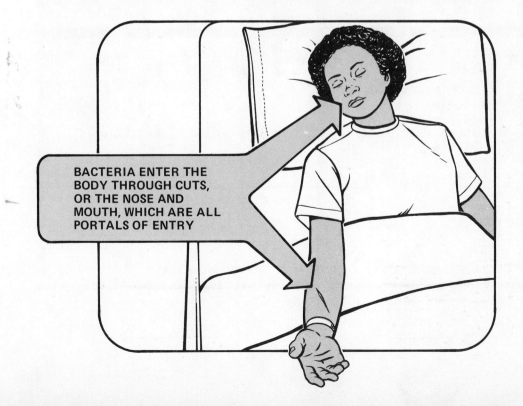

BACTERIA ENTER THE BODY THROUGH CUTS, OR THE NOSE AND MOUTH, WHICH ARE ALL PORTALS OF ENTRY

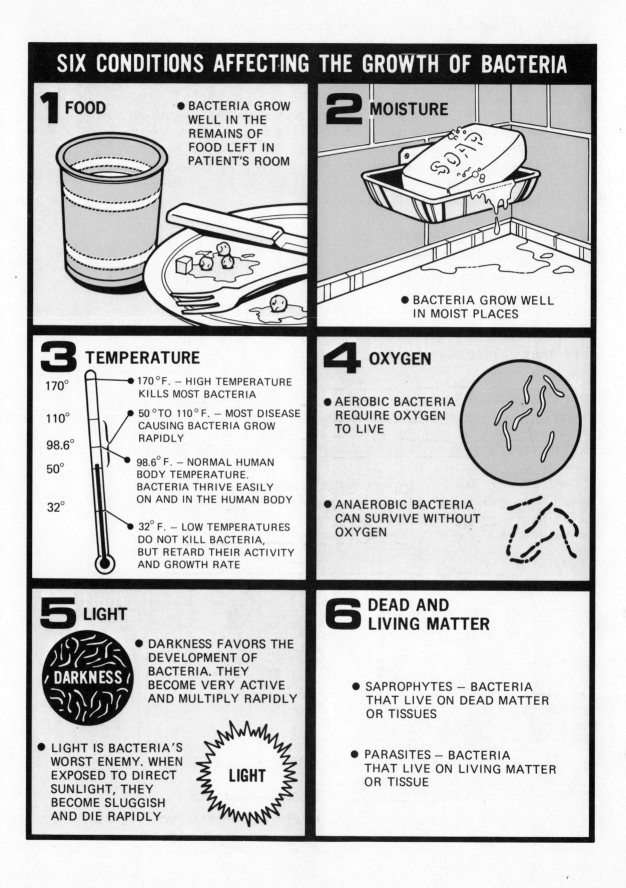

SIX CONDITIONS AFFECTING THE GROWTH OF BACTERIA

1 FOOD
- BACTERIA GROW WELL IN THE REMAINS OF FOOD LEFT IN PATIENT'S ROOM

2 MOISTURE
- BACTERIA GROW WELL IN MOIST PLACES

3 TEMPERATURE
- 170°F. — HIGH TEMPERATURE KILLS MOST BACTERIA
- 50° TO 110°F. — MOST DISEASE CAUSING BACTERIA GROW RAPIDLY
- 98.6°F. — NORMAL HUMAN BODY TEMPERATURE. BACTERIA THRIVE EASILY ON AND IN THE HUMAN BODY
- 32°F. — LOW TEMPERATURES DO NOT KILL BACTERIA, BUT RETARD THEIR ACTIVITY AND GROWTH RATE

170°
110°
98.6°
50°
32°

4 OXYGEN
- AEROBIC BACTERIA REQUIRE OXYGEN TO LIVE
- ANAEROBIC BACTERIA CAN SURVIVE WITHOUT OXYGEN

5 LIGHT
- DARKNESS FAVORS THE DEVELOPMENT OF BACTERIA. THEY BECOME VERY ACTIVE AND MULTIPLY RAPIDLY

DARKNESS

- LIGHT IS BACTERIA'S WORST ENEMY. WHEN EXPOSED TO DIRECT SUNLIGHT, THEY BECOME SLUGGISH AND DIE RAPIDLY

LIGHT

6 DEAD AND LIVING MATTER
- SAPROPHYTES — BACTERIA THAT LIVE ON DEAD MATTER OR TISSUES
- PARASITES — BACTERIA THAT LIVE ON LIVING MATTER OR TISSUE

food. They also give off waste products called toxins. These are absorbed into and poison the body.

In the hospital you will often hear the words *staph* or *staphylococcus* and *strep* or *streptococcus*. Staphylococcus and streptococcus are two types of bacteria. These pathogens are found in all health care institutions. They are usually found on the human skin. They enter the body through a portal of entry, for example, the nose, or the mouth, or a cut. When staphylococci (the microorganisms) get into the body, they may produce a local infection. There may be soreness and pus or a sty on the eyelid. Sometimes staphylococcus infections can affect the whole body. When streptococci enter the body, they can cause a septic sore throat, a local infection, or rheumatic fever, a general infection.

A virus is another form of microorganism. Viruses are much smaller than bacteria, and they cause many of man's diseases. Examples are measles, smallpox, and influenza. Viruses can survive only in living cells.

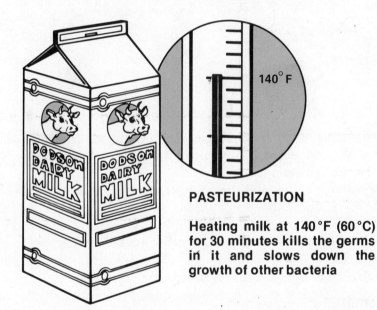

PASTEURIZATION

Heating milk at 140°F (60°C) for 30 minutes kills the germs in it and slows down the growth of other bacteria

History of Infection Control

The germ theory of disease was not actually proved until about 100 years ago. A French scientist named Louis Pasteur made two important discoveries about bacteria. First, he discovered that many diseases are caused by bacteria. Second, he discovered that bacteria could be killed by heat.

Pasteur's name has been used to refer to this method of killing germs. For example, *pasteurization* is the process of heating milk to about 140° F (60° C) and keeping it at that temperature for one-half hour. Pasteurization kills harmful bacteria and makes milk safe for us to drink.

A few years after Pasteur's discoveries, a British surgeon named Joseph Lister found that germs could also be killed by carbolic acid. Lister recognized that many deaths in hospitals seemed to be connected with unclean conditions. He was the first to want surgical wounds kept clean and the air in the operating room kept pure.

Lister changed things in hospitals by introducing the principles and methods of aseptic surgery. *Aseptic* means germ-free, without disease-producing organisms. Lister developed a technique to keep germs out of open wounds or to destroy them. His method was to spray the skin around the

MICROORGANISMS ARE EVERYWHERE

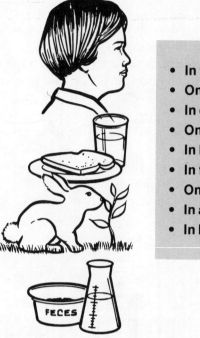

- **In the air we breathe**
- **On our bodies**
- **In our bodies**
- **On our clothing**
- **In liquids**
- **In food**
- **On animals**
- **In animals**
- **In human waste**

wound with carbolic acid. Also, surgical instruments were made aseptic by being dipped in a carbolic acid solution. This technique was a major advance in the battle against disease.

People working in hospitals began to realize that some disease-producing germs are everywhere. They are in the air, on the furniture, on and inside the patients' bodies, and on all the equipment. Doctors knew that germs multiply very rapidly. They also knew that if germs are not killed, they spread infection and disease from one person to another. Therefore, it was necessary to apply the principles of asepsis to the entire health care institution.

Disinfection and Sterilization

A continuous battle goes on in health care institutions to prevent the spread of pathogens. This battle is called *medical asepsis.* In spite of the best efforts of hospital personnel, there are always some harmful microorganisms around us. They can be made harmless, however, by ordinary cleanliness procedures. We can keep ourselves clean by bathing and frequent handwashing. We can keep the institution and its equipment clean with soap and water. Also, there are two very important methods for killing microorganisms or keeping them under control. These methods are disinfection and sterilization.

- *Disinfection* is the process of destroying as many harmful organisms as possible. It also means slowing down the growth and activity of the organisms that cannot be destroyed.
- *Sterilization* is the process of killing all microorganisms, including spores, in a certain area.

Spores are bacteria that have formed hard shells around themselves as a defense. These shells are like a protective suit of armor. Spores are very difficult to kill. Some can even live in boiling water. Spores can be destroyed, however, by being exposed to pressurized steam at a high temperature.

WAYS THAT MICROORGANISMS ARE SPREAD

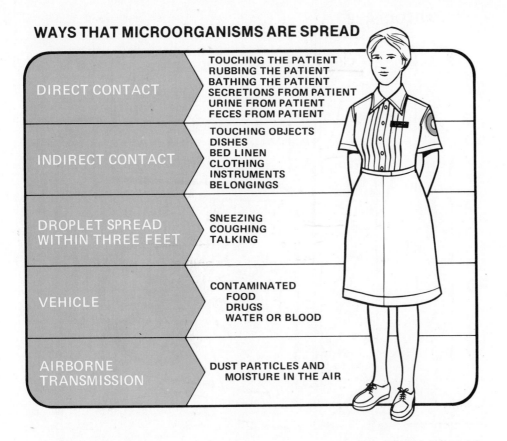

DIRECT CONTACT	TOUCHING THE PATIENT RUBBING THE PATIENT BATHING THE PATIENT SECRETIONS FROM PATIENT URINE FROM PATIENT FECES FROM PATIENT
INDIRECT CONTACT	TOUCHING OBJECTS DISHES BED LINEN CLOTHING INSTRUMENTS BELONGINGS
DROPLET SPREAD WITHIN THREE FEET	SNEEZING COUGHING TALKING
VEHICLE	CONTAMINATED FOOD DRUGS WATER OR BLOOD
AIRBORNE TRANSMISSION	DUST PARTICLES AND MOISTURE IN THE AIR

Machines called *autoclaves* can produce this high-temperature, pressurized steam. Autoclaves are used to kill spores and other disease-producing bacteria.

When an object is free of all microorganisms, it is called *sterile*. Bacteria are completely destroyed when enough heat is used, or when combined heat, moisture, and pressure are used. Using heat alone is not always the best method. Sometimes the amount of heat needed to kill all microorganisms on an article will burn the article itself. Therefore, scientists have developed a method of combining heat with moisture in the form of steam under pressure. This is an effective way of sterilizing objects used in the hospital, that is, of killing all microorganisms on and near the object.

Most supplies and equipment used in the care of patients can be disinfected to prevent them from spreading disease or infection. Sterilization is necessary if the article comes in direct contact with a wound, as in the case of surgical instruments.

Medical Asepsis

Medical asepsis means preventing the conditions that allow pathogens to live, multiply, and spread. As a nursing aide, you will share the responsibility for preventing the spread of disease and infection by using aseptic techniques.

The main purposes for medical asepsis in caring for patients are:

• Protecting the patient against becoming infected a second time by the same microorganism. This is called *reinfection*.

• Protecting the patient against becoming infected by a new or different type of microorganism from another patient or a member of the hospital staff. This is called *cross infection*.

AUTOCLAVE

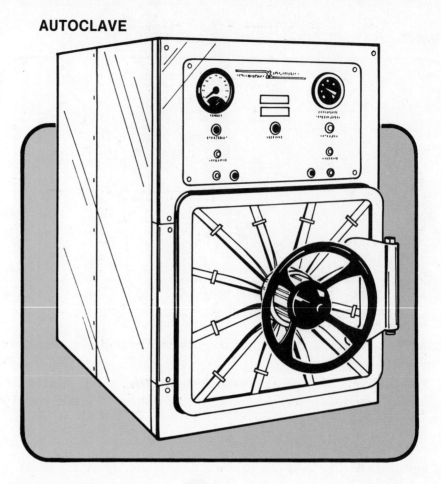

- Protecting all other patients and hospital staff against becoming infected by microorganisms passing from patient to patient, staff to patient, or patient to staff.

Handwashing

In your work you will be using your hands constantly. You will often be touching sick patients. You will handle supplies and equipment used in the treatment and care of patients. Germs will get on your hands.

They will come from the patient or from the things he or she has touched. Your hands could carry these germs to other persons and places. The germs could also be moved to your own face and mouth. Washing your hands will help to prevent this transfer of germs.

You must wash your hands before and after contact with each patient. This is the single most important way to prevent the spread of infection and disease.

Rules To Follow.   The following are rules and reasons for medical asepsis:

- Handwashing must be done before and after each nursing task and before and after direct patient contact.
- The water faucet is always considered contaminated. This means there are disease germs on it. This is why you use paper towels to turn the faucet on and off.

WASHING YOUR HANDS

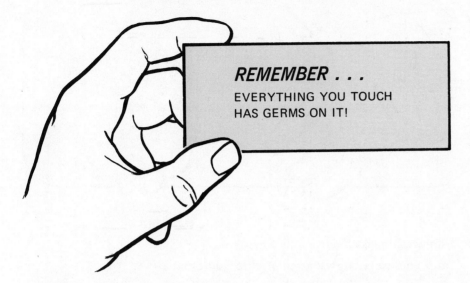

REMEMBER . . .
EVERYTHING YOU TOUCH
HAS GERMS ON IT!

- If your hands accidentally touch the inside of the sink, start over. Do the whole procedure again.
- Take soap from a dispenser, if possible, rather than use bar soap. Bar soap accumulates pools of soapy water in the soap dish, which is then considered contaminated.

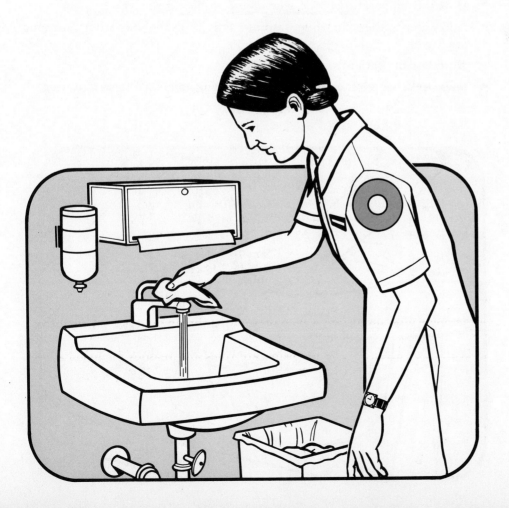

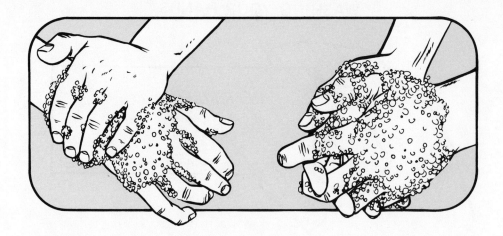

- Handwashing is effective only when:
  a. You use enough soap to produce lots of lather.
  b. You rub skin against skin to create friction, which helps to eliminate microorganisms.
  c. You rinse from the clean to the dirty parts of your hands. Rinse with running water from elbows to hands and then to the fingertips.
- Hold your hands lower than your elbows while washing. This is to prevent germs from contaminating your arms. Holding your hands down prevents backflow over unwashed skin.
- Have the temperature of the water comfortable for you.
- Add water to the soap while washing. This keeps the soap from becoming too dry.
- Never use the patient's soap for yourself.
- Rinse well. Soap left on the skin causes drying and can be very irritating.

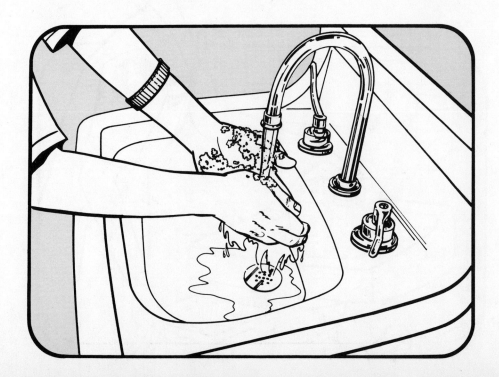

Procedure: Handwashing

1. <u>Assemble your equipment</u>. The equipment used for handwashing is found at all times at every sink in all health care institutions.
   a. <u>Soap or detergent</u>
   b. <u>Paper towels</u>
   c. <u>Warm running water</u>
   d. <u>Wastepaper basket</u>

2. Turn the faucet on with a paper towel held between your hands and the faucet. Adjust the water to a temperature comfortable for you.

3. Discard the paper towel in the wastepaper basket.

4. Completely wet your hands and wrists under the running water. Keep your fingertips pointed downward.

5. Apply soap or detergent.

6. Hold your hands lower than your elbows while washing.

7. Work up a good lather. Spread it over the entire area of your hands and wrists. Get soap under your nails and between your fingers.

8. Clean under your nails. Use an orange stick.

9. Use a rotating and rubbing (frictional) motion for one full minute:
   a. **Rub vigorously.**
   b. Rub one hand against the other hand and wrist.
   c. Rub between your fingers by interlacing them.
   d. Rub up and down to reach all skin surfaces on your hands and between your fingers.
   e. Rub the tips of your fingers against your palms to clean with friction around the nail beds.

10. Wash at least two inches above your wrists.

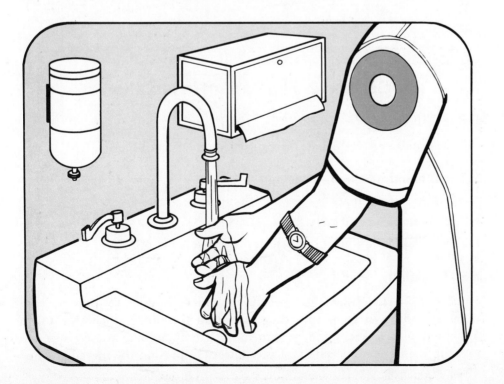

11. Rinse well. Rinse from your elbows to hands. Hold your hands and fingertips down, under running water.

12. Dry thoroughly with paper towels.

13. Turn off the faucet. Use a paper towel between your hands and the faucet. Never touch the faucet with your hands.

14. Throw the paper towel into the wastepaper basket. Don't touch the basket.

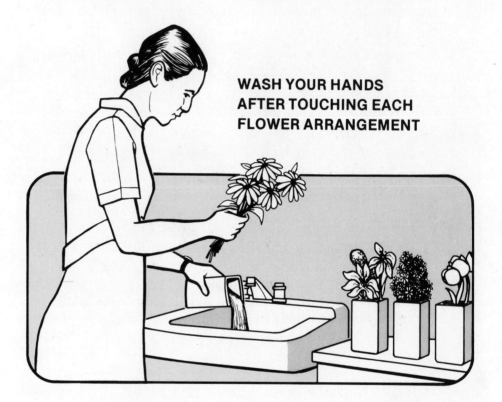

WASH YOUR HANDS AFTER TOUCHING EACH FLOWER ARRANGEMENT

Section 2: The Patient in Isolation

OBJECTIVES: WHAT YOU WILL LEARN

When you have completed this section, you should be able:

- To demonstrate double bagging
- To demonstrate mask and gown technique
- To define *clean* and *dirty*
- To explain isolation and reverse or protective isolation

KEY IDEAS

Aside from handwashing, special methods are used to prevent communicable diseases from spreading. Isolation technique, including use of masks and gowns, keeps disease germs away from equipment and personnel. Certain hospital areas need extra precautions to prevent the spread of infection and disease.

Communicable Diseases and Infections

Communicable diseases spread very quickly and easily from one person to another. Examples are measles and smallpox. Sometimes the more general term *communicable conditions* is used because it includes both diseases and infections. Ordinary cleanliness alone will not protect you and others from catching such diseases. When a patient has one of these diseases, special precautions are necessary. These safety measures are called *isolation technique.* The patient is separated (in isolation) from other patients and personnel.

The purpose of isolation technique is to keep the germs that cause the disease inside the isolated patient's unit. As you know, these disease germs are everywhere in the sick room. They are on the floor, furniture, bedding, articles brought to the bedside—and on the patient himself. The area, the articles, and the patient are said to be *contaminated.* When you touch or brush your clothes against any of them, disease germs are almost sure to contaminate your hands or clothing. Isolation technique is used to prevent the germs from leaving the unit on your hands, arms, or on clothing or articles used in the unit.

The special precautions and procedures outlined later tell you how to protect yourself from catching the patient's disease and how to avoid carrying it outside his unit to other persons.

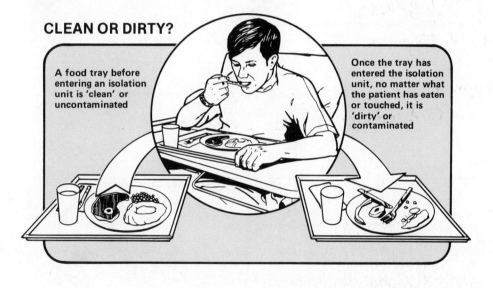

CLEAN OR DIRTY?

A food tray before entering an isolation unit is 'clean' or uncontaminated

Once the tray has entered the isolation unit, no matter what the patient has eaten or touched, it is 'dirty' or contaminated

Clean and *Dirty*

The words *clean* and *dirty* have a special meaning when we are talking about isolation technique. *Clean* means uncontaminated. It refers to those articles and places from which disease cannot spread. *Dirty* means contaminated. Articles or places near the patient who has a communicable condition are dirty. These are things and areas from which disease can spread. For example, before a patient receives his meal tray, the tray is clean. After the tray has been in his room, no matter what he has or has not touched or eaten, it is dirty and can spread disease.

Clean refers to all articles and places that have not been contaminated with or come in contact with pathogens.

Dirty refers to those articles and places that a patient has been near or touched. They may be "dirty" or contaminated with pathogens.

ISOLATION

PURPOSE OF ISOLATION

A HOSPITAL ISOLATES A PATIENT WITH A DISEASE THAT IS CATCHING TO REDUCE THE POSSIBILITY OF SPREADING THE DISEASE. THIS IS DONE TO PROTECT PATIENTS AND STAFF.

REGULAR ISOLATION

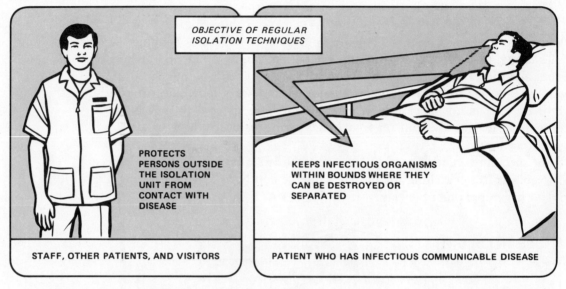

OBJECTIVE OF REGULAR ISOLATION TECHNIQUES

PROTECTS PERSONS OUTSIDE THE ISOLATION UNIT FROM CONTACT WITH DISEASE

KEEPS INFECTIOUS ORGANISMS WITHIN BOUNDS WHERE THEY CAN BE DESTROYED OR SEPARATED

STAFF, OTHER PATIENTS, AND VISITORS

PATIENT WHO HAS INFECTIOUS COMMUNICABLE DISEASE

IN REGULAR ISOLATION, CONTAMINATION IS PREVENTED FROM SPREADING FROM THE ROOM.

REVERSE OR PROTECTIVE ISOLATION

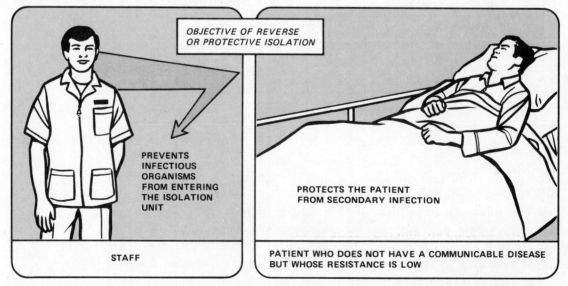

OBJECTIVE OF REVERSE OR PROTECTIVE ISOLATION

PREVENTS INFECTIOUS ORGANISMS FROM ENTERING THE ISOLATION UNIT

PROTECTS THE PATIENT FROM SECONDARY INFECTION

STAFF

PATIENT WHO DOES NOT HAVE A COMMUNICABLE DISEASE BUT WHOSE RESISTANCE IS LOW

SOMETIMES A PATIENT WHOSE RESISTANCE IS LOW AND WHO COULD EASILY CATCH A DISEASE IS ISOLATED FROM POSSIBLE INFECTIONS' THIS IS COMMONLY DONE FOR BURN PATIENTS. IT IS CALLED *REVERSE* OR *PROTECTIVE* ISOLATION. IN PROTECTIVE ISOLATION, CONTAMINATION MUST BE PREVENTED FROM ENTERING THE ROOM.

One good way to control the spread of disease is to have two areas:

- A *clean* utility room. Things are stored or prepared here that have never been near or had contact with a patient or any articles belonging to the patient.
- A *dirty* utility room. Things or articles are brought here after having been in contact with the patient or with the patient's belongings.

Equipment kept in these utility rooms varies greatly from one institution to another. In most hospitals there is a special area in the dirty utility room for items to be put that have to be returned to the central supply room (CSR) after having been used for a patient. Dirty linen hampers should be stored in the dirty utility room.

Protective Isolation Card: Color-coded Blue*

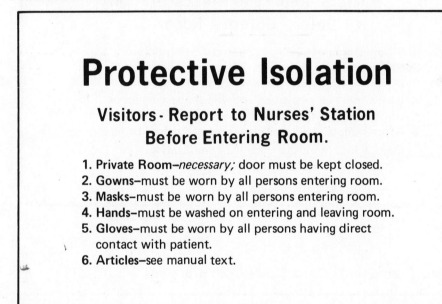

Protective Isolation

Visitors - Report to Nurses' Station Before Entering Room.

1. **Private Room**–*necessary;* door must be kept closed.
2. **Gowns**–must be worn by all persons entering room.
3. **Masks**–must be worn by all persons entering room.
4. **Hands**–must be washed on entering and leaving room.
5. **Gloves**–must be worn by all persons having direct contact with patient.
6. **Articles**–see manual text.

ONE OF THE FOLLOWING CARDS IS ALWAYS HUNG ON THE DOOR OF THE ISOLATED UNIT TO IDENTIFY THE TYPE OF ISOLATION AND TO GIVE INSTRUCTIONS TO EVERYONE ENTERING THE ISOLATED UNIT

*Public Health Service Publication no. 2054: Isolation technique for use in hospitals. Washington, DC, U.S. Government Printing Office.

Special Areas for Preventive Measures

Certain patient care areas in the hospital need special attention to ensure cleanliness. Precautions to prevent communicable conditions from spreading are more strict than in other areas. This is because the patients in these areas may have a low resistance to disease. However, they do not have any communicable conditions. These areas include:

- Newborn nursery
- Premature care nursery
- Postpartum patient care unit
- Surgical patient care unit (operating room)
- Delivery room
- Cardiac care unit
- Dialysis unit

Face Masks

When a patient's communicable condition can be spread by breathing, face masks are very important. Before you put on or take off a face mask, be sure your hands are thoroughly clean. Face masks are effective for 30 minutes only. If you stay in an isolated area longer, you must wash your hands and remove the old mask. Then you will put on a clean mask. Masks are used only once and then thrown away. If the mask gets wet, it must be changed.

Strict Isolation Card: Color-Coded Yellow*

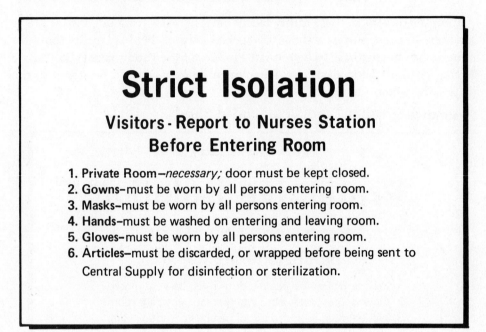

Strict Isolation

Visitors - Report to Nurses Station
Before Entering Room

1. **Private Room**—*necessary;* door must be kept closed.
2. **Gowns**–must be worn by all persons entering room.
3. **Masks**–must be worn by all persons entering room.
4. **Hands**–must be washed on entering and leaving room.
5. **Gloves**–must be worn by all persons entering room.
6. **Articles**–must be discarded, or wrapped before being sent to Central Supply for disinfection or sterilization.

Enteric Precautions Card: Color-Coded Brown*

Enteric Precautions

Visitors - Report to Nurses' Station
Before Entering Room

1. **Private Room**–*necessary for children only.*
2. **Gowns**–must be worn by all persons having direct contact with patient.
3. **Mask**–not necessary.
4. **Hands**–must be washed on entering and leaving room.
5. **Gloves**–must be worn by all persons having direct contact with patient.
6. **Articles**–special precautions necessary for articles contaminated with urine and feces. Articles must be disinfected or discarded.

*Public Health Service Publication no. 2054: Isolation technique for use in hospitals. Washington, DC, U.S. Government Printing Office

Wound and Skin Precautions Card: Color-Coded Green*

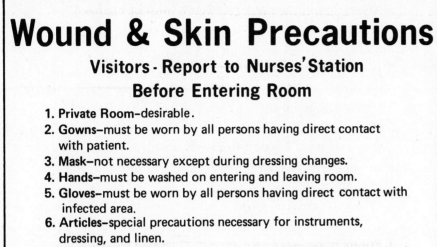

Wound & Skin Precautions
Visitors - Report to Nurses' Station
Before Entering Room

1. **Private Room**–desirable.
2. **Gowns**–must be worn by all persons having direct contact with patient.
3. **Mask**–not necessary except during dressing changes.
4. **Hands**–must be washed on entering and leaving room.
5. **Gloves**–must be worn by all persons having direct contact with infected area.
6. **Articles**–special precautions necessary for instruments, dressing, and linen.
7. **NOTE:** See manual for Special Dressing Techniques to be used when changing dressings.

Respiratory Isolation Card: Color-Coded Red*

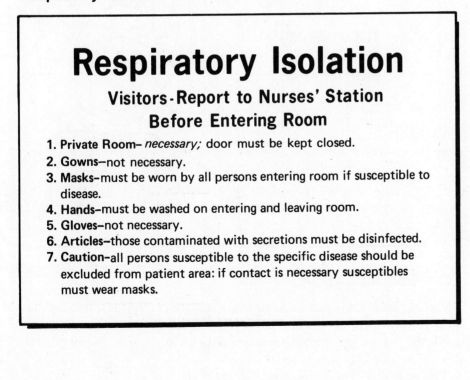

Respiratory Isolation
Visitors - Report to Nurses' Station
Before Entering Room

1. **Private Room**– *necessary;* door must be kept closed.
2. **Gowns**–not necessary.
3. **Masks**–must be worn by all persons entering room if susceptible to disease.
4. **Hands**–must be washed on entering and leaving room.
5. **Gloves**–not necessary.
6. **Articles**–those contaminated with secretions must be disinfected.
7. **Caution**–all persons susceptible to the specific disease should be excluded from patient area: if contact is necessary susceptibles must wear masks.

*Public Health Service Publications no. 2054: Isolation technique for use in hospitals. Washington, DC, U.S. Government Printing Office

Procedure: Mask Technique

1. Assemble your equipment: disposable paper mask.

2. Wash your hands.

3. Remove a clean mask from its container.

4. Hold the mask firmly, avoiding unnecessary handling. Do not touch the part of the mask that will cover your face. Hold the mask by the strings only.

5. Place the mask over your nose and mouth. Tie the top strings over your ears first. Then tie the lower strings.

6. Be sure the mask covers your nose and mouth during your task or procedure with the patient.

7. When you are ready to take off the mask, wash your hands.

8. Untie the bottom ties first, to avoid contamination. Hold the mask by the strings or loops only.

9. Untie the top strings. Remove the mask from your face. Discard it in the proper container inside the patient's room.

10. Wash your hands.

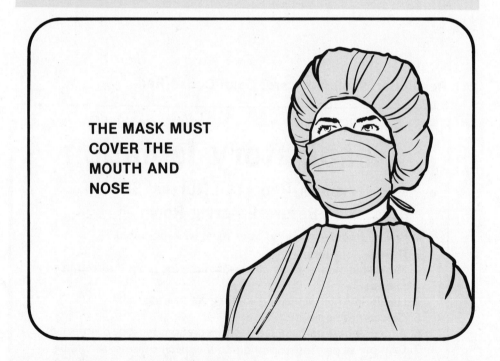

THE MASK MUST COVER THE MOUTH AND NOSE

KEY IDEAS: ISOLATION GOWNS

You will wear an isolation gown when you are caring for a patient in isolation. You will wear the gown if there is any possibility that your clothes could touch the patient or brush against any articles in the unit. Remember all of this is considered contaminated.

There are three types of isolation gowns:

- Cotton twill, which is reusable after proper washing
- A paper disposable gown, which is thrown away after one use
- A plastic disposable apron, which is worn once and thrown away

You will hear the expression, *individual gown technique*. This means that a gown should be used only once. It is then discarded in the proper dirty linen hamper or trash can. This is done before you leave the isolated room.

To be effective, the isolation gown must cover your uniform completely. Therefore, it is made wide enough to lap over in the back.

Put on a clean gown in the hall before you enter the patient's room. Take off the dirty gown in the patient's room before leaving.

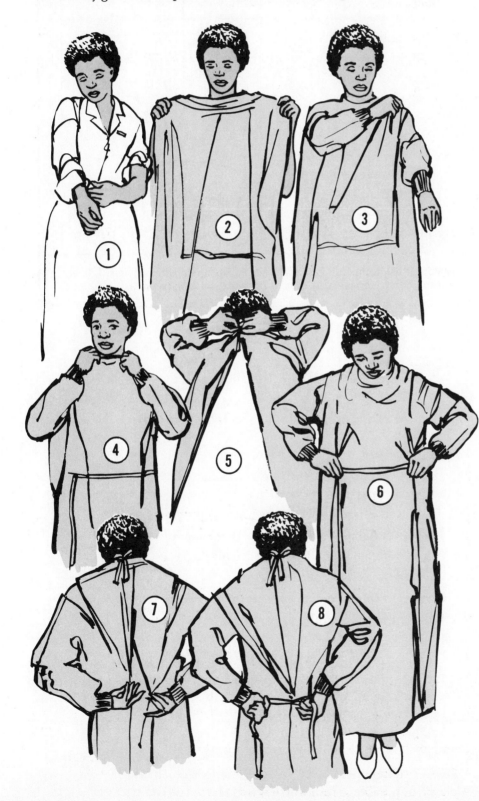

PROCEDURE: PUTTING ON AN ISOLATION GOWN IN THE HALL

1. With clean hands, roll long sleeves of uniform above the elbows.
2. Unfold gown so that opening is at back.
3. Put your arms in the sleeves.

4. Fit the gown at the neck making sure the uniform is covered.
5. Reach behind and tie the neck band with a simple shoelace bow.
6. Grasp edges of gown and pull to back.

7. Overlap edges of gown; roll gown edges together in back.
8. Tie waist tapes in a bow.

SOILED, CONTAMINATED LINEN
DOUBLE-BAGGING TECHNIQUE

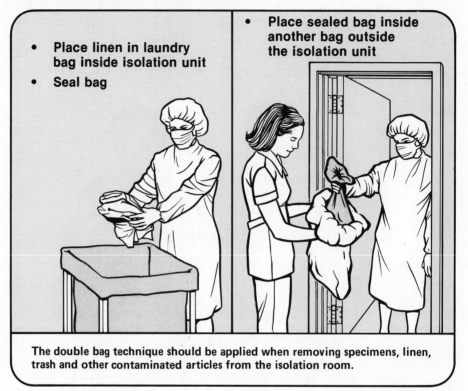

- **Place linen in laundry bag inside isolation unit**
- **Seal bag**

- **Place sealed bag inside another bag outside the isolation unit**

The double bag technique should be applied when removing specimens, linen, trash and other contaminated articles from the isolation room.

Procedure: Removing an Isolation Gown

1. Untie the waist-tapes and loosen the gown.
2. Use a paper towel to turn on the faucet. Don't touch the faucet with your fingers.
3. Throw the paper towel into the wastepaper basket.
4. Wash your hands and dry them with a paper towel.
5. Again, with a dry paper towel, turn off the faucet.
6. Open the neck band of the gown.
7. Place your fingers under one cuff to pull the sleeve over your hand.
8. Pull your arm out of the sleeve by grasping the opposite sleeve with your gown-covered hand.
9. Roll the gown in half, with the contaminated part inside.
10. If the gown is washable, put it in the dirty linen hamper inside the patient's room. If the gown is disposable, place it in a trash container inside the patient's room.
11. Wash your hands.
12. Use a paper towel to open the door to leave the room. Put the towel in the wastepaper basket inside the patient's room as you leave.

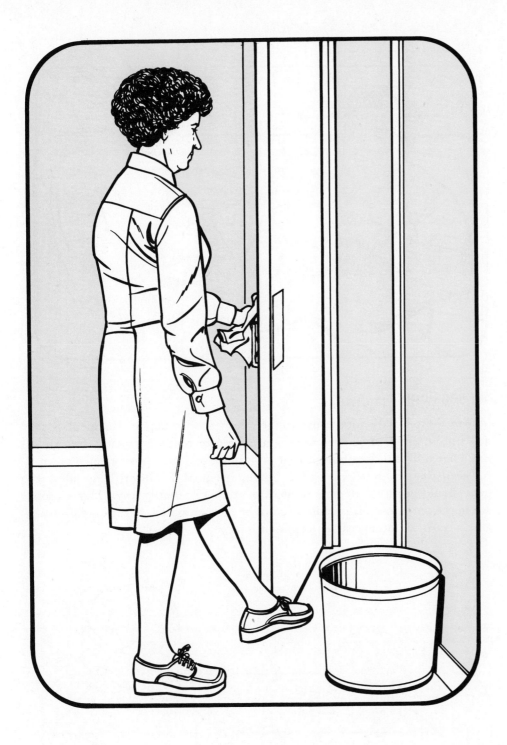

KEY IDEAS: PERSONAL CARE OF THE PATIENT IN ISOLATION

The patient in isolation needs the same personal care as any other patient. It is very important to combine normal patient care with good isolation technique. These tasks should be performed in your usual efficient and pleasant manner. You will make continuous observations to note any pattern of change in the patient's appearance or behavior.

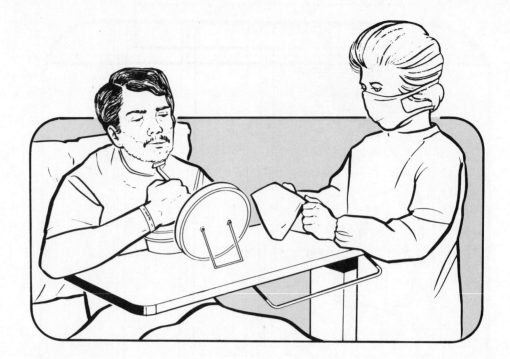

Serving Food

Many hospitals do not require you to wear a gown when serving meals to patients in isolation. If you are serving a patient or removing a tray, be careful that your uniform does not become contaminated. You must wear a gown if you feed a patient or stay with him during his meal. Food for the isolated patient should be served in disposable dishes on a disposable tray. Uneaten food left in the patient's unit is considered to be contaminated. Scraps are disposed of in a trash container inside the patient's room.

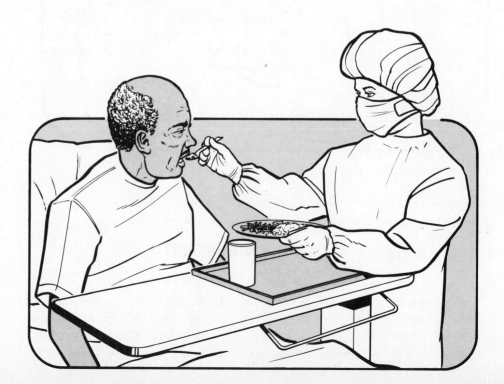

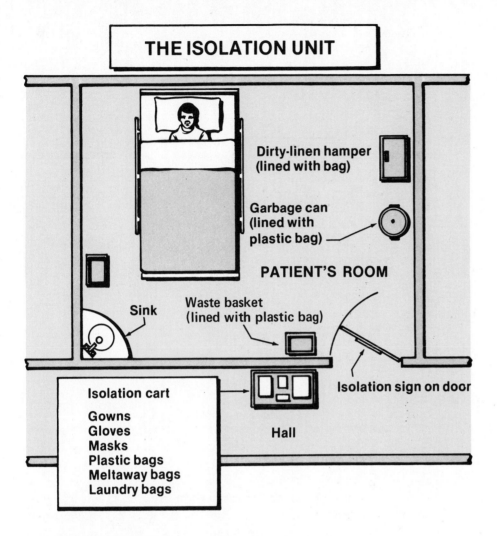

THE ISOLATION UNIT

Dirty-linen hamper (lined with bag)

Garbage can (lined with plastic bag)

PATIENT'S ROOM

Sink

Waste basket (lined with plastic bag)

Isolation sign on door

Isolation cart

Gowns
Gloves
Masks
Plastic bags
Meltaway bags
Laundry bags

Hall

Contaminated Articles and Excreta

For some patients in isolation it is necessary to take special precautions with articles contaminated by urine or feces. For example, it may be necessary to disinfect (or discard) a bedpan and excreta. Follow your hospital's procedure and the instructions of your head nurse or team leader.

WHAT YOU HAVE LEARNED

Diseases are caused by microorganisms. The spread of pathogens is reduced by keeping everything clean. Being extra careful to avoid contamination is a way of keeping the hospital environment safe.

Isolation technique is especially important. Each step in every isolation procedure must be done carefully.

Washing your hands before and after contacts with patients is probably the best example of protection for people—personnel as well as patients.

Your Working Environment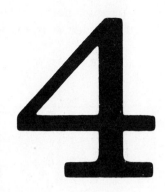

Section 1: The Patient's Unit and Equipment

OBJECTIVES: WHAT YOU WILL LEARN

When you have completed this section you should be able:

- To describe the patient's unit
- To check the unit
- To define disposable equipment
- To list the equipment contained in the unit
- To identify and describe the purpose of each piece of large equipment

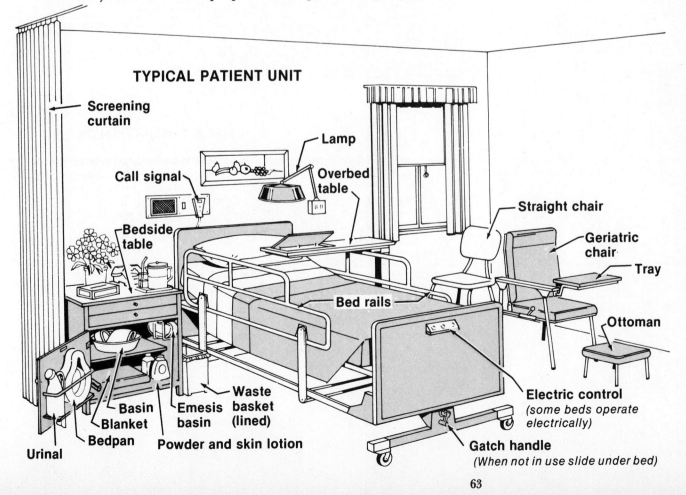

TYPICAL PATIENT UNIT

Screening curtain

Lamp

Call signal

Overbed table

Straight chair

Geriatric chair

Tray

Bedside table

Bed rails

Ottoman

Electric control *(some beds operate electrically)*

Waste basket (lined)

Basin

Emesis basin

Blanket

Bedpan

Powder and skin lotion

Urinal

Gatch handle *(When not in use slide under bed)*

KEY IDEAS

A patient's unit consists of all of the room space and furniture and equipment provided by the hospital for one patient. Each unit can be screened off

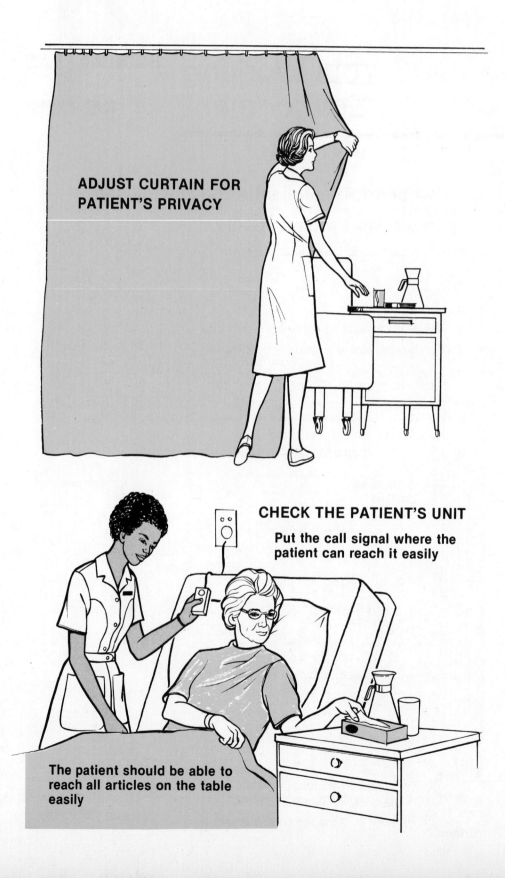

ADJUST CURTAIN FOR PATIENT'S PRIVACY

CHECK THE PATIENT'S UNIT

Put the call signal where the patient can reach it easily

The patient should be able to reach all articles on the table easily

for privacy by movable screens or draw curtains.

After a patient has been assigned to the unit for which you are responsible, make sure everything that belongs in the unit is there, and in its proper place.

A hospital unit designed for children may be different from an adult unit. A child's age and the reason he is in the hospital will determine how his unit is arranged and the equipment that will be needed.

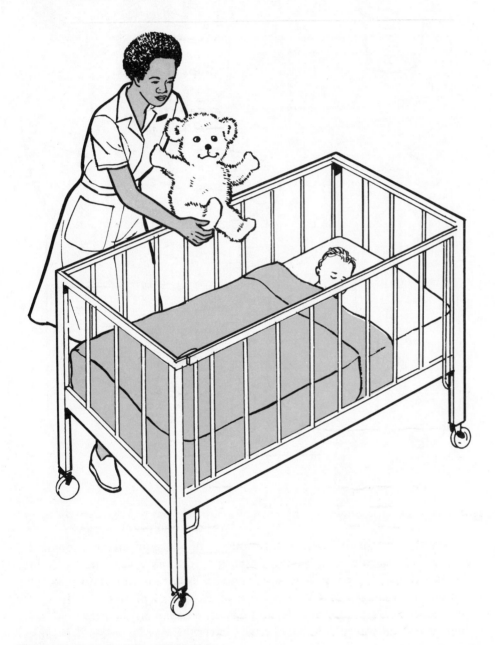

If the Patient Is a Small Child

Before you leave the unit:

- Be sure the bedside rails are pulled up and locked in place.
- Be sure there are no small toys or objects in the patient's bed that he can swallow.
- Remove larger objects that the child could stand on. He might fall out of bed. Also, remove toys or objects with which the child could injure himself.

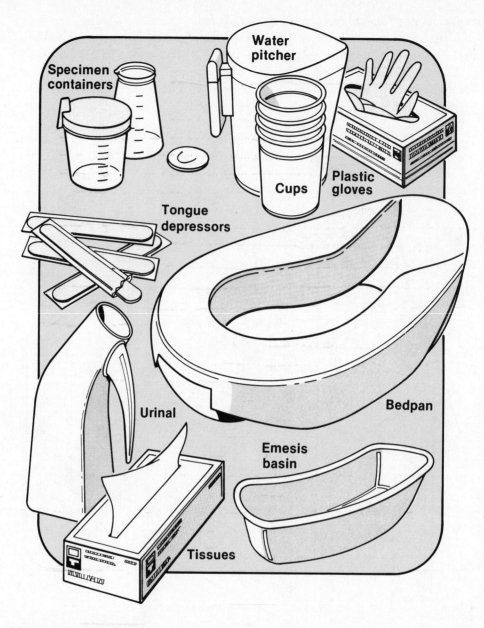

Disposable Equipment

Today in most health care institutions standard equipment is being replaced by disposable equipment. *Standard equipment* requires washing, disinfecting, and sterilizing. *Disposable equipment* needs almost no care. This equipment is usually prepackaged. It may be made of plastic, styrofoam, or paper. Some of this equipment is used only one time and then thrown away. Other disposable equipment may be used several times for *one patient only*. The equipment is cleaned between uses and thrown away when that patient is discharged from the hospital. Nursing aides usually get disposable equipment from the central supply room (CSR) as needed. (Central supply may also be called SPD—Special Purchasing Department, or CSD—Central Supply Department.) This is a central place for storing supplies and equipment. You will need a requisition slip to get equipment from CSR.

Large Equipment

The modern health care institution has many pieces of large equipment needed for patient care and treatment. This equipment might include:

- Intravenous poles. These are often called *IV poles, IV standards,* or a *standard*. These support the containers or tubes used in various

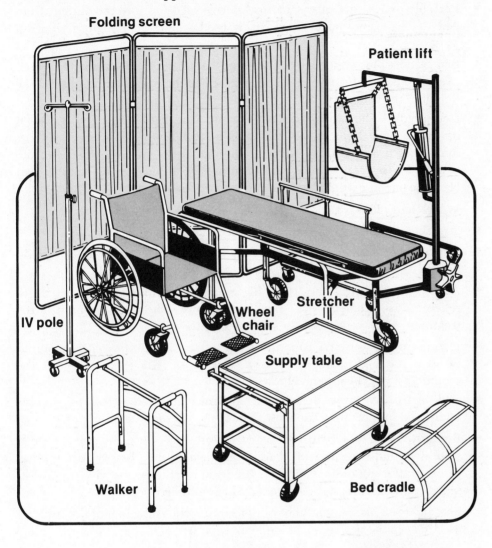

Folding screen

Patient lift

IV pole

Wheel chair

Stretcher

Supply table

Walker

Bed cradle

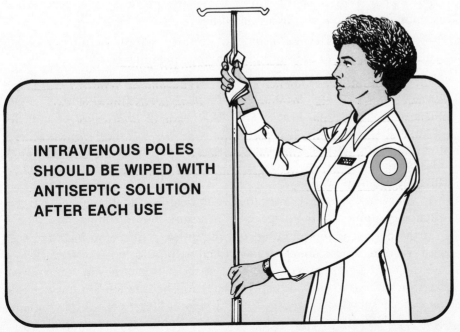

INTRAVENOUS POLES SHOULD BE WIPED WITH ANTISEPTIC SOLUTION AFTER EACH USE

treatments. Some IV poles are on casters or rollers for easy movement. Other IV poles fit right into the bed frame.

- Portable patient lift. A mechanical device used to move the patient from bed to chair and back again. It is used when the patient needs full assistance.

- Bed cradle. This cradle looks like a half barrel cut the long way. It is used to cover a part of the patient's body where he is having great pain. Even the weight of the bedspread and top sheet would cause more pain.

- Heat cradle. The heat cradle is the same as a regular bed cradle. But it has an electric light in it. It acts as a heat lamp. The heat cradle is sometimes ordered alone (dry). Sometimes it is ordered when the patient is having continuous warm compresses applied to an arm or leg. Here the purpose would be to keep the compress warm.

- Wheelchair. This is a chair with wheels used to transport patients.

- Stretcher. This is a narrow table on wheels used to transport patients.

- Walker. The walker is an aluminum frame used by the patient to help himself to walk.

- Air or rubber rings. These look like small inner tubes. They are used to relieve pressure on the lower back or buttocks. The rings are used in the treatment or prevention of bedsores (decubiti).

- Alternating-pressure (A-P) mattress. A device like an air mattress placed beneath the bedridden or elderly patient. It reduces pressure on the shoulders, back, heels, and elbows.

- Bed board. A large board placed beneath the mattress to provide additional support for patients with back muscle or bone problems.

- Binders. These are strips of heavy cotton cloth. Binders are wrapped securely around the patient's body over the abdomen to give support and comfort after abdominal surgery. Binders are also used to give support to female patients' breasts or abdomen after childbirth.

- Foot board. This is a small board placed upright at the foot of the bed and used to keep the patient's feet aligned properly.

- Lamb's wool. Wide strips of lamb's wool cloth (or soft synthetic materials) used for the same purpose as air or rubber rings.

- Protective devices. Devices, usually of cotton, used to restrain a patient's arms, legs, or body to prevent him from injuring himself.

- Traction equipment. Plaster casts are used to protect broken or injured bones while they heal. Traction is often used for the same purpose when injuries are very severe. Traction refers to both a procedure and an apparatus of ropes, weights, and metal. This device is attached to the bed and also to the part of the patient's body that must be kept immobilized. This means the body part must be kept in one position, without moving, so the bone will heal properly.

In your work you must never touch the weights, ropes, or metal parts of traction equipment without special permission from the nurse.

If the patient is complaining, tell the nurse. Often sand bags are used with traction. These are cloth bags filled with sand to make them heavy. Ask the nurse before moving the bags. If she tells you they may be moved, carry on with your work. When you have finished, be sure to put the bags back in the same position they were in before. Never change the patient's body position without permission from the head nurse or team leader.

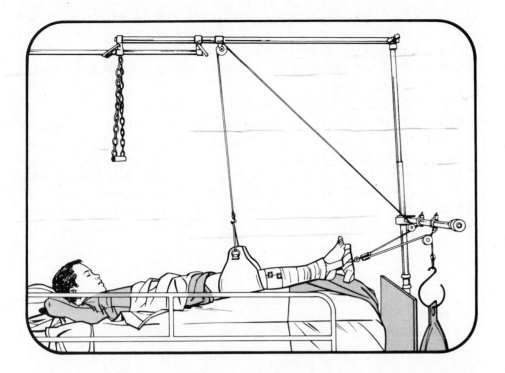

• Turning frame, manually operated. This frame is a hospital bed designed for the patient whose position in bed must be changed very carefully and under controlled conditions. The equipment has two frames on which the patient can lie. The anterior frame is for the patient to lie prone. The posterior frame is for him to lie flat on his back. At the bottom is a rack for storing the frames when not in use. Other parts are the arm boards, the reading board, and the bedpan rack. By using a rotating-frame type of bed, we accomplish several things:

    a.   The patient may be turned with ease.
    b.   Turning does not alter the position of the patient.

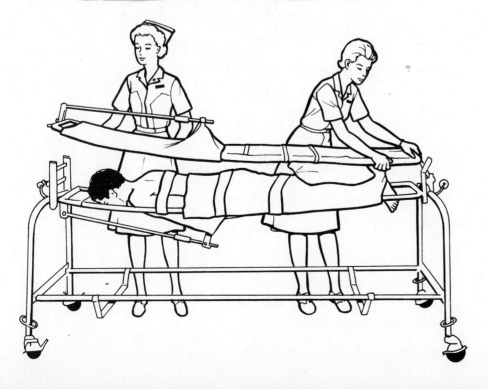

c. The danger of pressure areas is reduced (decubitus ulcers are avoided).

d. The bedpan is handy for the patient.

e. The patient can eat, read, and write in the prone position.

f. Bathing is easier.

g. The bed is at the right height for nursing care.

- Circular turning frame, electrically powered. As a nursing aide, you will have very little contact with this orthopedic device. It is a circular double-frame turning bed. The turning is done by an electric motor controlled from a panel. The controls are similar to those on standard hospital beds. The machine can be controlled either by an attendant or by the patient himself. The circular turning frame bed is used for a patient who must stay completely still but who still should keep a normal posture and position.

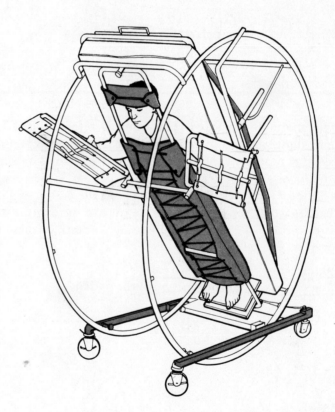

Section 2: Bedmaking

OBJECTIVES: WHAT YOU WILL LEARN

When you have completed this section, you should be able:

- To make the closed bed
- To make the open fan-folded or empty bed
- To make the operating room (OR) bed
- To make the occupied bed

KEY IDEAS

When the average person is a hospital patient, he spends more time in a bed than he is used to. Therefore, the way a patient's bed is made is very important to his comfort and well-being. Making hospital beds is done with much greater care than is necessary at home.

A patient is often not allowed to get up and move around. All his activities are carried on while he is in bed. He is fed and bathed there. His bodily functions (urination, defecation) are taken care of. And medical treatments are given. During these activities, the bed should be as comfortable as possible. There should be no wrinkles in the bedclothes. Wrinkles are uncomfortable for the patient. They also restrict his circulation, and this can cause painful bed sores (decubitus ulcers), which are often hard to heal.

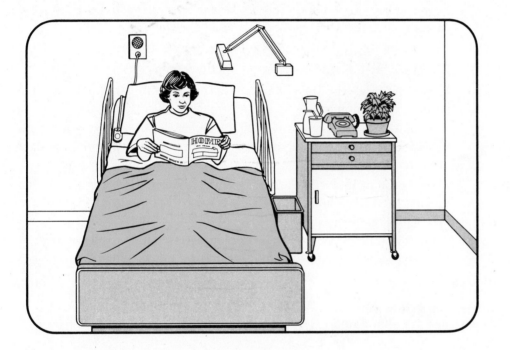

Beds should always be made with clean linen that is drawn smooth and fastened firmly at the corners. There should always be enough blankets and pillows for the patient's comfort.

There are four basic ways of making a bed in a patient's unit:

1. *The closed bed.* This bed is made after environmental service personnel have cleaned the unit following a patient's discharge. The bed is made up *closed* so it will stay clean until a new patient is assigned to it.

2. *The open bed.* When a patient is assigned to a unit, the closed bed is made into an *open* bed by fan folding the top sheets.

3. *The occupied bed.* Sometimes a patient is completely bedridden. His bed must be made while he is in it.

4. *The postoperative bed.* This also may be called the OR bed, surgical bed, recovery bed, or stretcher bed. A special method is used to make this bed for a patient who is returning to his unit after surgery.

Rules To Follow

1. Return torn linen to a "repair box" in the linen closet for repair. Never use a torn piece of linen. It will probably tear even more.

2. Never use a pin on any item of linen.

3. Never use bed linen for any purpose other than that for which it was intended.

4. Report to the head nurse if you see patients or visitors trying to remove articles of linen from the hospital for any reason.

5. Most hospitals that use wool blankets have special rules for their use. Be sure to learn and follow these rules at all times.

6. Don't shake the bed linen. Shaking would spread germs to everything and everyone in the room, including you.

7. Never bring extra linen into a patient unit. It will be considered contaminated (or dirty) and can't be used elsewhere.

8. Never allow any linen to touch your body or your uniform.

9. Dirty used linen should never be put on the floor.

10. In most hospitals the linen hamper is in the dirty utility room. Used linen is put into this hamper.

11. Some hospitals use melt-away plastic bags for laundry bags. These bags dissolve during the washing process. The dirty linen is put into the bags at the patient's bedside. Then it is carried to the laundry hamper.

12. Many hospitals make the bed without the blanket. However, the person making the bed should always leave a folded blanket at the foot of the bed to be used later.

13. Some hospitals today use fitted bottom sheets. Others still use regular (flat) sheets where the nursing aide has to make mitered corners. A

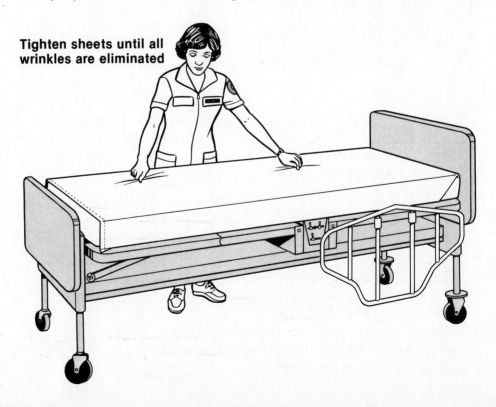

Tighten sheets until all wrinkles are eliminated

mitered corner is also called a hospital corner. The sheet is held tightly in place. The mitered corner keeps the sheets firm and smooth and makes the bed neat and attractive.

14. The bottom sheet must be firm and smooth under the patient. This is very important for the patient's comfort. Always make sure that the bottom sheet is tight and unwrinkled.

15. A fan fold makes it easy for the patient to get back into his bed.

16. Fan fold a bed that is being made ready to receive a patient.

17. Some hospitals use a disposable draw sheet made of plastic and paper rather than the plastic draw sheet covered by a cotton draw sheet.

18. Some hospitals do not use a draw sheet at all. Instead, small disposable bed protectors are placed on the bed under the patient as necessary.

19. Plastic should never touch a patient's skin. When using a plastic draw sheet, be sure to cover it entirely with a cotton draw sheet.

20. The cotton draw sheet is about the size of half of a regular sheet. When cotton draw sheets are not available, a large sheet can be folded in half widthwise (with hems together) and used to cover plastic draw sheets. The fold must always be placed toward the head of the bed and the hems toward the foot of the bed.

21. The plastic draw sheet and disposable bed protectors protect the hospital mattress.

22. *Bottom of the bed* refers to the mattress pad, the bottom sheet, and the draw sheets.

23. *Top of the bed* refers to the top sheet, blanket, and bedspread.

24. Remember that you save time and energy by first making as much of the bed as possible on one side before going to the other side.

The Closed Bed

In some hospitals the environmental service personnel make up the closed bed after they finish washing the unit. In other hospitals the nursing aide

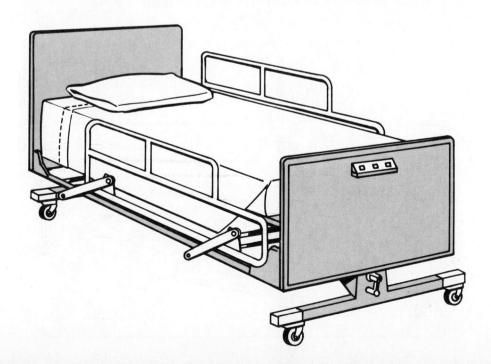

makes up the closed bed after the environmental service personnel have finished washing the bed.

Procedure: Making the Closed Bed

1. Assemble your equipment: Mattress cover, bottom sheet, cotton or plastic drawsheet (or disposable bed protector), top sheet, blanket, bedspread, pillowcase, and pillow.

2. Wash your hands.

3. Put a chair near the bed.

4. Put the pillow on the chair.

5. Stack the bedmaking items on the chair in the order that you will use them. First things on top, last things on the bottom. (See the list of equipment in the illustration.)

6. Adjust the bed to its highest position. Lock it in place.

7. Pull the mattress to the head of the bed. The mattress touches the headboard.

8. Place the mattress pad on the mattress. Make it even with the head of the mattress.

9. Fold the bottom sheet lengthwise and place it on the bed.
   a. Have the center fold of the sheet at the center of the mattress from head to foot.
   b. Put the hem at the foot of the bed, even with the foot of the mattress.
   c. Have the large hem at the head of the bed.

10. Open the sheet from the fold. The sheet now hangs evenly the same distance over each side of the bed. The rough edges of the hem are facing down.

11. There should be about 18 inches of the sheet to tuck smoothly under the head of the mattress. Tuck it in tightly.

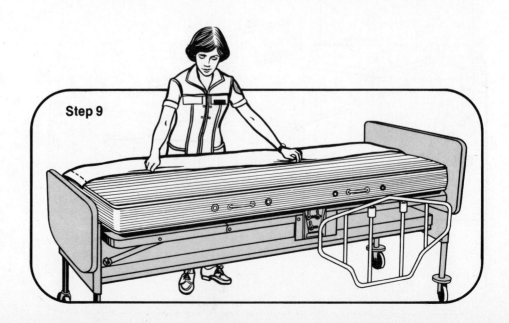

Step 9

12. Make a mitered corner. Here's how:

    a. Pick up the edge of the sheet at the side of the bed 12 inches from the head.

    b. Place the triangle (the folded corner) on top of the mattress

    c. Tuck the hanging portion under the mattress.

    d. While you hold the fold at the edge of the mattress, bring the triangle down over the side of the mattress.

    e. Tuck the sheet under the mattress from head to foot.

13. Stand and work entirely on one side of the bed until that side is finished.

14. Place the plastic draw sheet about 14 inches (two open hand spans) down from the head of the bed. Tuck it in.

15. Cover the plastic draw sheet with the cotton draw sheet and tuck it in.

16. Fold the top sheet lengthwise and place it on the bed.

    a. Have the center fold on the center of the bed from head to foot.

    b. Put the large hem at the head of the bed. Make it even with the top of the mattress.

    c. Open the sheet. Have the rough edge of the hem up.

    d. Tightly tuck the sheet under at the foot of the bed.

    e. Make a mitered corner at the foot of the bed.

    f. Do not tuck in at the sides of the bed.

17. Fold the blanket lengthwise and place the blanket on the bed.

    a. Have the center fold on the center of the bed from head to foot.

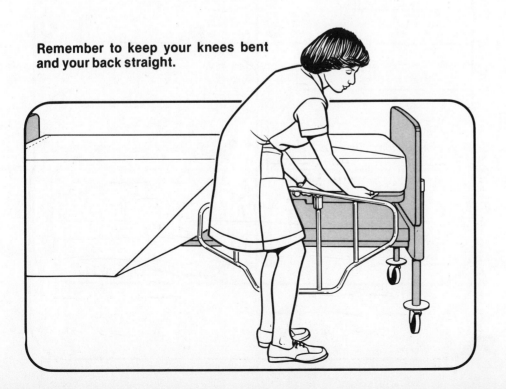

Remember to keep your knees bent and your back straight.

Step 12

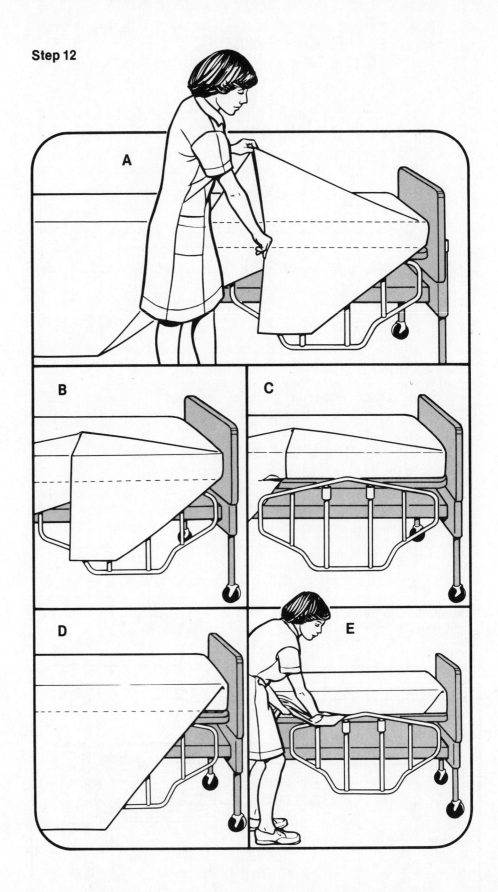

  b. Put the upper hem about 6 inches from the head of the bed.

  c. Open the blanket.

  d. Tuck it under at the foot of the bed tightly.

  e. Make a mitered corner at the foot of the bed.

  f. Do not tuck in at the sides of the bed.

Step 14

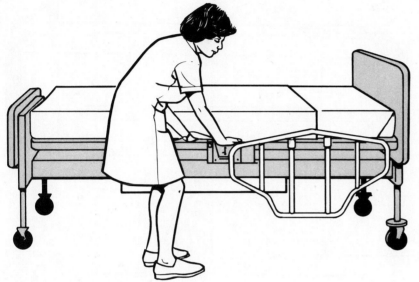

18. Fold the bedspread lengthwise and place it on the bed.

  a. Have the center fold on the center of the bed from head to foot.

  b. Put the upper hem even with the head of the mattress.

  c. Have the right side up.

Step 15

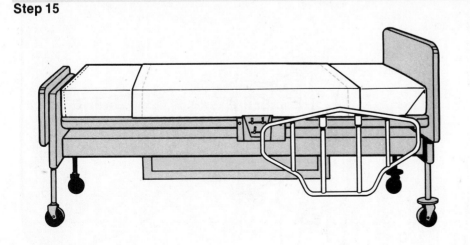

Step 19

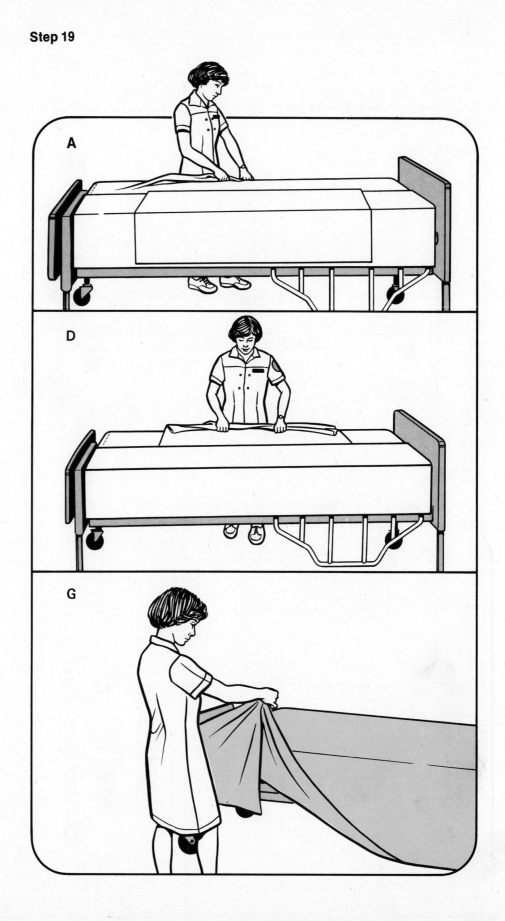

    d.   Open the spread.

    e.   Tuck it under at the foot of the bed tightly.

    f.   Make a mitered corner at the foot of the bed.

    g.   Do not tuck in at the sides of the bed.

19.   Now go to the other side of the bed. Start with the bottom sheet.

    a.   Pull the sheet tight to get rid of all wrinkles.

    b.   Miter the top corner.

    c.   Pull the plastic sheet tight and tuck it in.

    d.   Pull the cotton draw sheet tight and tuck it in.

    e.   Straighten out the top sheet, making the mitered corner at the foot of the bed.

    f.   Miter the corner of the blanket.

    g.   Miter the corner of the bedspread.

20.   Make a cuff.

    a.   Fold the top hem of the spread under the top hem of the blanket.

    b.   Fold the top hem of the sheet back over the edge of the spread and the blanket to form a cuff. Have the rough edge of the sheet away from where the patient will lie.

21.   Put the pillowcase on the pillow.

    a.   Hold the pillowcase at the center of the end seam.

    b.   With your hand outside of the case, turn the case back over your hand.

    c.   Grasp the pillow through the case at the center of one end.

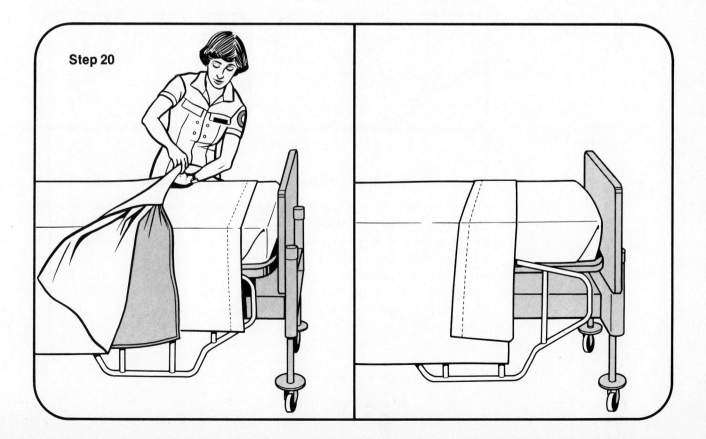

Step 20

d. Bring the case down over the pillow.
e. Fit the corner of the pillow into the seamless corner of the case.
f. Fold the extra material from the side seam under the pillow.
g. Place the pillow on the bed with the open end away from the door.

PUTTING A PILLOWCASE ON A PILLOW

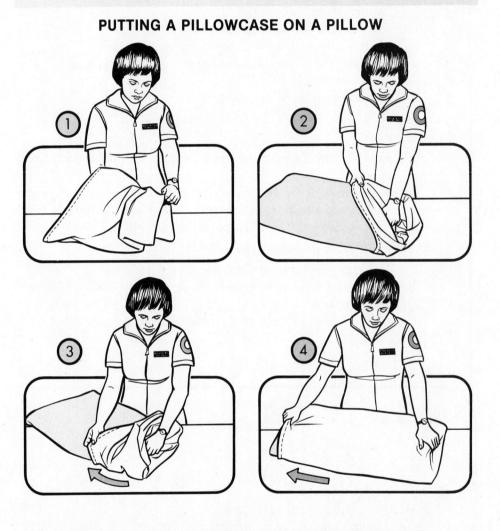

KEY IDEAS: THE OPEN BED, FAN-FOLDED BED, EMPTY BED

The procedures for making the open bed, the fan-folded bed, and the empty bed are all basically the same. You will be making an open bed when a new patient has been assigned to a unit. You will also be making an open bed when a unit is already occupied but the patient is able to get out of bed and move around while you are arranging the unit.

The open bed is made exactly like the closed bed except for one thing: The bedding is opened so that the patient can easily get into bed.

This is done after you finish making the cuff at the head of the bed.

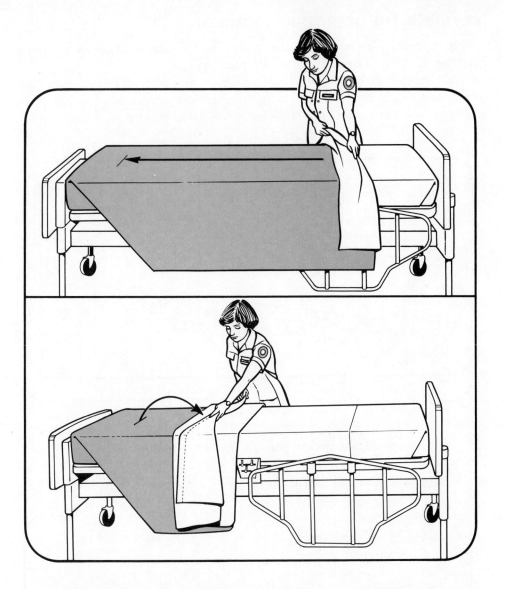

Procedure: Making the Open Fan-Folded Empty Bed

1. Assemble your equipment: closed bed.

2. Wash your hands.

3. Grasp the cuff of the bedding in both hands.

4. Pull it to the foot of the bed.

5. Fold the bedding back on itself toward the head of the bed. Make the edge of the cuff meet the fold.

6. Smooth the hanging parts on each side neatly into the folds you have made.

7. Wash your hands.

KEY IDEAS: THE OPERATING ROOM BED

The operating room bed is also known as the postoperative bed, or the stretcher bed, or, in some hospitals, the recovery bed.

The operating room bed is used by patients returning from the postoperative recovery room or the postdelivery recovery room. The patient is brought in on a stretcher. The stretcher will be lined up alongside the bed.

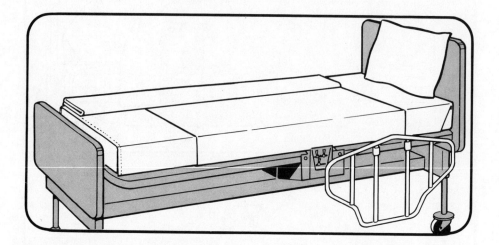

Procedure: Making the OR Bed or Stretcher Bed

1. Assemble your equipment:
    a. Mattress cover
    b. Bottom sheet
    c. Plastic draw sheet
    d. Cotton draw sheet
    e. Top sheet
    f. Blanket
    g. Pillowcase
    h. Pillow
    i. Bedspread
    j. Two cotton bath blankets
    k. Disposable paper pillow, if used in your hospital
    l. Plastic laundry bag
2. Wash your hands.
3. Strip all used linen from the bed and place in the plastic laundry bag.
4. Make the bottom part of the bed. Follow the instructions for making a closed bed.
5. Spread one bath blanket across the bed, on top of the draw sheet and bottom sheet. The bottom end of the bath blanket should be even with the foot of the mattress. Tuck the edge under the mattress on your side of the bed.

6. Go to the other side of the bed. Tuck the bath blanket under the mattress.

7. Spread the second bath blanket across the bed. The upper edge should be about 6 inches from the head of the bed. This blanket gives the patient extra warmth.

8. Put the top sheet, the regular blanket, and the spread on the bed. Do this the same way as when making the closed bed. But do not tuck them in at the foot of the bed. Instead, all the bedding at the foot end should be folded back on the bed so the folded edge is even with the foot of the mattress.

9. Go to the side of the bed where the stretcher will be brought.

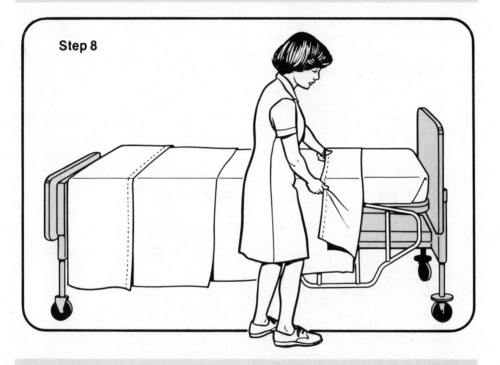

Step 8

10. Grasp the top bedding at the side with both hands. Fold the bedding across the bed so the folded edge is even with the far side of the mattress. Fold the bedding to the edge again.

11. Put the pillow into the pillowcase. Put the pillow upright against the headboard. Place it so as to protect him from hitting his head on a hard surface. You will later place the pillow under the patient's head.

12. Move the bedside table, the chair, and any other furniture out of the way to make room for the stretcher.

13. Remove everything from the bedside table except a box of tissue and an emesis basin.

14. Bring an IV standard into the room and place it near the head of the bed, out of the way.

15. Wash your hands.

PREPARING BEDDING FOR A STRETCHER PATIENT

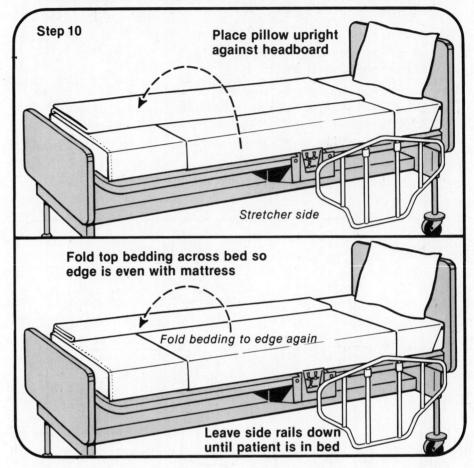

Step 10

Place pillow upright against headboard

Stretcher side

Fold top bedding across bed so edge is even with mattress

Fold bedding to edge again

Leave side rails down until patient is in bed

KEY IDEAS: THE OCCUPIED BED

Making the occupied bed is necessary when the patient can't get out of bed or is not allowed to get out of bed. The hardest part of making an occupied bed is to get the sheets smooth and tight under the patient. This is so there will be no wrinkles to rub against the patient's skin. When you are making the bottom of this bed, you must keep in mind how important it is to divide the bed in two parts—the side the patient is lying on and the side you are making. Always keep the side rail up on the side of the bed where the patient is. Usually you make the occupied bed after giving the patient a bed bath. The patient should always be covered with the bath blanket while you are making his bed.

Procedure: Making the Occupied Bed

1. Assemble your equipment:
    a. Two large sheets
    b. One plastic draw sheet, if used

    c.   One cotton draw sheet, if used

    d.   Bath blanket

    e.   Pillowcase

    f.   Blanket

    g.   Bedspread

    h.   Plastic laundry bag.

2. Wash your hands.

3. Identify the patient by checking the identification bracelet.

4. Ask all visitors to step out of the room.

5. Tell the patient you are going to make his bed.

6. Pull the curtain around the bed for privacy.

7. Put the linens on the chair in the order in which you will use them. That is, the last item to be put on the bed should be on the bottom of the pile.

8. Lower the backrest and kneerest until the bed is flat, if that is allowed.

9. If the patient can't sit up, lock arms with him and raise him, to remove the pillow. (You may leave the pillow under the patient's head. If you do, move it over to the side of the bed with the patient. This method is more comfortable for him.)

10. Put the pillow on the chair with the linen on top of it.

11. Loosen all sheets around the entire bed.

12. Take the blanket and spread off the bed and fold them over the back of the chair.

13. Cover the patient with the bath blanket. Ask him to hold the blanket, and, without exposing him, remove the top sheet from under the bath blanket. Fold the top sheet and place cover over the back of the chair.

14. If the mattress has slipped out of place, move it to its proper position. Ask another nursing aide to help if necessary.

15. Raise the bedside rail on the opposite side from where you will be working.

16. Ask the patient to turn on his side toward the side rail. Help the patient to turn, if necessary. The patient is now on the far side of the bed.

17. Fold all bottom sheets toward the patient and tuck them against his back. This strips your side of the bed down to the mattress pad.

18. Take the large clean sheet from the chair and fold it in half lengthwise.

19. Put it on the bed, still folded, with the fold running along the middle of the bed. The small hem end of the sheet should be even with the foot of the mattress. Fold the top half of the sheet toward the patient. Tuck the folds against his back, below the plastic draw sheet. Miter the corner at the head of the mattress. Tuck in the clean bottom sheet on your side from head to foot of the mattress.

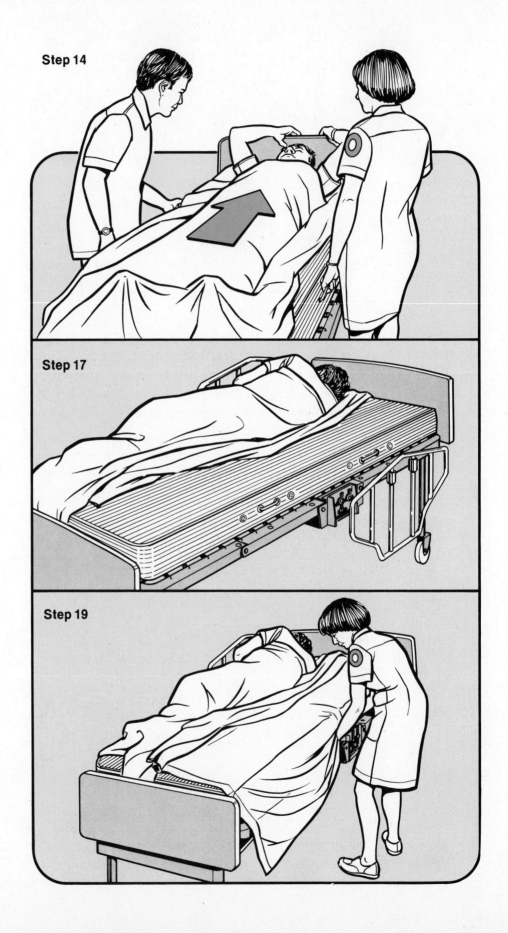

Step 14

Step 17

Step 19

20. Pull the plastic draw sheet toward you, over the clean bottom sheet, and tuck in. Put on the clean cotton draw sheet, folded in half. Fold the top half toward the patient, tucking the folds under his back, as you did with the bottom sheet. Tuck in the draw sheet under the mattress. Raise the bedside rail on your side.

21. Go to the opposite side of the bed. Lower the bedside rail on this side of the bed. Ask the patient, or help him, to roll over the "hump" onto the clean sheets.

22. Remove the old bottom sheet and cotton draw sheet from the bed. Pull the fresh bottom sheet toward the edge of the bed. Tuck it under the mattress at the head of the bed and make a mitered corner. Then tuck the bottom sheet under the mattress from the head to the foot.

23. Pull the rubber or plastic sheet and clean cotton draw sheet toward you.

24. Then, one at a time, tuck the draw sheets under the mattress along the side.

25. Be sure to pull all the sheets tight as you tuck them in.

26. Have the patient turn on his back, or turn him yourself.

27. Change the pillowcase and put the pillow under the patient's head. If necessary, lock arms with the patient and raise him to put the pillow in place.

28. Spread the clean top sheet over the bath blanket with the wide hem at the top. The middle of the sheet should run along the middle of the bed. Make sure the wide hem is even with the head of the mattress. Ask the patient to hold the hem of the clean sheet, if he can, while you take off the bath blanket, moving toward the foot of the bed. Tuck the clean top sheet under the mattress at the foot of the bed. Make sure you leave enough room for the patient to move his feet freely. Miter the corner of the sheet.

29. Spread the blanket on the top of the sheet. Be sure the middle of the blanket runs along the middle of the bed. Make sure the blanket is high enough to cover the patient's shoulders.

30. Tuck the blanket in at the foot of the bed. Make a mitered corner on the blanket. Put the spread on the bed in the same way. Make a mitered corner with the spread.

31. Fold the spread under the blanket at the head of the bed. Fold the sheet back over the blanket and spread, to form a cuff.

32. Raise the backrest and kneerest to suit the patient, if this is allowed.

33. Before you leave, be sure to put the signal cord where the patient can reach it. Move the bedside table back into place.

34. Put used linen in the plastic laundry bag.

35. Wash your hands.

36. Report to your head nurse or team leader that you have made the occupied bed. Also report your observations of anything unusual.

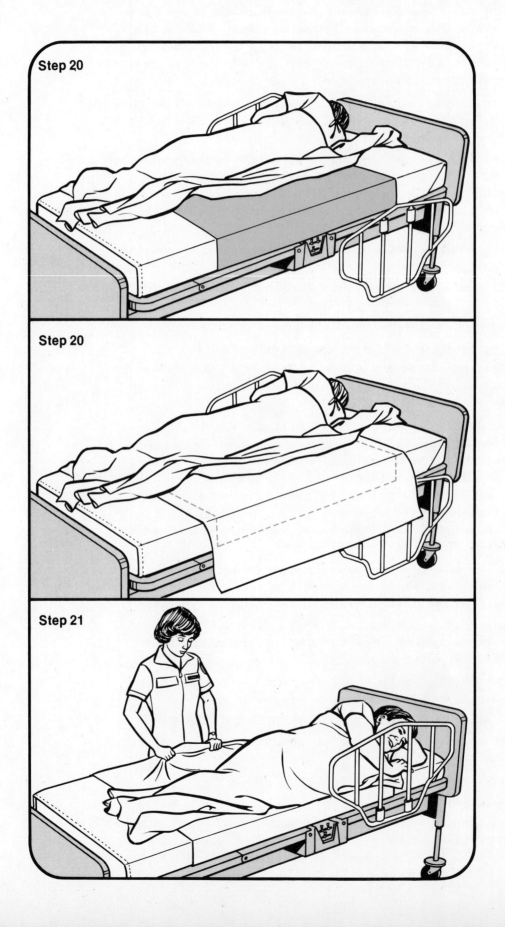

Step 20

Step 20

Step 21

Section 3: Safety and Fire Prevention

OBJECTIVES: WHAT YOU WILL LEARN

When you have completed this section, you should be able:

- To list the general rules of hospital safety
- To describe the special safety precautions necessary when oxygen is being used
- To explain what you can do to prevent fires
- To explain what to do in case of fire

KEY IDEAS

Patients are handicapped by illness, disabilities, worries, and medications. Many of them cannot take care of themselves in an emergency. Patients must be looked after and protected in an emergency. Therefore, hospital personnel must be especially careful to guard against accidents, to prevent fires and other kinds of emergencies, and to know what to do if an emergency arises.

Rules To Follow: General Hospital Safety

Following are general rules for safety in the hospital:

- Report immediately any unsafe conditions you may notice.

A SAFETY MEASURE

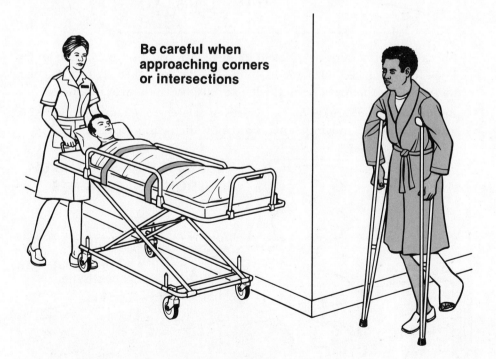

Be careful when approaching corners or intersections

- When you see something on the floor that doesn't belong there, pick it up. If you see spilled liquid, wipe up the area.

- If you are injured, even slightly, report this and get first aid immediately.

- Walk, never run, especially in halls or on stairs. Keep to the right. Use the handrails on stairways and avoid collisions. Use special care at intersections.

- Watch out for swinging doors.

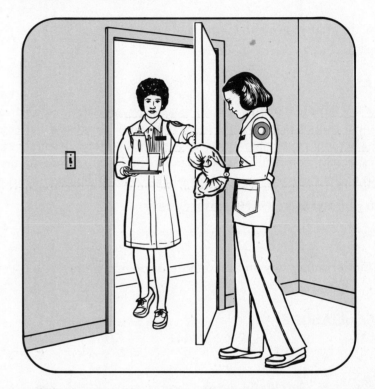

- Check soiled linen for overlooked items before you send it to the laundry. Look for misplaced instruments, pins, needles, or other articles. Remove these and put them where they belong or dispose of them as instructed.

- Be sure to set the brakes on the wheels of stretchers, examining tables, or wheelchairs when moving patients on or off such equipment.

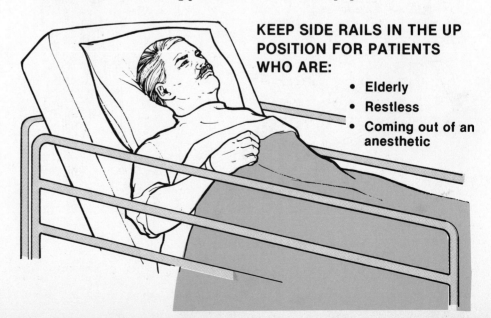

KEEP SIDE RAILS IN THE UP POSITION FOR PATIENTS WHO ARE:

- **Elderly**
- **Restless**
- **Coming out of an anesthetic**

- Never use the contents of an unlabeled bottle. Take the bottle to your head nurse or team leader. If you do not understand what is written on the label of a container, take it to your head nurse or team leader and ask for an explanation.

Safety for Children

People who work with children must always be alert to things that may cause accidents.

Following are some special measures to take in a pediatrics department or a children's hospital to make accidents less likely to happen:

- Small children should never be left unattended when they are awake.
- Every child in a protective device should be checked frequently.
- Articles used in the child's care should be kept out of reach of a toddler when they are not being used. Watch especially for needles, water, safety pins, medications, matches, electrical equipment, syringes, or thermometers.
- Toys should never be left carelessly on the floor. Be especially alert to pick them up—they could cause someone to fall. Also, remember to clean up spills and messes—such as food, urine, and feces—right away.
- The sides of a child's crib should be up at all times except when someone is giving direct care to the child.
- Doors to stairways, utility rooms, and the kitchen should always be closed immediately after use. They should be locked whenever possible.
- Linen chutes should be kept locked except when they are being used by hospital personnel.
- Venetian blind cords should be kept out of the reach of children.

KEEP ITEMS FOR CHILD'S CARE OUT OF REACH

REMEMBER. . . A CHILD CAN REACH FAR AND IS QUICK

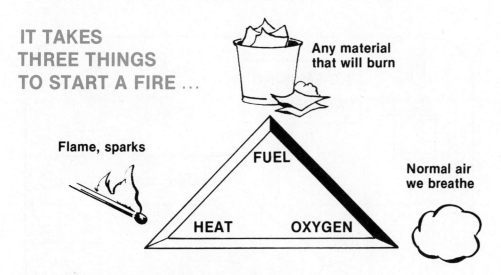

IT TAKES THREE THINGS TO START A FIRE ...

Any material that will burn

Flame, sparks

FUEL

Normal air we breathe

HEAT   OXYGEN

Fire Safety and Prevention

Fire safety means two things: preventing fires and doing the right things if a fire breaks out.

Smoking is the number-one cause of fires in hospitals. You can help by observing these rules:

- See that ashtrays are provided and that they are used.

- Never empty ashtrays into plastic bags, plastic wastebaskets, or containers of rubbish that can burn. Smoking materials should be collected in a separate metal container. A pail with water or sand in the bottom should be used to make sure that cigarette and cigar butts are out.
- Smoke only where it is permitted.
- A patient who has been given a sedative should not be allowed to smoke.

SMOKING AND MATCHES

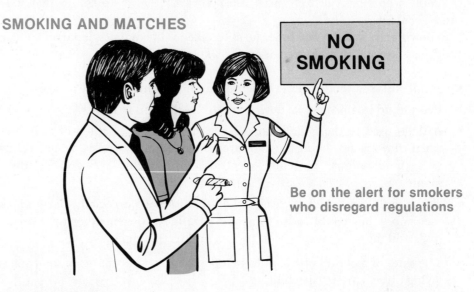

NO SMOKING

Be on the alert for smokers
who disregard regulations

Oxygen Safety

A special device is necessary when large, portable oxygen tanks are used. This device is called a "regulator." It <u>controls, or regulates,</u> <u>the flow of oxy-</u><u>gen.</u> Special procedures are to be followed in the care and use of portable oxygen tanks and regulators. Oxygen therapy departments take care of this equipment.

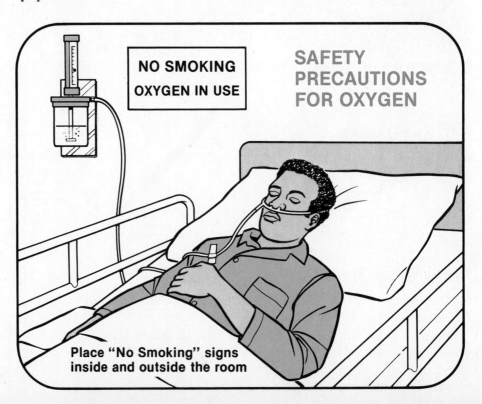

NO SMOKING
OXYGEN IN USE

SAFETY
PRECAUTIONS
FOR OXYGEN

Place "No Smoking" signs
inside and outside the room

Special precautions must be observed when more than the normal amount of oxygen is present in a particular area, such as the patient's unit. Extra oxygen can make things catch fire and burn much more rapidly than they would in normal air. To prevent fires when a patient is being given extra oxygen, the following rules must be strictly observed:

- Whenever possible, electrical appliances such as heating pads and electric shavers should be taken out of the room.
- The signal cord is replaced by a bell.
- If some electrical appliances are still in the room, they should be turned off or the plugs should be pulled from the outlets *before* the oxygen is started. If a plug is pulled from an outlet while the oxygen is being given, a spark could cause an explosion because there is live electricity in the outlet.
- Remove cigarettes and matches from the bedside table.
- Oil, alcohol, or anything else that might burn readily should not be used for rubbing patients while oxygen is being given.
- Never comb a patient's hair while he is in an oxygen tent. Because of static electricity, combing hair actually can create an electrical spark that could set off an explosion.
- Wool blankets and anything else that could cause static electricity should be removed from the bed when oxygen is being used. Patients should wear cotton hospital nightgowns. Other fabrics might generate static electricity.

MISUSES OF ELECTRICITY

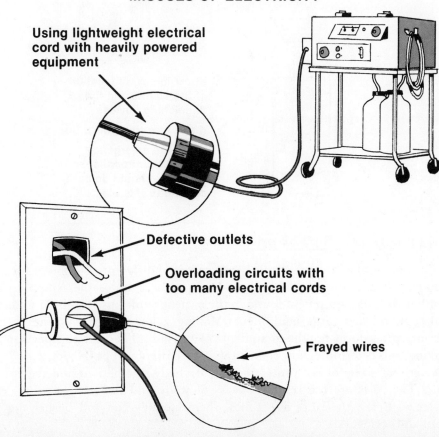

Using lightweight electrical cord with heavily powered equipment

Defective outlets

Overloading circuits with too many electrical cords

Frayed wires

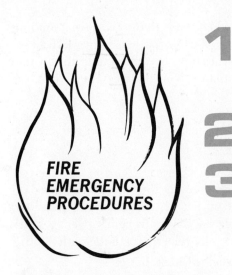

FIRE EMERGENCY PROCEDURES

1 PULL NEAREST FIRE ALARM BOX.

NOTIFY MAIN SWITCHBOARD AS TO EXACT LOCATION AND NATURE OF FIRE AS SOON AS POSSIBLE.

2 IF FIRE OCCURS IN PATIENT AREA, ASSIST PATIENTS TO SAFETY.

3 FOLLOW FIRE EMERGENCY PROCEDURES FOR YOUR DEPARTMENT.

DO NOT PANIC. . . MANY LIVES MAY DEPEND UPON YOUR ACTIONS IN AN EMERGENCY.

FIRE SAFETY PLANNING

- **Know the floor plan of your department and the hospital as a whole**
- **Pay particular attention to exit routes**

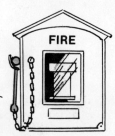

- **Know the exact location of fire alarms and fire extinguishing devices**
- **Know how to report a fire**
- **Know the emergency plan of your hospital and what you should do according to this plan**

WHAT YOU HAVE LEARNED

The modern health care institution uses lots of different equipment for patient care and treatment. Much of this equipment is disposable. You must be familiar with the equipment found in the patient's unit, disposable equipment and supplies, and large equipment. Making a bed properly is one of the primary procedures taught to students of nursing. The skill you develop in making beds determines how comfortable the patient will be in bed.

Safety rules are for the protection of everybody, the patient and the entire staff. The rules are the result of years of study and research based on experience. Learn the rules and follow them closely. You will be helping to eliminate accidents.

Lifting, Moving, and Transporting Patients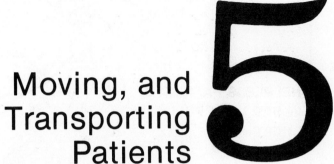

Section 1: Body Mechanics

OBJECTIVES: WHAT YOU WILL LEARN

When you have completed this section, you should be able:

- To lift, hold, or move an object or patient using good body mechanics
- To lock arms with a patient to raise his head and shoulders
- To help a patient to stand from a sitting position
- To move the helpless patient up in bed
- To move a patient to the head of the bed with his help
- To move the mattress to the head of the bed with the patient's help
- To roll the patient like a log
- To move a helpless patient to one side of the bed on his back
- To turn a patient on either side

KEY IDEAS

The term *body mechanics* refers to special ways of standing and moving one's body. The purpose is to make the best use of strength and avoid fatigue. You should understand the rules of good body mechanics and learn to apply them to your work. Then you will find that you will be less tired and will feel better at the end of the day.

Rules for Good Body Mechanics

- When an action requires physical effort, try to use as many muscles or groups of muscles as possible. For example, use both hands rather than one hand to pick up a heavy piece of equipment.
- Get yourself into a good posture. Keep your body aligned properly. Keep your back straight. Have your knees bent. Keep your weight evenly balanced on both feet.
- Check your feet when you are going to lift something. They should be 12 inches apart. This will give you a broad base of support and good balance.
- Get close to the load that is being lifted. Don't reach very far for it.
- When you have to move a heavy object, it is better to push it, pull it, or roll it rather than lift and carry it.

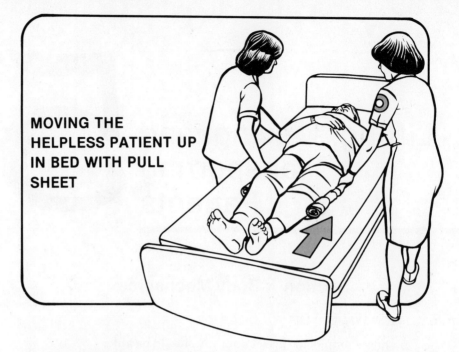

MOVING THE HELPLESS PATIENT UP IN BED WITH PULL SHEET

- Use your arms to support the object. The muscles of your legs actually do the job of lifting, not the muscles of your back.

- When you are doing work such as giving a back rub, making a corner on a bed, or moving the patient, work with the direction of your efforts, not against it. Avoid twisting your body as much as you can.

- When you lift an object:
  a. Kneel or squat close to the load.
  b. Keep your back straight.
  c. Grip the object firmly.
  d. Hold the load as close to your body as possible.
  e. Lift by pushing up with your strong leg muscles.

- If you think you may not be able to lift the load—if it seems too large or heavy—then get help. Don't try to lift it alone.

- Two or more people are needed to move a patient who is completely helpless or who is not allowed to move by himself.

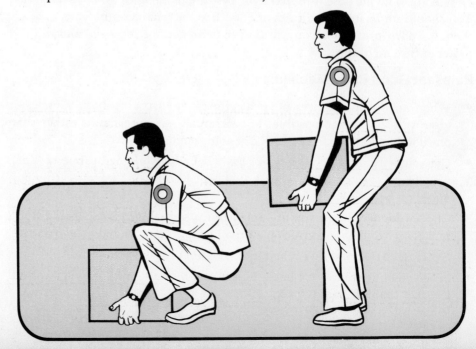

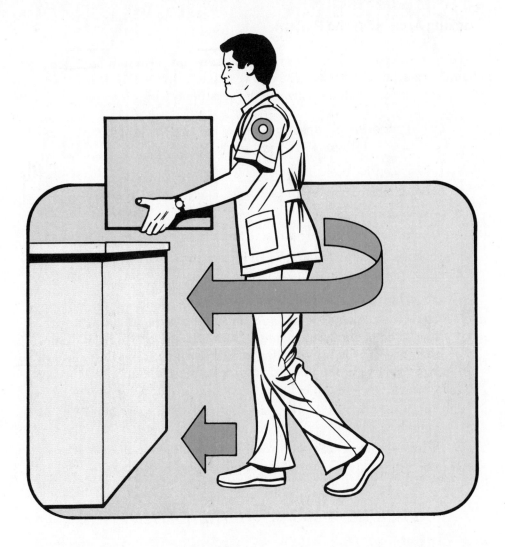

- Lift smoothly to <u>avoid strain</u>. Always count "one, two, three" with the person you are working with, your partner. Or say "ready" and "go" so you work in unison. Do this with both the patient and with other nursing aides.

- When you want to change the direction of movement:
    a. <u>Pivot</u> (turn) <u>with your feet</u>.
    b. <u>Turn with short steps</u>.
    c. <u>Turn your whole body</u> without twisting your back and neck.

KEY IDEAS: LIFTING AND MOVING PATIENTS

Many of your tasks require lifting and moving helpless or nearly helpless patients. A bedridden patient must have his position changed often. Proper support and alignment of the patient's body are important.

The patient's body should be straight and properly supported because otherwise his safety and comfort might be affected. The correct positioning of the patient's body is referred to as body alignment. Body alignment means arrangement or adjustment of the patient's body so that all parts of the body are in their proper positions in relation to each other.

Many conditions and injuries, as well as special patient care treatments, make it difficult or even dangerous for a patient to be in a certain position. As a member of the nursing team, you will be responsible for making sure that a patient you are caring for is in the position ordered by his doctor.

Locking Arms with the Patient

To turn the patient's pillow over, or to raise his head and shoulders, you should lock arms with the patient who is able to help. For the helpless patient two nursing aides should lock arms with the patient to lift him.

Procedure: Locking Arms with the Patient To Raise His Head and Shoulders

1. Wash your hands.
2. Identify the patient by checking the identification bracelet.
3. Ask visitors to step out of the room.
4. Tell the patient you are going to lock arms to raise him.
5. Pull the curtain around the bed for privacy.
6. Lock the wheels on the bed.
7. Face the head of the bed. Bend your knees.
8. Have the patient put his arm under your arm (the arm next to him), and behind your shoulder, with his hand over the top of your shoulder. (If you are standing at his right side, his right hand will be on your right shoulder. If you are on his left, you will be locking your left arm with his left arm.)
9. Put your arm under the patient's arm with your hand on his shoulder.
10. When you say "one, two, three," help the patient pull himself up as you support him. This will raise his head and shoulders.

LOCKING ARMS WITH THE PATIENT

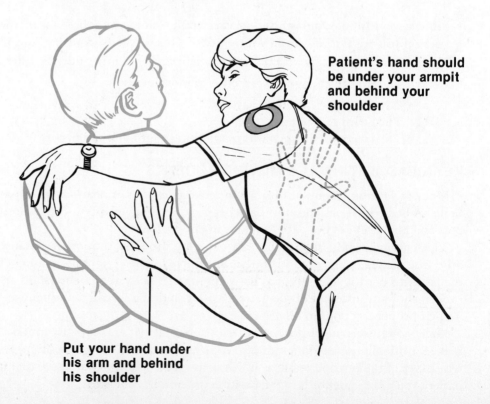

Patient's hand should be under your armpit and behind your shoulder

Put your hand under his arm and behind his shoulder

11. Turn or replace the pillow with your free hand.

12. To help the patient lie down again, continue supporting him with your locked arm and your free hand. Help the patient gently ease himself down.

13. Make the patient comfortable.

14. Wash your hands.

15. Report to your head nurse or team leader that you have changed the patient's position. Also report your observations of anything unusual.

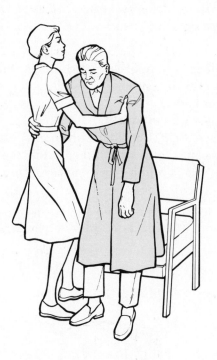

Procedure: Helping the Patient To Stand from a Sitting Position

1. Assemble your equipment, depending on the needs of the patient:
    a. Chair
    b. Walker
    c. Wheelchair

2. Wash your hands.

3. Identify the patient by checking the identification bracelet.

4. Ask visitors to step out of the room.

5. Tell the patient you are going to help him to stand up.

6. Pull the curtain around the bed for privacy.

7. Encourage the patient to help as much as he can, if his effort is permitted.

8. Move the chair, walker, or wheelchair very close to the bed. Then all the patient has to do is stand, pivot (turn), and sit.

9. Lock the wheels on the bed or wheelchair.

10. First method:

    a. Grasp the patient under both arms.

    b. Have the patient put his arm around your waist.

    c. Keep your back straight.

    d. Bend your knees before you start lifting.

    e. Place your right foot firmly on the floor, between the patient's feet. Place your left foot firmly on the floor next to the patient's right foot.

    f. Use your leg muscles to do most of the work.

    g. On your signal "one, two, three," lift the patient gently but firmly to a standing position.

11. Second method:

    a. Put one foot in front of the patient's feet. Put your other foot in back of the patient's feet.

    b. Bend your knees.

    c. Lock arms with the patient.

    d. Grasp the patient's shoulder with your free hand.

    e. On your signal "one, two, three," while the patient leans on your shoulder, lift him gently but firmly into a standing position.

12. Report to your head nurse or team leader that you have helped the patient to stand. Also report your observations of anything unusual.

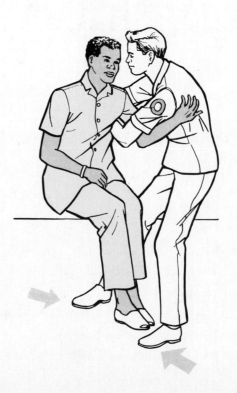

Procedure: Moving the Helpless Patient Up in Bed

1. Ask another nursing aide to work with you.

2. Wash your hands.

3. Identify the patient by checking the identification bracelet.

4. Ask visitors to step out of the room.

5. Tell the patient that you and your partner are going to move him up in the bed. Say this even if he appears to be unconscious.

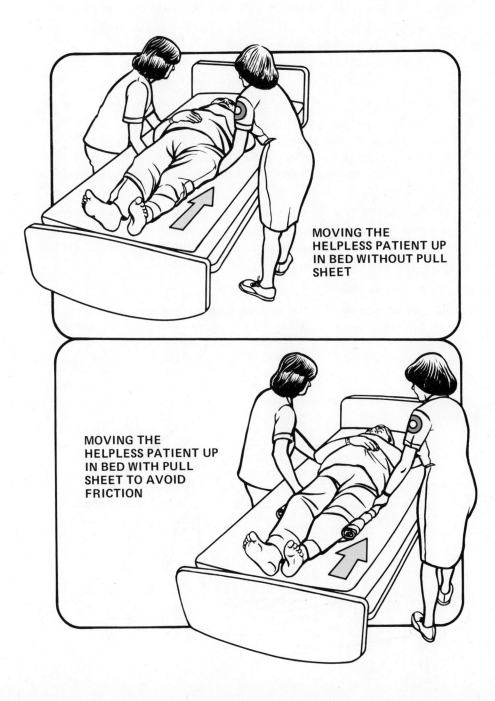

MOVING THE
HELPLESS PATIENT UP
IN BED WITHOUT PULL
SHEET

MOVING THE
HELPLESS PATIENT UP
IN BED WITH PULL
SHEET TO AVOID
FRICTION

6. Pull the curtain around the bed for privacy.

7. Remove the pillow from the bed. Put it on a chair.

8. Lock the wheels on the bed.

9. Stand on one side of the bed. The other nursing aide will stand on the other side.

10. You both should stand straight, turned slightly toward the head of the bed. Your feet should be 12 inches apart. The foot closest to the head of the bed should be pointed in that direction. Bend your knees. Keep your back straight.

11. Use of a "draw" or "pull" sheet is always preferred for moving a patient up in bed. This is to avoid friction between the patient's skin and bedding.

12. When a pull sheet is not used, you will:
    a. Put one arm under the patient's shoulder nearest you.
    b. Put your other arm under the patient's buttocks.

13. The other nursing aide will do the same from the other side.

14. You will be sliding the patient's body when you move him up in bed. Straighten your knees as you start to slide the patient. Your body is in the correct position for the direction in which you will move. Therefore, you can shift your weight easily from one foot to the other.

15. When you say "one, two, three" in unison, you and your partner will move together to slide the patient gently and move him toward the head of the bed, or to the position he should be in.

16. Make the patient comfortable.

17. Wash your hands.

18. Report to your head nurse or team leader that you have changed the patient's position. Also report your observations of anything unusual.

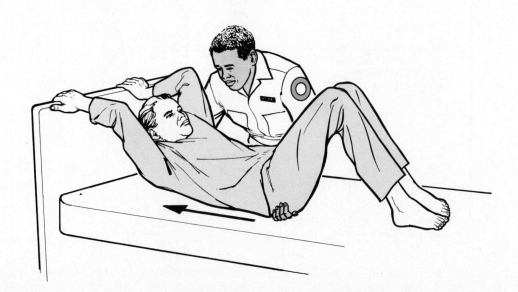

Procedure: Moving a Patient to the Head of the Bed with His Help

1. Wash your hands.
2. Identify the patient by checking the identification bracelet.
3. Ask visitors to step out of the room.
4. Tell the patient you are going to move him up in the bed. Before you begin, be sure the patient is allowed to exert himself as much as is necessary for this move.
5. Pull the curtain around the bed for privacy.
6. Lock the wheels on the bed.
7. Lower the backrest, if this is allowed.
8. Lock arms with the patient and remove the pillow with your free hand.
9. Put the pillow on a chair, or at the foot of the bed.
10. Put the side rails in the up position on the far side of the bed.
11. Put one hand under the patient's shoulder. Put your other hand under the patient's buttocks.
12. Ask the patient to bend his knees and brace his feet firmly on the mattress.
13. Ask the patient to grasp the head of the bed.
14. Have your feet 12 inches apart. The foot closest to the head of the bed should be pointed in that direction.
15. Bend your knees. Keep your back straight.
16. Bend your body from your hips facing the patient and turned slightly toward the head of the bed.
17. At the signal "one, two, three," have the patient pull with his hands toward the head of the bed and push with his feet against the mattress.
18. At the same time, help him move toward the head of the bed by sliding him with your hands and arms.
19. Lock arms with the patient and put the pillow back in place, under his head and shoulders.
20. Make the patient comfortable.
21. Wash your hands.
22. Report to your head nurse or team leader that you have changed the patient's position. Also report your observations of anything unusual.

Procedure: Moving the Mattress to the Head of the Bed with the Patient's Help

1. Wash your hands.
2. Identify the patient by checking the identification bracelet.
3. Ask visitors to step out of the room.
4. Tell the patient you are going to move his mattress to the head of the bed.

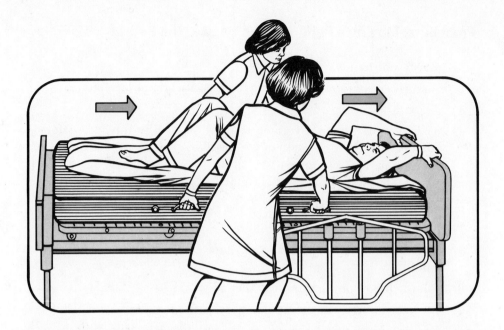

5. Pull the curtain around the bed for privacy.

6. Lock the wheels on the bed.

7. Lower the backrest, if allowed.

8. Put the side rail in the up position on the far side of the bed.

9. Lock arms with the patient and remove the pillow.

10. Put the pillow on the chair.

11. Ask the patient to grasp the headboard with both hands.

12. Stand at the side of the bed. The sheets should be loosened.

13. Ask the patient to bend his knees and brace his feet firmly on the mattress.

14. Grasp the mattress loops, or grasp the sides of the mattress if there are no loops.

15. On the signal "one, two, three," have the patient pull with his hands toward the head of the bed and push with his feet against the mattress.

16. At the same time, you will slide the mattress toward the head of the bed. Keep your knees bent and your back straight as you move the mattress.

17. Lock arms with the patient and put the pillow back in place.

18. Make the patient comfortable.

19. Wash your hands.

20. Report to your head nurse or team leader that you have moved the mattress. Also report your observations of anything unusual.

Procedure: Rolling the Patient Like a Log (Log Rolling)

1. Wash your hands.

2. Identify the patient by checking the identification bracelet.

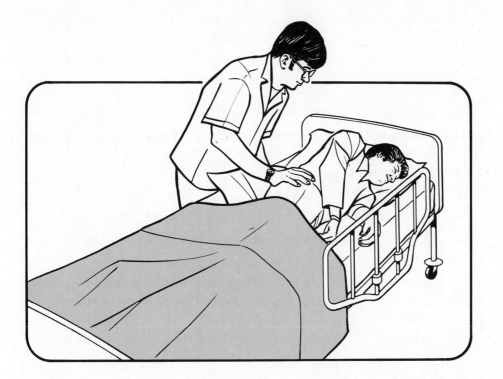

3. Ask visitors to step out of the room.

4. Tell the patient you are going to roll him to his side as if he were a log.

5. Pull the curtain around the bed for privacy.

6. Get help from a second nursing aide, if necessary.

7. Lock the wheels on the bed. Raise the side rails on the far side of the bed.

8. Remove the pillow from under the patient's head, if allowed.

9. Put a pillow between the patient's knees and cross the patient's legs in the direction of movement.

10. Use pull sheets when necessary.

11. Keep your knees bent, your back straight, and your weight balanced evenly on both feet.

12. Roll the patient onto his side like a log. Turn his body as a whole unit, without bending his joints. Turn him gently.

13. Replace the pillow under the patient's head, if allowed.

14. Use pillows against the patient's back to keep his body in proper alignment.

15. Reverse the procedure to turn the patient on his opposite side.

16. Wash your hands.

17. Report to your head nurse or team leader that you have changed the patient's position. Also report your observations of anything unusual.

Procedure: Moving a Helpless Patient to One Side of the Bed on His Back

1. Wash your hands.
2. Identify the patient by checking the identification bracelet.
3. Ask visitors to step out of the room.
4. Tell the patient you are going to move him to one side of the bed on his back without turning him.
5. Pull the curtain around the bed for privacy.
6. Lock the wheels on the bed.
7. Lower the backrest and footrest, if this is allowed.
8. Put the side rail in the up position on the far side of the bed.
9. Loosen the sheets, but don't expose the patient.
10. Push both your hands under the patient's back until they are under his far shoulder. Then slide the patient's shoulders toward you on your arms.
11. Push both hands as far as you can under the patient's buttocks and slide his body toward you. Use a pull sheet whenever possible.

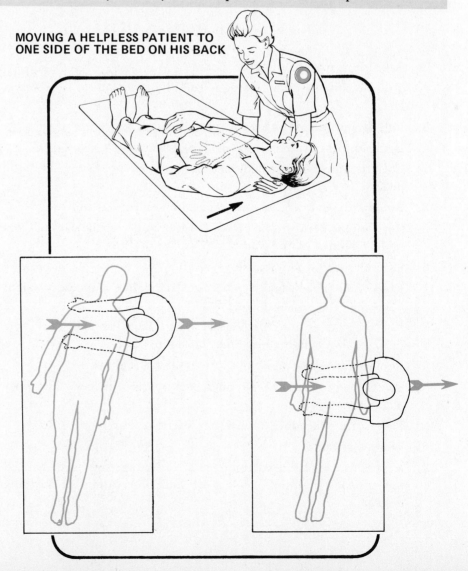

MOVING A HELPLESS PATIENT TO
ONE SIDE OF THE BED ON HIS BACK

12. Keep your knees bent and your back straight as you slide the patient.

13. Place both hands under the patient's feet and slide them toward you.

14. Lock arms with the patient and put the pillow back in place.

15. Make the patient comfortable.

16. Report to your head nurse or team leader that you have changed the patient's position. Also report your observations of anything unusual.

Procedure: Turning a Patient onto His Right Side Toward You

1. Wash your hands.

2. Identify the patient by checking the identification bracelet.

3. Ask visitors to step out of the room.

4. Tell the patient you are going to turn him on his side.

5. Pull the curtain around the bed for privacy.

6. Lock the wheels on the bed.

7. Lower the backrest and footrest, if this is allowed.

8. Put the side rail in the up position on the far side of the bed.

9. Loosen the top sheets, but don't expose the patient.

10. When you are turning the patient to the right side, cross his left leg over his right foot.

11. Cross the patient's arms over his chest.

12. Reach across the patient and put one hand behind his far shoulder.

13. Place your other hand behind his far hip. Gently roll him toward you.

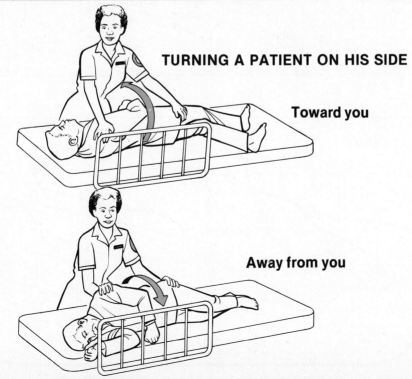

TURNING A PATIENT ON HIS SIDE

Toward you

Away from you

TURNING A PATIENT ONTO HIS RIGHT SIDE TOWARD YOU

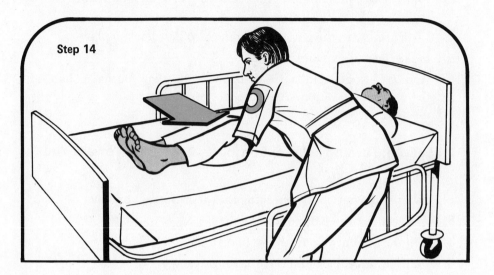

Step 14

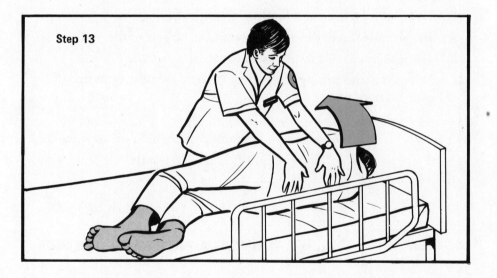

Step 13

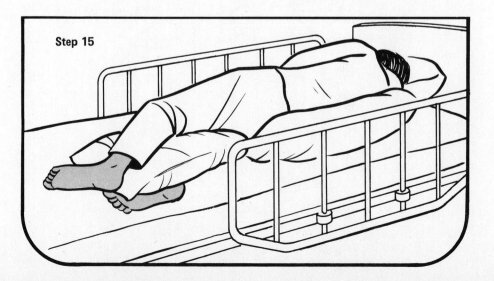

Step 15

14. Raise the side rail, if the patient is close to the edge of the bed. Go to the opposite side of the bed. Lower the side rail. Then carefully move his body by sliding it to the center of the bed—first the shoulders, then the hips, and then the legs.

15. Fold a pillow lengthwise and place it against the patient's back for support.

16. Support the patient's head with the palm of one hand. With your other hand slide a pillow under his head and neck.

17. See that the patient's arms and legs are in a comfortable position.

18. Check to make sure the signal cord is within easy reach of the patient. Be sure both side rails are up.

19. Wash your hands.

20. Report to your head nurse or team leader that you have changed the patient's position. Also report your observations of anything unusual.

Procedure: Turning a Patient onto His Left Side Away from You

1. Wash your hands.

2. Identify the patient by checking the identification bracelet.

3. Ask visitors to step out of the room.

4. Tell the patient you are going to turn him onto his other side.

5. Pull the curtain around the bed for privacy.

6. Lock the wheels on the bed.

7. Lower the backrest and footrest.

8. Put the side rail in the up position on the far side of the bed.

9. Loosen the top sheets, but don't expose the patient.

10. Cross the patient's arms over his chest.

11. When turning a patient to the left side, cross his right leg over his left foot.

12. Slide one arm under the patient's back with your hand under his far shoulder.

13. Put your other hand under his buttocks.

14. Draw your arms toward you, sliding the patient's body close to your side of the bed. At the same time roll him gently on his side, facing away from you.

15. Fold a pillow lengthwise. Place it against the patient's back for support.

16. Support the patient's head with the palm of one hand. With your other hand slide a pillow under his head and neck.

17. Make sure the patient's arms and legs are in a comfortable position. Put a pillow between his knees, if this helps to make the patient comfortable.

18. Check to make sure the signal cord is within easy reach of the patient.

19. Raise the second side rail to the up position.

20. Wash your hands.

21. Report to your head nurse or team leader that you have changed the patient's position. Also report your observations of anything unusual.

Section 2: Transporting a Patient

OBJECTIVES: WHAT YOU WILL LEARN

When you have completed this section, you should be able:

• To transport a patient by wheelchair or stretcher

• To move a patient from the bed to a wheelchair and back into bed

• To move the helpless patient using a portable mechanical patient lift

• To move a patient from the bed to a stretcher and back into bed

TRANSPORTING THE PATIENT BY WHEELCHAIR

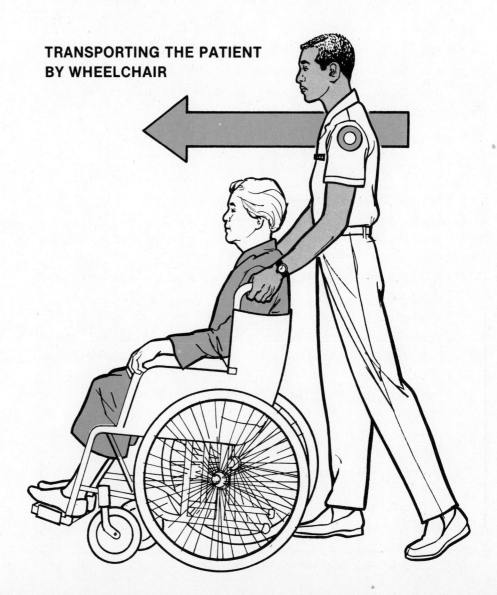

KEY IDEAS: TRANSPORTING A PATIENT BY WHEELCHAIR

The patient in a wheelchair should be well covered, even if he is dressed in a robe and slippers. You may cover his feet as well as his shoulders with a blanket. Make sure the blanket does not get caught in the wheels. The seat of the wheelchair should be covered with a disposable bed protector or a piece of clean linen. The wheelchair should be wiped off with an antiseptic solution after it has been used by each patient.

When you are moving a patient in a wheelchair, you should push the wheelchair from behind, except when going into or out of elevators. When you are entering an elevator, pull the wheelchair into the elevator backwards. When you are leaving an elevator, ask everyone to step out. Push the button marked "open." Turn the chair around, and pull it out of the elevator backwards. Don't move the wheelchair while the elevator is in motion.

When you are moving a patient down a steep ramp, you should take the chair down backwards. To do this, stand behind the chair with your back facing the direction you want to go. Walk backwards, holding the chair and moving it carefully down the ramp. Glance back now and then to make sure of your direction and to avoid collisions, as if you were driving a car in reverse.

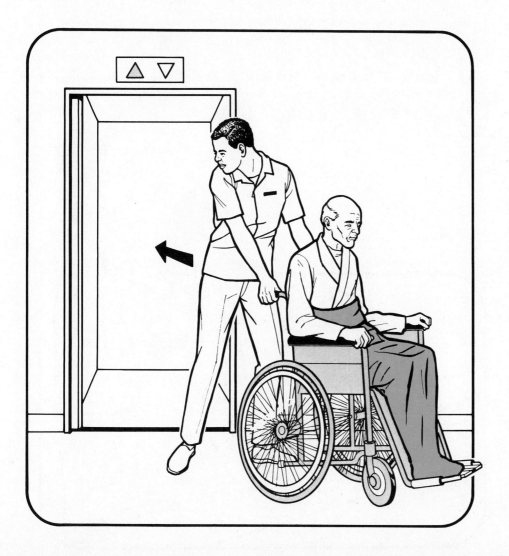

Procedure: Helping a Patient Who Can Stand into a Chair or a Wheelchair

1. Assemble your equipment:
   a. Wheelchair or chair
   b. Blanket or sheet
2. Wash your hands.
3. Identify the patient by checking the identification bracelet.
4. Ask visitors to step out of the room.
5. Tell the patient you are going to help him into a chair or wheelchair.
6. Pull the curtain around the bed for privacy.
7. Lock the wheels on the bed.
8. Bring the chair or wheelchair into the room and put it at the bedside. Have the back of the chair near the head of the bed.
9. Fold the footrests of the wheelchair up so they are out of the way. If the chair or wheelchair has leg rests, adjust them to hang straight down.
10. Set the brakes on the wheelchair so it can't roll. If you are using an armchair, place the back of the chair against the wall so it can't slide.
11. Spread a blanket or sheet on the chair. Have a blanket corner between the handles over the back so the opposite corner will be at the patient's feet.

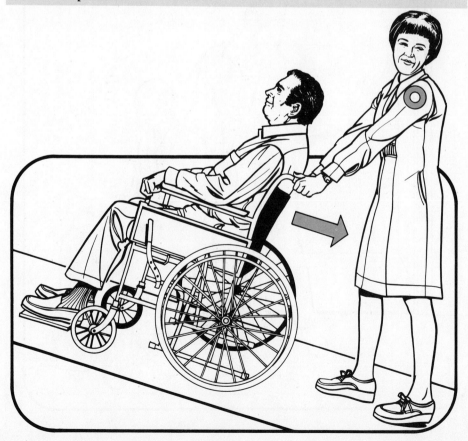

12. If the bed can be lowered and raised, lower it to a level that allows the patient's feet to touch the floor when he sits up.

13. If you can't lower the bed, put a footstool in a position where the patient will be able to step onto it.

14. Help the patient put his robe and slippers on while he is in bed.

15. Slide the patient to your side of the bed.

16. Raise the side rail.

17. Raise the backrest so the patient is in a sitting position.

18. Lower the side rail.

19. Turn the patient so he is sitting on the side of the bed. His feet will be dangling over the side of the bed.

20. Stand at the patient's side. Put your arm around his waist and help him to stand on the floor.

21. Help the patient to sit down in the chair or wheelchair.

22. Fasten the safety straps.

23. Adjust the footrests so the patient's feet are resting on them.

24. Arrange the blanket snugly but firmly around the patient. Make sure that no part of the blanket can possibly get caught in the wheels.

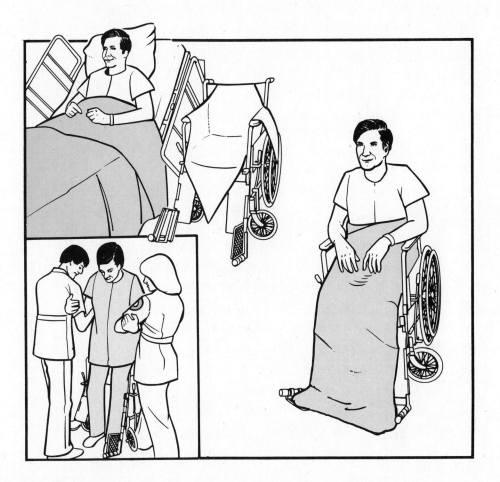

OBSERVE THE PATIENT

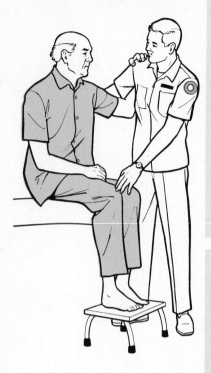

25. Observe the patient's color. Use the signal cord to call your team leader or the head nurse and take the patient's pulse if you observe any of the following:
    a. The patient becomes very pale.
    b. The patient is perspiring a lot.
    c. The patient says something like "I feel weak" or "I feel dizzy" or "I feel faint."
26. Adjust the chair to a comfortable angle.
27. Put a pillow behind the patient's back or shoulders, if needed.
28. Wash your hands.
29. Report to your head nurse or team leader that you have helped the patient out of bed and into a wheelchair. Also report your observations of anything unusual.

Procedure: Moving the Helpless Patient into a Wheelchair

1. Assemble your equipment:
   a. Wheelchair
   b. Blanket or sheet
   c. Mechanical patient lift
2. Wash your hands.
3. Identify the patient by checking the identification bracelet.
4. Ask visitors to step out of the room.
5. Tell the patient you are going to help him into a wheelchair.
6. Pull the curtain around the bed for privacy.
7. Lock the wheels on the bed.
8. Bring the wheelchair into the room. Put it at the bedside with the back of the chair near the head of the bed.
9. Fold the footrests up so they are out of the way. If the wheelchair has legrests, adjust them to hang straight down.
10. Set the brakes on the wheelchair so it cannot roll.
11. Spread a blanket or sheet on the chair. Have a corner of the blanket between the handles over the back so the opposite corner will be at the patient's feet.
12. If the bed can be lowered and raised, lower it to a level that allows the patient's feet to touch the floor when he sits up.
13. Ask another nursing aide to help you. You should work in unison.
14. Put robe and slippers on the patient while he is in the bed.
15. Move the patient to your side of the bed.
16. Raise the side rail.
17. Raise the backrest so the patient is in a sitting position.
18. Lower the side rail.
19. Each nursing aide locks arms with the patient. Together you lift him gently from the bed to the chair, or use a portable mechanical patient lift.

20. Fasten the safety straps around the patient to keep him from falling out of the chair.

21. Arrange the blanket snugly but firmly around the patient. Make sure that no part of the blanket can possibly get caught in the wheels.

22. Adjust the footrests so that the patient's feet are resting on them.

23. Observe the patient's color. Use the signal cord to call your team leader or the head nurse and take the patient's pulse if you observe any of the following:

    a. The patient becomes very pale.
    b. The patient seems to be perspiring a lot.
    c. The patient says something like "I feel weak" or "I feel dizzy" or "I feel faint."

24. Adjust the chair to a comfortable angle.

25. Put a pillow behind the patient's back or shoulders, if needed.

26. Wash your hands.

27. Report to your head nurse or team leader that you have moved the helpless patient out of bed. Also report your observations of anything unusual.

Procedure: Helping a Patient Back into Bed from a Chair or a Wheelchair

1. Wash your hands.

2. Identify the patient by checking the identification bracelet.

3. Ask visitors to step out of the room.

4. Tell the patient you are getting him back into bed.

5. Pull the curtain around the bed for privacy.

6. Lock the wheels on the bed.

7. Bring the wheelchair very close to the bed.

8. Lock the wheels of the wheelchair.

9. Raise the footrests.

10. Raise the headrest of the bed to a sitting position.

11. Lower the bed to its lowest position. If the bed can't be lowered, bring a footstool to the bedside.

12. Open the safety straps on the wheelchair.

13. Help the patient out of the wheelchair. Have him in a sitting position on the side of the bed. His legs should be hanging down.

14. Lean the patient against the backrest.

15. Put one arm around the patient's shoulders for support. Put the other arm under his knees.

16. Swing his body slowly around, helping him to lift his legs onto the bed.

17. Lower the backrest.

18. Help the patient move to the center of the bed.

**HELPING A PATIENT
OUT OF OR INTO THE BED**

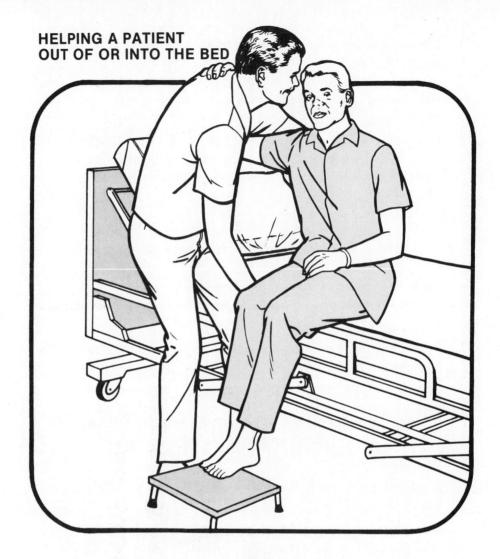

19. Make the patient comfortable. Take off his robe and slippers.
20. Fold and put the blanket in its proper place.
21. Return the wheelchair to its proper place and wash it with an antiseptic solution.
22. Wash your hands.
23. Report to your head nurse or team leader that you have helped the patient back into bed. Also report your observations of anything unusual.

Procedure: Using a Portable Mechanical Patient Lift to Move the Helpless Patient

1. Assemble your equipment:
    a. Mechanical patient lift
    b. Sling
2. Wash your hands.
3. Identify the patient by checking the identification bracelet.

4. Ask visitors to step out of the room.

5. Tell the patient that you are going to get him out of bed by using the portable mechanical patient lift. (You may need the help of a second nursing aide as a partner.)

6. Pull the curtain around the bed for privacy.

7. Position the chair to receive the patient very near to the bed.

8. Cover the chair with a blanket or sheet.

9. By turning the patient from side to side on the bed, slide the sling under the patient.

10. Attach the sling to the mechanical lift with the hooks in place through the metal frame.

11. Have the patient fold both arms across his chest, if possible.

12. Using the crank, lift the patient from the bed.

13. Have your partner—a second nursing aide—guide the patient's legs.

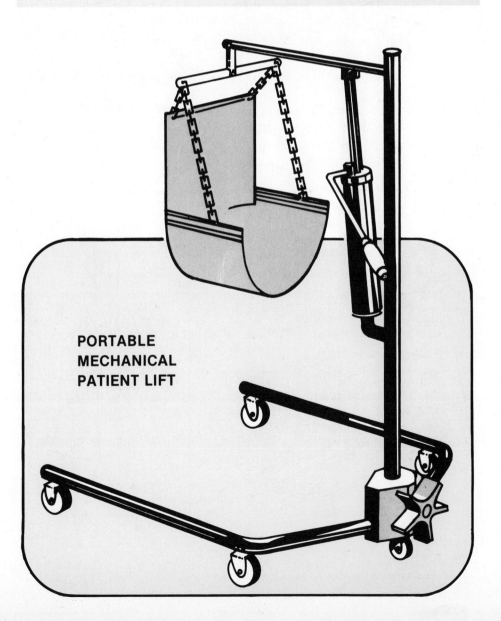

**PORTABLE
MECHANICAL
PATIENT LIFT**

14. Lower the patient into the chair.

15. Remove the hooks from the frame of the portable mechanical patient lift.

16. Leave the patient safe and comfortable in the chair for the proper amount of time, according to your instructions.

17. To get the patient back to bed, put the hooks through the metal frame of the sling, which is still under the patient.

18. Raise the patient by using the crank on the mechanical patient lift. Lift him from the chair into the bed. Have your partner guide the patient's legs.

19. Remove the hooks from the frame.

20. Remove the sling by having the patient turn from side to side on the bed.

21. Raise the side rails to the up position.

22. Leave the patient safe and comfortable.

23. Wash your hands.

24. Make your report and record your observations:

    a. The patient was taken out of bed by means of the portable mechanical patient lift.

    b. The patient was left in a chair for the prescribed length of time.

    c. The patient was put back into bed by means of the mechanical patient lift.

    d. Any unusual observations that you have noted.

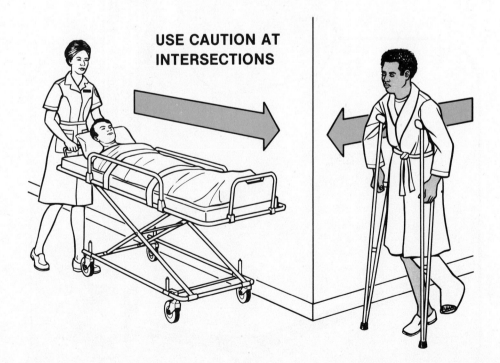

USE CAUTION AT INTERSECTIONS

KEY IDEAS: USING A STRETCHER

A hospital stretcher, sometimes called a litter or gurney, is a wheeled cart on which patients remain lying down while they are moved from one place to another. For moving a helpless patient from his bed to a stretcher, you will need a second nursing aide working as your partner. Whenever you are moving the stretcher, you should stand at the end where the patient's head is and push the stretcher so the patient is moving feet first. Be careful to protect the patient's head at all times. When entering an elevator, stand at the patient's head. Pull the stretcher into the elevator with the head end first. Stand at the patient's head while the elevator is in motion. When you leave the elevator, push the stretcher out of the elevator foot end first.

Use restraining straps whenever you move a patient on a stretcher. Check the straps before you move the stretcher. Guide the vehicle from the foot end when going down a ramp.

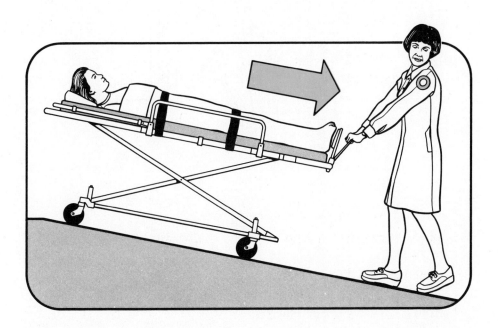

Procedure: Moving a Patient from the Bed to a Stretcher

1. Assemble your equipment:
   a. Stretcher
   b. Sheet or blanket
2. Ask another nursing aide to help you. The two of you should work in unison to move the patient from the bed to a stretcher.
3. Wash your hands.
4. Identify the patient by checking the identification bracelet.
5. Tell the patient you are going to move him from the bed to a stretcher.
6. Ask visitors to step out of the room.

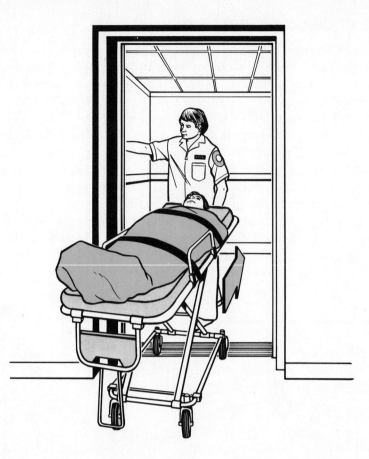

7. Pull the curtain around the bed for privacy.

8. Raise the bed so that it is even with the stretcher. Lock the wheels on the bed.

9. Loosen the top sheets.

10. Cover the patient with a blanket or sheet. Remove the top sheets without exposing the patient.

11. Bring the stretcher next to the bed.

12. Lock the wheels on the stretcher.

13. You will stand on the far side of the bed using your body to hold the bed in place.

14. Your partner will stand on the far side of the stretcher using his body to hold the stretcher in place.

15. You should both have your knees bent, your backs straight, and your weight balanced on both feet.

16. At the signal "one, two, three," push, pull, and slide the patient from the bed to the stretcher. Use a pull sheet whenever possible.

17. Support the patient's head and feet, keeping his body covered with a loose blanket or sheet.

18. Fasten the stretcher straps around the patient at his hips and shoulders.

19. Put the side rails of the stretcher in the up position for the patient's safety.

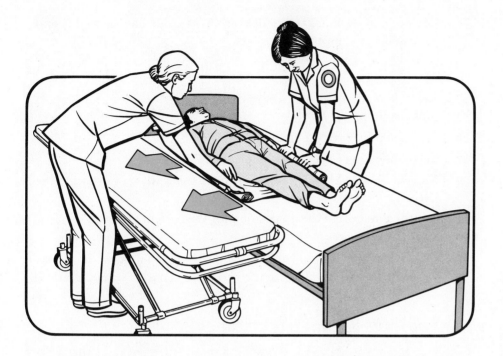

20. Wash your hands.

21. Report to your head nurse or team leader that you have moved the patient to the stretcher. Also report your observations of anything unusual.

Procedure: Moving a Patient from a Stretcher to the Bed

1. Assemble your equipment:
   a. Stretcher
   b. Sheet or blanket

2. Ask another nursing aide to help. You should work in unison to move the patient from a stretcher to the bed.

3. Wash your hands.

4. Identify the patient by checking the identification bracelet.

5. Tell the patient you are going to move him from the stretcher to the bed.

6. Ask visitors to step out of the room.

7. Pull the curtain around the bed for privacy.

8. Lock the wheels on the bed.

9. Fan fold the top sheet to the bottom of the bed.

10. Bring the stretcher next to the bed.

11. Lock the wheels on the stretcher.

12. One nursing aide stands on the far side of the bed using his body to hold the bed in place.

13. One nursing aide stands on the far side of the stretcher using his body to hold the stretcher in place.

14. Open the stretcher straps.

15. Both of you should have your knees bent, your back straight, and your weight balanced on both feet.

16. At the signal "one, two, three," slide the patient from the stretcher to the bed. Use a pull sheet.

17. Keep the patient covered with a loose blanket or sheet and support his head and feet.

18. Slide the patient to the center of the bed.

19. Make the patient as comfortable as possible.

20. Replace the top sheets, removing the blanket without exposing the patient.

21. Put the side rails in the up position for the patient's safety.

22. Wash your hands.

23. Report to your head nurse or team leader that you have moved the patient from the stretcher to the bed. Also report your observations of anything unusual.

WHAT YOU HAVE LEARNED

Every day in your work you will be doing many different tasks that will require muscular exertion. Understanding and using the principles of good body mechanics will help you in your work. You will save your energy and lessen strain and fatigue. Also your work will go better—more smoothly and efficiently. You will feel less awkward.

Proper body alignment for the patient can add to his comfort and well-being. Changing the patient's position frequently will reduce the dangers of bed sores caused by pressure, that is, decubitus ulcers.

Personal Care of the Patient

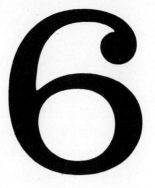

Section 1: Daily Care of the Patient

OBJECTIVES: WHAT YOU WILL LEARN

When you have completed this section, you should be able:

- To care for the patient's mouth using good oral hygiene techniques
- To bathe the patient
- To help the patient use the bedpan or urinal

KEY IDEAS: SCHEDULE OF DAILY CARE

Early Morning Care—Before Breakfast

1. Offer the bedpan or urinal.
2. Wash the patient's hands and face.
3. Help with oral hygiene.
4. Pass fresh drinking water.

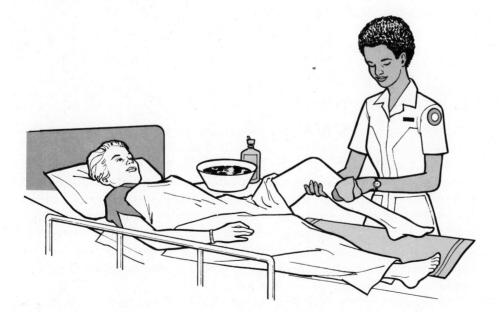

Morning Care—After Breakfast

1. Offer the bedpan or urinal.
2. Assist with oral hygiene.
3. Help the patient to bathe. Follow instructions from your head nurse or team leader. Give the patient a complete bed bath, or partial bed bath, or shower, or tub bath.
4. Change the patient's gown.
5. Help the male patient to shave his face.
6. Give the patient a back rub, if allowed.
7. Help the patient comb his hair.
8. Make the bed.
9. Straighten the unit.

Afternoon Care

1. Change the patient's gown, if necessary.
2. Straighten the unit.
3. Pass fresh drinking water.
4. Offer the bedpan or urinal.

Evening Care

1. Offer the bedpan or urinal.
2. Wash the patient's hands and face.
3. Assist with oral hygiene.
4. Give each patient a back rub, if allowed.
5. Change the draw sheet, if necessary.
6. Smooth and tighten the sheets.

KEY IDEAS: ORAL HYGIENE

A person's mouth and teeth need even more care when he is sick than when he is well. This care is called "oral hygiene." A sick person's mouth often has a bad taste. Sometimes it feels "fuzzy" because of his illness. His tongue may be covered with a grayish coating that spoils his appetite. On the other hand, with good care the patient's mouth will feel fresh and clean. Cleaning the patient's teeth and mouth—that is, giving oral hygiene—is an essential part of daily patient care. Teeth should be brushed every morning and evening and after each meal. In your work you will be giving oral hygiene to conscious and unconscious patients. When necessary, you will be cleaning their false teeth (dentures).

Oral hygiene is given to unconscious patients every two hours. The purpose is to keep the tissues moist. Unless this is done, tissues tend to dry out and develop a mucous coating much more rapidly.

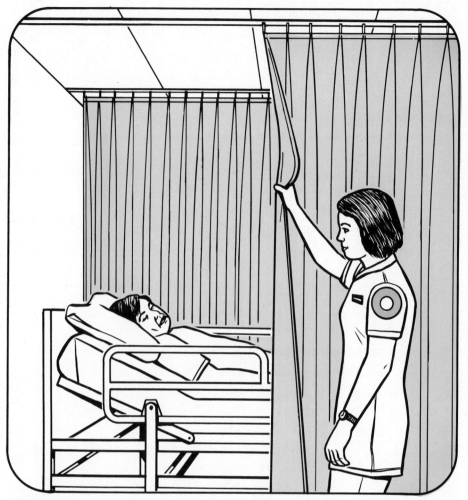

Before giving personal care always pull the curtain around the bed to give the patient privacy.

GIVING THE PATIENT ORAL HYGIENE

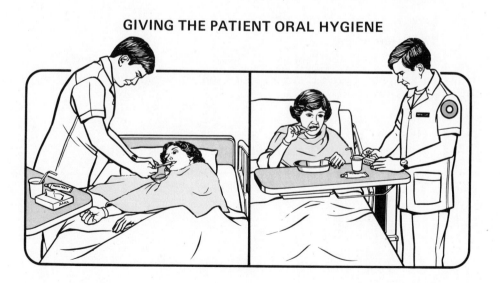

Procedure: Giving Oral Hygiene to the Conscious Patient

1. Assemble your equipment:
    a. Mouthwash
    b. Fresh water
    c. Disposable cup
    d. Straw
    e. Toothbrush
    f. Toothpaste
    g. Emesis basin
    h. Face towel
2. Wash your hands.
3. Identify the patient by checking the identification bracelet.
4. Ask visitors to step out of the room.
5. Tell the patient you will help him clean his teeth and mouth.
6. Pull the curtain around the bed for privacy.
7. Spread the towel across the patient's chest to protect the gown and top sheets.
8. Mix one-half cup of water with one-half cup of mouthwash.
9. Let the patient take a mouthful of the mixture and rinse his mouth.
10. Hold the emesis basin under the patient's chin so he can spit out the mouthwash solution.
11. Put toothpaste on the wet toothbrush.
12. If the patient can do it, let him brush his own teeth. If he can't, brush his teeth for him. Use an up-and-down motion.
13. Help the patient wash the toothpaste out of his mouth. Use the mouthwash solution.
14. Clean and put your equipment in its proper place. Throw away all disposable supplies and equipment.
15. Make the patient comfortable.
16. Wash your hands.
17. Report to your head nurse or team leader that you have given the patient oral hygiene. Also report your observations of anything unusual.

Procedure: Cleaning Dentures (False Teeth)

1. Assemble your equipment:
    a. Tissues
    b. Mouthwash
    c. Disposable cup
    d. Emesis basin
    e. Toothbrush or denture brush
    f. Towel
2. Wash your hands.
3. Identify the patient by checking the identification bracelet.
4. Ask visitors to step out of the room.

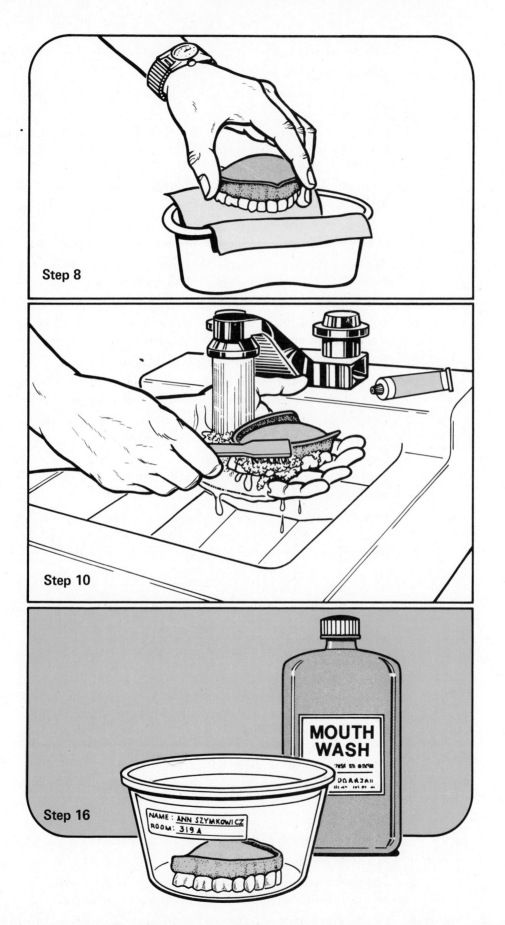

Step 8

Step 10

Step 16

5. Tell the patient you wish to clean his dentures.

6. Pull the curtain around the bed for privacy.

7. Spread the towel across the patient's chest to protect the gown and top sheets.

8. Ask the patient to remove his dentures. Have tissue in the emesis basin ready to receive them. Help the patient who is unable to remove his own dentures.

9. Take the dentures to the sink in the lined emesis basin. Hold the dentures securely in the basin.

10. Line the sink with a paper towel or fill the sink with water to guard against breaking the dentures if you accidentally drop them.

11. Apply toothpaste or denture cleanser. With the dentures in the palm of your hand, brush until they are clean.

12. Rinse thoroughly under running water.

13. Fill the clean denture cup with water and mouthwash. Or use water and salt—a saline solution. Place the dentures in the cup.

14. Help the patient to rinse his mouth with mouthwash.

15. Have the patient replace dentures in his mouth if that is what he wants. Be sure dentures are moist before replacing them.

16. Leave the labeled denture cup with the clean solution on the bedside table where the patient can reach it easily.

17. Clean all your equipment and put it in its proper place. Throw away used disposable supplies and equipment.

18. Wash your hands.

19. Report to your head nurse or team leader that you have cleaned the patient's dentures. Also report your observations of anything unusual.

Procedure: Giving Oral Hygiene to the Unconscious Patient

1. Assemble your equipment:
   a. Towel
   b. Emesis basin
   c. Special disposable mouth care kit from the central supply room (CSR) of commercially prepared swabs. Or, if such a kit is not available:
   d. Tongue depressor
   e. Applicators or gauze sponges
   f. Lubricant such as glycerine, petroleum jelly, or solution of lemon juice and glycerine

2. Wash your hands.

3. Identify the patient by checking the identification bracelet.

4. Ask visitors to step out of the room.

5. Tell the patient what you are going to do. Even though a patient seems to be unconscious, he still may be able to hear you.

6. Pull the curtain around the bed for privacy.

7. Stand at the side of the bed. Turn the patient's head to the side facing you.

8. Put a towel on the pillow under the patient's head and partly under his face.

9. Put the emesis basin on the towel under the patient's chin.

10. Ask the patient to open his mouth. If he is in a coma, he may not be able to respond. In this case you will have to hold his mouth open. Press on his cheeks and hold his tongue in place with a tongue depressor.

11. Open the commercial package of swabs. Wipe the patient's entire mouth: roof, tongue, and inside the cheeks and lips with the prepared swabs.

12. Put used swabs into the emesis basin. Commercial swabs leave a coating of glycerine solution on the entire inside of the mouth, tongue, and teeth.

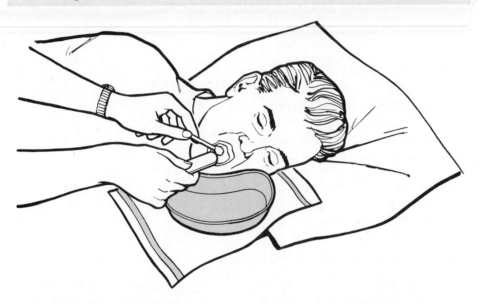

If a disposable mouth care kit of commercially prepared swabs is not available:

13. Moisten the applicators with mouthwash solution.

14. Use your free hand to insert the applicators in the patient's mouth. Thoroughly wipe the roof of the mouth, the teeth, and the tongue.

15. Change applicators frequently.

16. Place the used applicators and other supplies in the emesis basin.

17. Use clear water on more applicators to rinse out the patient's mouth.

18. Dry the patient's face with the towel.

19. Using an applicator, put a small amount of the lubricant on the patient's lips and tongue and the inside of his mouth.

20. Clean your equipment and put it in its proper place. Discard used disposable supplies and equipment.

21. Wash your hands.
22. Report to your head nurse or team leader that you have given the patient special oral hygiene. Also report your observations of anything unusual.

KEY IDEAS: HELPING THE PATIENT TO BATHE

There are several important reasons for bathing the patient. Bathing gets rid of dirt on the patient's body. It eliminates body odors and cools and refreshes the patient. The bath stimulates circulation and helps to prevent bedsores. Bathing requires movements of certain parts of the body: the patient's legs and arms are lifted and his head and torso are turned. This activity exercises muscles that might otherwise remained unused. A patient may be bathed in one of four ways, depending on his condition. He may be given a complete bed bath, a partial bed bath, a tub bath, or a shower.

The Complete Bed Bath. The patient who is too weak or sick to leave his bed at any time is given a complete bed bath. When you are giving this bath, you will get little or no help from the patient.

The Partial Bath. A patient may be able to take care of most of his own bathing needs. In this case you bathe only the areas that are hard for him to reach such as his back. A partial bath is given while the patient is in bed.

The Tub Bath. The tub bath might be ordered by the doctor for therapeutic reasons.

The Shower. Showers may be permitted for convalescent patients—patients who are recovering from their illness. These patients have been judged by their doctor to be strong enough to get out of bed and walk around.

Rules To Follow When Bathing the Patient

1. Usually the complete bed bath is given as part of morning care. After the bath, the occupied bed is made, the hair is combed, and the gown is changed.
2. Take everything you will need to the bedside before you start the bath. Clear off the bedside table and put the items you will be using on it.
3. Always cover the patient with a bath blanket before giving the complete bed bath.
4. Have the patient move or help him to move close to you, so you can work easily without strain on your back.
5. Use good body mechanics. Keep your feet separated. Stand firmly, bend your knees, and keep your back straight.
6. Make a mitten for your hand out of the washcloth. This will prevent it from dragging roughly across the patient's skin.
7. Change the water during the bed bath as necessary. For example, change the water whenever it becomes soapy, dirty, or cold. Change it before washing the patient's legs and before washing his back.
8. Only one part of the body is washed at a time. Wash, rinse, and dry each body part or area very well. Then cover it right away with the bath blanket.

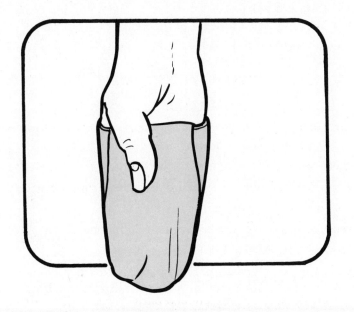

9. Soap will have a drying effect on the patient's skin. Be sure to rinse off all of the soap.

10. When you are not using the soap, keep it in the soap dish instead of the basin. In this way, the water will not dissolve the soap and get too soapy.

11. Putting the patient's hands and feet into the water makes the patient feel relaxed.

12. Observe the condition of the patient's skin when you are giving the bath. Report any redness, rashes, broken skin, or tender places you see on the patient's body.

13. Never trim or cut toenails without special instructions from your head nurse or team leader.

14. Lotion for the back rub should be warmed in your hand. Put the bottle in the bath water to keep it warm.

15. Powder and deodorant should be used only if the patient asks for it. They should be applied after the bath has been completed and after the clean bed has been made.

16. Check the patient's gown for valuables before putting it in the laundry hamper.

Procedure: Giving the Complete Bed Bath

1. Assemble your equipment:
   a. Soap and soap dish
   b. Washcloth
   c. Wash basin
   d. Bath thermometer
   e. Face and bath towels
   f. Talcum powder
   g. Clean gown

h.   Bath blanket

i.   Orange stick for care of the nails

j.   Lotion for back rub

k.   Comb or hair brush

l.   Disposable plastic laundry bags for dirty linen, if used in your hospital, or linen laundry bag. A pillowcase is sometimes used for dirty linen.

m.   Clean bed linen, stacked on chair in order of use, if the bed is to be made following the bed bath.

2.   Wash your hands.

3.   Identify the patient by checking the identification bracelet.

4.   Ask visitors to step out of the room.

5.   Tell the patient you are going to give him a bed bath.

6.   Pull the curtains around the bed for privacy.

7.   Assist the patient with oral hygiene, if this has not already been done. (Oral hygiene should follow each meal, in addition to morning and evening care, whenever possible.)

8.   Offer the bedpan or urinal.

9.   Arrange your equipment conveniently on the bedside table. Put the linen on the chair close to the bed. Put the laundry bag on a chair close by.

10.   Pull out all the bedding from under the mattress. Leave it hanging loosely at all four sides of the bed.

11.   Take the bedspread and regular blanket off the bed. Fold them loosely over the back of the chair, leaving the patient covered with the top sheet.

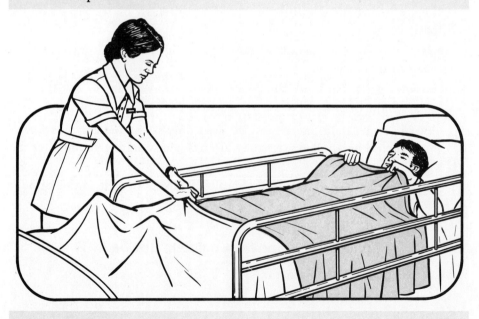

12.   Place the bath blanket over the top sheet. Ask the patient to hold the blanket in place.

13.   Remove the top sheet from underneath without uncovering (exposing) the patient. Fold the sheet loosely over the back of the chair if it is to be used again. Or put it in the laundry bag.

14. Lower the headrest and kneerest of the bed, if permitted. The patient should be in a flat position, as flat as is comfortable for him.

15. Ask the patient to remove any jewelry and put it in the drawer of the bedside table.

16. Take off the patient's gown. Keep the patient covered with the bath blanket. If the gown belongs to the patient, put it away as requested. Put a hospital gown into the laundry bag.

17. Fill the wash basin two-thirds full of water at 115° F (46.1° C). Use the bath thermometer to test the temperature of the water.

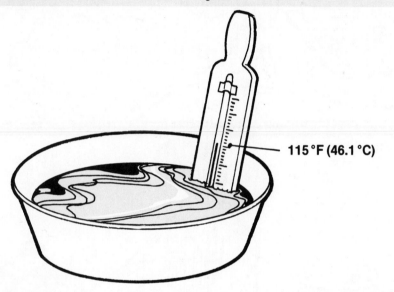

115°F (46.1°C)

18. Help the patient to move to the side of the bed closest to you. Use good body mechanics.

19. Put a towel across the patient's chest and make a mitten with the washcloth. Wash the patient's eyes from the nose to the outside of his face. Ask the patient if he wants soap used on his face. Wash the face. Be careful not to get soap in his eyes. Rinse and dry by patting gently.

20. Put a towel lengthwise under the patient's arm farthest from you. This is to keep the bed from getting wet. Support the patient's arm with the palms of your hand under his wrist. Then wash his shoulder, armpit (axilla), and arm. Use long, firm, circular strokes. Rinse and dry the area well.

21. Put the basin of water on the towel. Put the patient's hand into the water. Wash, rinse, and dry the hand well. Place it under the bath blanket.

22. Wash, rinse, and dry the arm, hand, axilla, and shoulder closest to you in the same way.

23. Clean the patient's fingernails with an orange stick.

24. Place a towel across the patient's chest. Fold the bath blanket down to the patient's abdomen. Wash and rinse the patient's ears, neck, and chest. Take note of the condition of the skin under the female patient's breasts. Dry the area thoroughly.

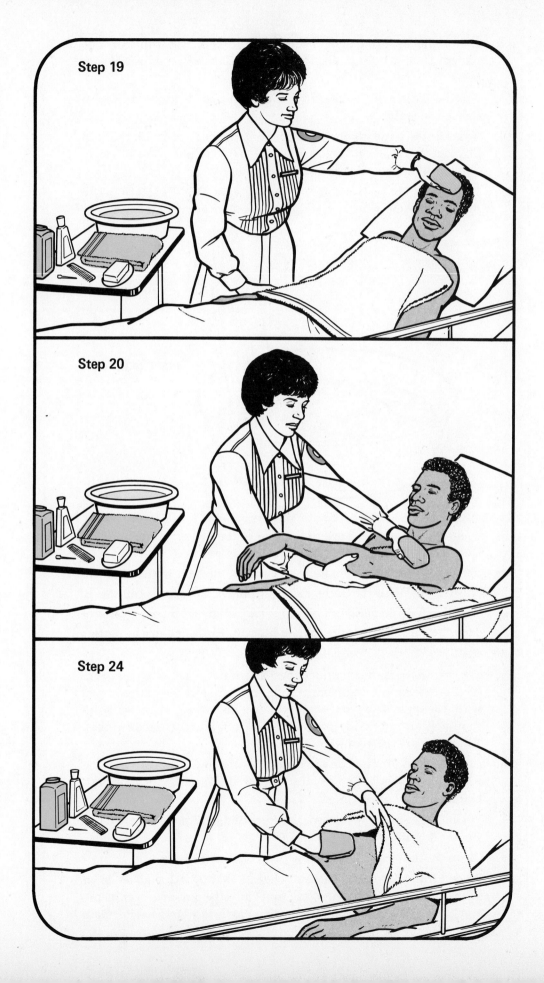

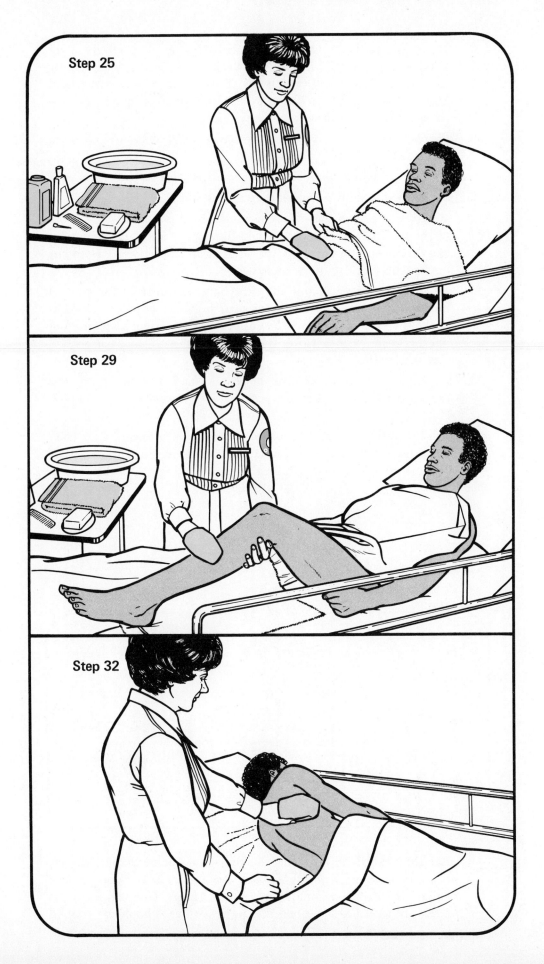

Step 25

Step 29

Step 32

25. Cover the patient's entire chest with the towel. Fold the bath blanket down to the pubic area. Wash the patient's abdomen. Be sure to wash the navel (umbilicus) and in any creases of the skin. Dry the patient's body. Then pull the bath blanket up over the abdomen and chest and remove the towels.

26. Empty the dirty water. Rinse the basin. Fill the basin with clean water at 115° F (46.1° C)

27. Fold the bath blanket back from the patient's leg farthest from you.

28. Put a towel lengthwise under that leg and foot.

29. Bend the knee and wash, rinse, and dry the leg and foot. Take hold of the heel for more support when flexing the knee. If the patient can easily bend his knee, put the wash basin on the towel. Then put his foot directly into the basin to wash it.

30. Observe the toenails and the skin between the toes for general appearance and condition. Look especially for redness and cracking of the skin. Take away the basin. Dry the patient's leg and foot and between the toes. Cover the leg and foot with the bath blanket and remove the towel.

31. Repeat the entire procedure for the leg and foot closest to you. Empty the basin. Rinse and refill it with clean water at 115° F (46.1° C).

32. Ask the patient to turn on his side with his back toward you. If he needs help in turning, assist him. Raise the side rail to the up position so the patient is safe. Return to your working side of the bed.

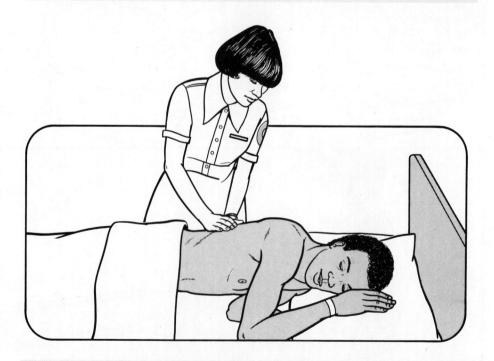

33. Put the towel lengthwise on the bottom sheet near the patient's back. Wash, rinse, and dry his back, buttocks, and back of the neck behind the ears with long firm circular strokes. Give the patient a back rub with warm lotion. The patient's back should be rubbed

for about a minute and a half. Give special attention to bony areas (shoulder blades, hips, elbows, for example). Look for red areas. Dry the patient's back, remove the towel, and turn him on his back.

34. Offer the patient a soapy washcloth to wash his genital area. Give him a clean wet washcloth to rinse himself well. Give him a dry towel for drying himself. If he is unable to do this for himself, get a pair of disposable gloves, put them on, and wash the patient's genital area. Allow for privacy at all times.

35. Put a clean gown on the patient without exposing him.

36. Comb the patient's hair if he cannot do this for himself.

37. Make the patient's bed. Straighten the bedside table. Remove any unneeded articles. Replace the items the patient wants on the table.

38. Raise the backrest and kneerest to suit the patient, if this is allowed.

39. Be sure the signal cord is in its proper place, where the patient can easily reach it.

40. Clean your equipment and put it in its proper place. Throw away used disposable supplies and equipment.

41. Wipe off the bedside table. Discard soiled linen in the dirty linen hamper in the utility room.

42. Make the patient comfortable.

43. Wash your hands.

44. Report to your head nurse or team leader that you have given the patient a bed bath. Also report your observations of anything unusual.

Procedure: Giving the Partial Bed Bath

1. Assemble your equipment:
   a. Soap and soap dish
   b. Washcloth
   c. Wash basin
   d. Bath thermometer
   e. Face and bath towels
   f. Talcum powder
   g. Clean gown
   h. Bath blanket
   i. Orange stick for care of the nails
   j. Lotion for back rub
   k. Comb or hair brush
   l. Disposable plastic laundry bag for dirty linen or a linen laundry bag. (A pillowcase is sometimes used for this purpose.)
   m. Clean bed linen, stacked on the chair in order of use, if the bed is to be made following the bed bath

2. Wash your hands.

3. Identify the patient by checking the identification bracelet.

4. Ask visitors to step out of the room.

5. Tell the patient you are going to help him with a bath.

6. Pull the curtains around the bed for privacy.

7. Assist the patient with oral hygiene, if this has not already been done. (Oral hygiene should follow each meal, in addition to morning and evening care, whenever possible.)

8. Offer the bedpan or urinal.

9. Arrange the equipment conveniently on the bedside table. Place the linen on the chair close to the bed. Have the laundry bag on the chair close by.

10. Pull out all of the bedding from under the mattress. Leave it hanging loosely at all-four sides of the bed.

11. Take the bedspread and regular blanket off the bed. Fold them loosely over the back of the chair, leaving the patient covered with the top sheet.

12. Place the bath blanket over the top sheet. Ask the patient to hold the blanket in place. Remove the top sheet from underneath without uncovering (exposing) the patient. Fold the sheet loosely over the back of the chair if it is to be used again. Or put it into the laundry bag. Ask the patient to remove any jewelry and put it in the drawer of the bedside table.

13. Take off the patient's gown, keeping him covered with the bath blanket. If the gown belongs to the patient, put it away as requested. Put a hospital gown into the laundry bag.

14. Fill the wash basin two-thirds full of water at 115° F (46.1° C). Use the bath thermometer to test the temperature.

15. Ask the patient to wash the areas of his body that he can reach easily.

16. Place the signal cord where the patient can easily reach it. Instruct him to signal when he is finished washing himself.

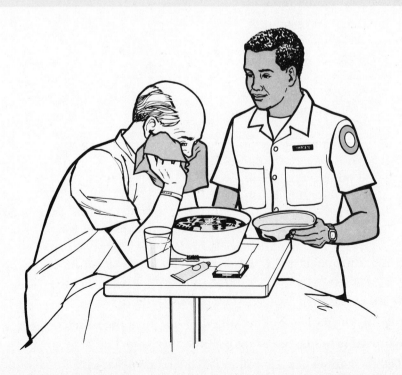

17. Wash your hands and leave the room.

18. When the patient signals that he is finished, go back into the room.

19. Wash your hands.

20. Empty the water. Rinse the basin and fill it with clean water at 115° F (46.1° C).

21. Wash the areas of the body that the patient was unable to reach. Follow the procedure you learned for a complete bed bath. The body parts washed by the patient plus the body parts washed for the patient by the nursing aide should equal a complete bed bath.

22. Put a clean gown on the patient without exposing him.

23. If the patient is allowed out of bed, assist him to a chair.

24. Make the empty bed.

25. Place the signal cord in its proper place.

26. Clean your equipment and put it in its proper place. Throw away used disposable supplies and equipment.

27. Wipe off the bedside table. Discard all soiled linen in the dirty linen hamper in the utility room.

28. Wash your hands.

29. Report to your head nurse or team leader that you have given the patient a partial bath. Also report your observations of anything unusual.

Procedure: Giving the Tub Bath

1. Assemble your equipment:
   a. Bath towels
   b. Washcloths
   c. Soap
   d. Bath thermometer
   e. Chair
   f. Clean gown
   g. Disinfectant solution

2. Wash your hands.

3. Identify the patient by checking the identification bracelet.

4. Ask visitors to step out of the room.

5. Tell the patient that you are going to give him a tub bath.

6. Pull the curtain around the bed for privacy.

7. Help the patient out of bed. Get him into a bathrobe and slippers and to the tub room, either walking or by wheelchair.

8. For safety, remove all electric appliances from the tub room.

9. Place a chair next to the bathtub. Assist the patient into the chair.

10. Wash the bathtub with the disinfectant solution.

11. Fill the bathtub one-half full of water at 105° F (40.5° C). Test the temperature of the water with a bath thermometer.

12. Place one towel in the bathtub for the patient to sit on.

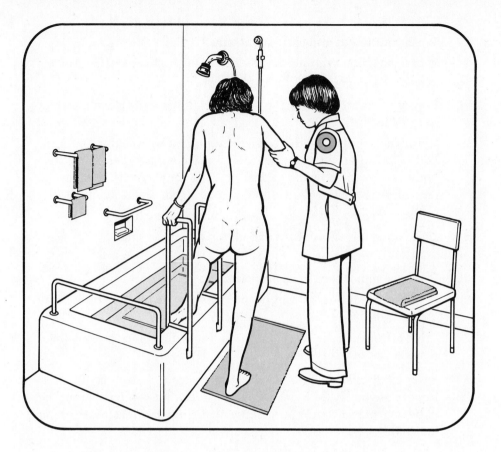

13. Place one towel on the floor where the patient will step out of the bathtub. This will prevent him from slipping.

14. Assist the patient to get undressed and into the bathtub.

15. Let the patient stay in the bathtub as long as permitted, according to your instructions.

16. Help the patient wash himself, if help is needed.

17. Put one towel across the chair.

18. Help the patient out of the bathtub. Seat him on the towel-covered chair, if he needs assistance.

19. Dry the patient well by patting gently. Help him put on pajamas or gown.

20. Help the patient return to his room and into bed.

21. Make the patient comfortable.

22. Return to the tub room. Clean the bathtub with disinfectant solution.

23. Remove all used linen. Put it in the dirty linen hamper in the utility room.

24. Wash your hands.

25. Report to your head nurse or team leader that you have given the patient a tub bath and the time and length of the bath. Also report your observations of anything unusual.

Procedure: Helping the Patient Take a Shower

1. Assemble your equipment:
   a. Towels
   b. Soap
   c. Shower cap
   d. Washcloth
   e. Clean gown
   f. Disinfectant solution

2. Wash your hands.

3. Identify the patient by checking the identification bracelet.

4. Ask visitors to step out of the room.

5. Tell the patient that you will assist him with taking a shower.

6. Pull the curtain around the bed for privacy.

7. Help the patient out of bed. Help him into a bathrobe and slippers. Help him to the shower room, as necessary.

8. For safety, remove all electrical appliances from the shower room.

9. Place one towel on the floor outside the shower.

10. Place one towel on a chair close to the shower. Assist the patient into the chair.

11. Wash the floor of the shower with disinfectant solution.

12. Turn on the shower and adjust the water temperature.

13. Assist the patient into the shower.

14. Give the patient soap and washcloth so he can wash himself.

15. Turn off the water and assist the patient out of the shower. Seat him on the towel-covered chair.

16. Dry the patient well by patting gently.

17. Assist him with putting on pajamas or nightgown.

18. Help the patient back to his room and into bed.

19. Make the patient comfortable.

20. Return to the shower room. Remove all used linen and put it in the dirty-linen hamper in the dirty utility room.

21. Wash your hands.

22. Report to your head nurse or team leader that you have helped the patient with a shower. Also report your observations of anything unusual.

KEY IDEAS: THE BACK RUB

Rubbing a patient's back refreshes him, relaxes his muscles, and stimulates circulation. Because of pressure caused by the bedclothes and the lack of movement to stimulate circulation, the skin of a bedridden patient needs special care.

Back rubs are usually given during morning care, right after the patient's bath. They also are given: (a) as part of evening care, (b) when changing the position of a helpless patient, (c) for very restless patients who need relaxing, and (d) on doctor's orders for "special back care."

Procedure: Giving the Patient a Back Rub

1. Assemble your equipment:
   a. Towels
   b. Lotion
2. Wash your hands.
3. Identify the patient by checking the identification bracelet.
4. Ask visitors to step out of the room.
5. Tell the patient you are going to give him a back rub.
6. Pull the curtain around the bed for privacy.
7. Ask the patient to turn on his side so his back is toward you. Or have him turn on his abdomen. Use the position that is most comfortable for the patient and yourself.
8. The side rail should be in the up position on the far side of the bed.
9. Lotion should be warmed by placing the container in a basin of warm water. Warm your hands, too, by running warm water over them.

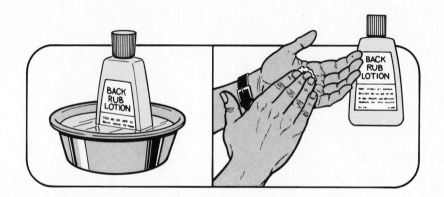

10. Open the ties on the gown. Put a towel lengthwise on the mattress close to the patient's back.
11. Pour a small amount of lotion into the palm of your hand.
12. Rub your hands together to warm the lotion more.
13. Apply lotion to the entire back with the palms of your hands. Use long, firm strokes from the buttocks to the shoulders and back of the neck.
14. Keep your knees slightly bent and your back straight.
15. Exert firm pressure as you stroke upward from the buttocks to shoulders. Use gentle pressure as you stroke downward from shoulders to buttocks.
16. Use a circular motion on each bony area.
17. This rhythmic rubbing motion should be continued for from one and one-half minutes to three minutes.
18. Dry the patient's back by patting gently with a towel.

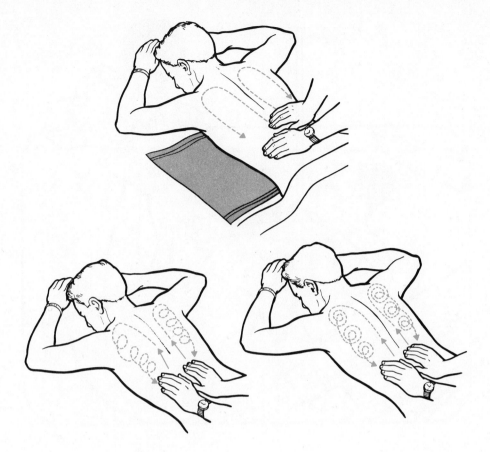

19. Close and retie the gown.

20. Remove the towels.

21. Assist the patient to turn back to a comfortable position.

22. Arrange the top sheets of the bed neatly.

23. Put your equipment back in its proper place.

24. Wash your hands.

25. Report to your head nurse or team leader that you have given the patient a back rub, and the time, if necessary. Also report your observations of anything unusual.

KEY IDEAS: CHANGING THE PATIENT'S GOWN

It is important when you change a patient's gown not to expose his body unnecessarily. In this way you avoid chills caused by drafts. You will also prevent embarrassment for the patient.

When you want to change the gown of the patient who has an IV, regard the bottle and tube as part of the patient's arm. Carefully lift the bottle from the hook. Then quickly slip the sleeve of the gown over the bottle. Replace the bottle on the hook. Slip the gown down the tube and then over the patient's arm. To take off the gown, reverse this procedure.

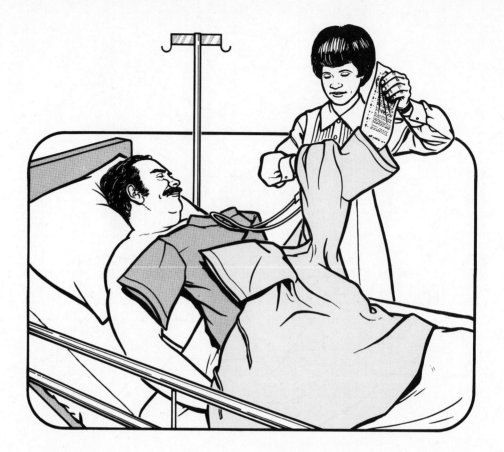

Procedure: Changing the Patient's Gown

1. Assemble your equipment: a clean gown.

2. Wash your hands.

3. Identify your patient by checking the identification bracelet.

4. Ask visitors to step out of the room.

5. Tell the patient you are going to change his gown.

6. Pull the curtain around the bed for privacy.

7. Have the patient turn on his side with his back toward you so you can untie the tapes.

8. If the patient cannot be turned, you will have to reach under his neck to untie the tapes.

9. Loosen the soiled gown around the patient's body.

10. Get the clean gown ready to put on the patient. Unfold it and lay it across the patient's chest on top of the bath blanket.

11. Take off one sleeve at a time, leaving the old gown in place on the patient.

12. Slide each arm through one sleeve of the clean gown. .

13. If the patient can't hold his arm up, put your hand through the sleeve. Take his hand in yours and slip the sleeve up the patient's wrist and arm. Do this for both arms. Then pull the body of the

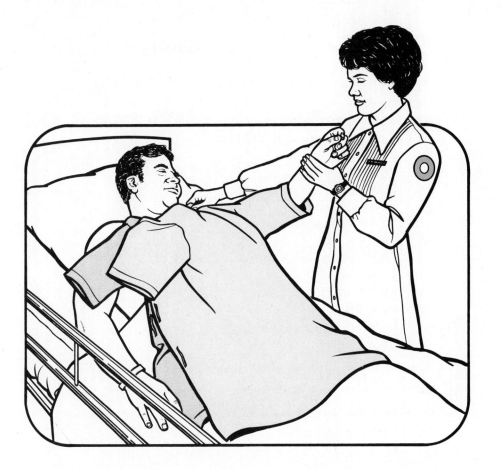

gown down over the patient's chest. If the patient has a sore arm, remove the sleeve on the well arm first. Then remove the sleeve on the sore arm. To put a clean gown on, put the sleeve on the sore arm first. Then slide the well arm through the second sleeve.

14. Remove the soiled gown from under the bath blanket.

15. Tie the tapes on the clean gown. Some patients want only the tapes at the neck tied so that they won't be lying on knots.

16. Put the soiled gown in the dirty-linen hamper in the dirty utility room.

17. Wash your hands.

18. Report to your head nurse or team leader that you have replaced the patient's soiled gown with a clean one. Also report your observations of anything unusual.

KEY IDEAS: SHAMPOOING THE PATIENT'S HAIR

Patients who will be in the health care institution for a long time may need to have their hair shampooed from time to time. The doctor must write the order for a shampoo. And your head nurse or team leader must give you instructions for giving the shampoo. The patient must be in bed when the shampoo is given.

Procedure: Shampooing the Patient's Hair

1. Assemble your equipment:
    a. Chair
    b. Basin of water at 105° F (40.5° C).
    c. Pitcher of water at 115° F (46.1° C).
    d. Bath thermometer
    e. Wastepaper basket
    f. Water trough or plastic sheet
    g. Disposable bed protector
    h. Pillow with waterproof case
    i. Bath towels
    j. Washcloth, to cover the patient's eyes
    k. Paper cup
    l. Bath blanket
    m. Small towel
    n. Cotton

2. Wash your hands.

3. Identify the patient by checking the identification bracelet.

4. Ask visitors to step out of the room.

5. Tell the patient that you will give him a shampoo.

6. Pull the curtain around the bed for privacy.

7. Clear the bedside table to make room for your equipment.

8. Put a chair at the side of the bed near the patient's head. The chair should be lower than the bed.

9. Place the small towel on the chair. Put the empty wastepaper basket on the towel.

10. Put cotton in the patient's ears for protection.

11. Ask the patient to move across the bed so that his head is close to where you are standing.

12. Remove the pillow from under the patient's head. Cover the pillow with the waterproof case. Have the pillow under the small of the patient's back, so that when he lies down, his head is tilted back.

13. Put the bath blanket on the bed. From underneath, fan fold the top sheets to the foot of the bed without exposing the patient.

14. Place the disposable bed protector on the mattress under the patient's head.

15. Place the shampoo trough under the patient's head. A trough can be made by rolling up the sides of the plastic sheet. This makes a channel for the water to run off. Three sides must be rolled over three times to make the channel. Put the end of the channel under the patient's head. Have the other open end hanging over the side of the bed. This free end of the plastic sheet should be put into the wastepaper basket.

16. Loosen the patient's gown at the neck and turn the neckband under.

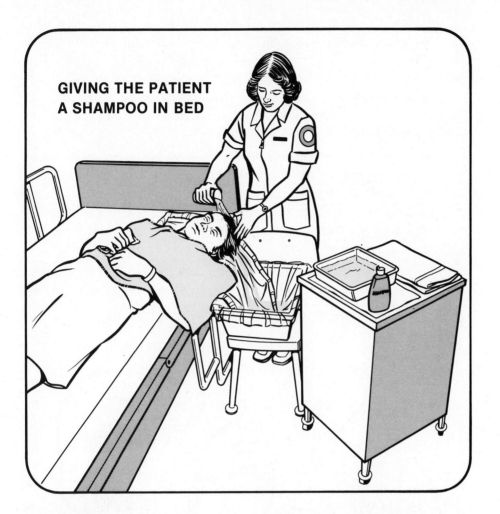

GIVING THE PATIENT A SHAMPOO IN BED

17. Ask the patient to hold the washcloth over his eyes.

18. Fill the basin with water at 105° F (40.5° C). Put the basin on the bedside table with the paper cup.

19. Fill the pitcher with water at 115° F (46.1° C). Have the pitcher on the bedside table, for extra water, if needed.

20. Brush the patient's hair. Have him turn his head from side to side so the hair can be brushed one exposed side at a time.

21. Fill the paper cup with water from the basin. Pour it over the hair until completely wet.

22. Apply shampoo and, using both hands, wash the hair and massage the patient's scalp with your fingertips. Avoid using fingernails as they could scratch the scalp.

23. Rinse the soap off the hair by pouring water from the cup over the hair. Have the patient turn his head from side to side. Repeat this until the hair is clear of shampoo.

24. Dry the patient's forehead and ears with the face towel.

25. Remove the cotton from the ears.

26. Raise the patient's head and wrap the hair with a bath towel.

27. Rub the patient's hair with the towel to dry it as much as possible.

28. Remove your equipment from the bed. Change the patient's gown if necessary.

29. Comb the patient's hair. Then leave a towel wrapped around the head. Or spread a towel out over the pillow under the head until the hair is completely dry. If a dryer is available, use it to dry the patient's hair.

30. Make the patient comfortable.

31. Remove the bath blanket and at the same time bring the top sheets back up to cover the patient.

32. Clean your equipment and put it in its proper place. Throw away used disposable supplies and equipment.

33. Wash your hands.

34. Report to your head nurse or team leader that you have given the patient a shampoo. Also report your observations of anything unusual.

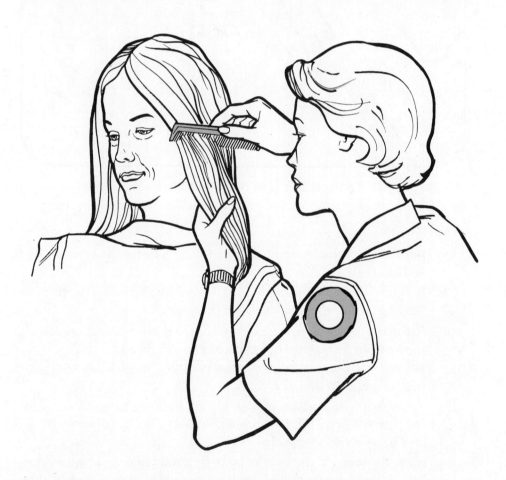

KEY IDEAS: COMBING THE PATIENT'S HAIR

As with other types of personal care, a patient may be too weak or sick to take care of his own hair. It may be difficult for him to raise his arms. Almost always, however, combing and brushing a patient's hair, which makes him look better, will make him feel better.

Procedure: Combing the Patient's Hair

1. Assemble your equipment:

    a. Towel
    b. Comb or brush
    c. Hand mirror, if available

2. Wash your hands.
3. Identify the patient by checking his identification bracelet.
4. Ask visitors to step out of the room.
5. Tell the patient you are going to brush or comb his hair.
6. Pull the curtain around the bed for privacy.
7. If possible, comb the patient's hair after the bath and before you make the bed.
8. Lay a towel across the pillow, under the patient's head. If the patient can sit up in bed, drape the towel around his shoulders.
9. If the patient wears glasses, ask him to take them off before you begin. Be sure to put the glasses in a safe place.
10. Part the hair down the middle to make it easier to comb.
11. Brush or comb the patient's hair carefully, gently, and thoroughly in his usual style.
12. For the patient who cannot sit up, separate the hair into small sections. Then comb each section separately, using a downward motion. Ask the patient to turn his head from side to side. Or turn it for him so you can reach the entire head.
13. Arrange the patient's hair the way he wants you to.
14. If the patient has very long hair, suggest braiding it to keep it from getting tangled.
15. Be sure you brush the back of the head.
16. Remove the towel when you are finished.
17. Let the patient use the mirror.
18. Put your equipment back in its proper place.
19. Wash your hands.
20. Report to your head nurse or team leader that you have combed the patient's hair. Also report your observations of anything unusual.

KEY IDEAS: SHAVING THE PATIENT'S FACE

A regular morning activity for most men is shaving the beard. A patient is often well enough to shave himself. In this case, you will give him only the help that is necessary, such as being sure he has the equipment he needs. Sometimes patients are too ill or weak to shave themselves. In such cases, you will do it. Before shaving any patient's face, be sure to get permission from the head nurse or team leader. Certain patients may not be permitted to shave or be shaved.

Shaving can be done with an electric razor or a safety razor. Often, the patient will have his own electric razor. You will be able to use it to shave him.

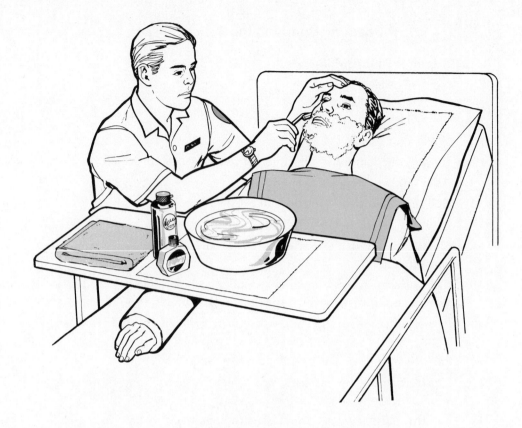

Electric razors are never used while the patient is being given oxygen. If oxygen is being given to any patient in the room, electric razors cannot be used.

Procedure: Shaving the Patient's Face

1. Assemble your equipment:
   a. Basin of water at 115° F (46.1° C)
   b. Shaving brush and shaving cream
   c. Safety razor
   d. Face towel
   e. Mirror
   f. Tissues
   g. After-shave lotion, if available
   h. Face powder, if available
2. Wash your hands.
3. Identify the patient by checking the identification bracelet.
4. Ask visitors to step out of the room.
5. Tell the patient that you are going to shave his face.
6. Pull the curtain around the bed for privacy.
7. Adjust a light so that it shines on the patient's face.
8. Raise the head of the bed, if allowed.
9. Put your equipment on the bedside table.

10. Spread the face towel under the patient's chin. If the patient has dentures, be sure they are in his mouth.

11. Pat some warm water on the patient's face to soften his beard.

12. Apply shaving soap generously to the face.

13. With the fingers of one hand, hold the skin taut (tight) as you shave in the direction that the hairs grow. Start under the sideburns and work downward over the cheeks. Continue carefully over the chin. Work upward on the neck under the chin. Use short firm strokes.

14. Rinse the razor often.

15. Areas under the nose and around the lips are sensitive. Take special care in these areas.

16. If you nick the patient's skin, report this to your head nurse or team leader.

17. Wash off the remaining soap when you have finished shaving.

18. Apply after-shave lotion or powder as the patient prefers.

19. Clean your equipment and put it in its proper place. Throw away used disposable supplies and equipment.

20. Wash your hands.

21. Report to your head nurse or team leader that you have shaved the patient's face. Also report your observations of anything unusual.

KEY IDEAS: GIVING THE BEDPAN OR URINAL

Some patients are unable to get out of bed to use the bathroom. For these patients a urinal and a bedpan are required. The urinal is a container into which the male patient urinates. The bedpan is a pan into which he defecates. You should always cover the bedpan and remove it from the patient's bedside to the bathroom as quickly as possible after use. At this time you would collect a specimen if required. You would also measure the urine if the patient is on *intake and output*.

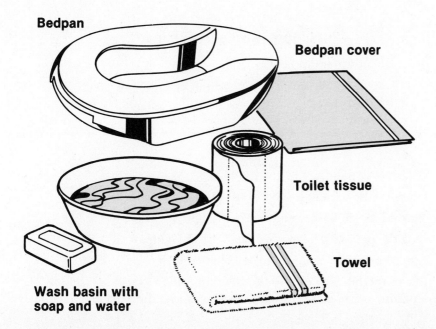

Bedpan

Bedpan cover

Toilet tissue

Towel

Wash basin with soap and water

BEDPANS

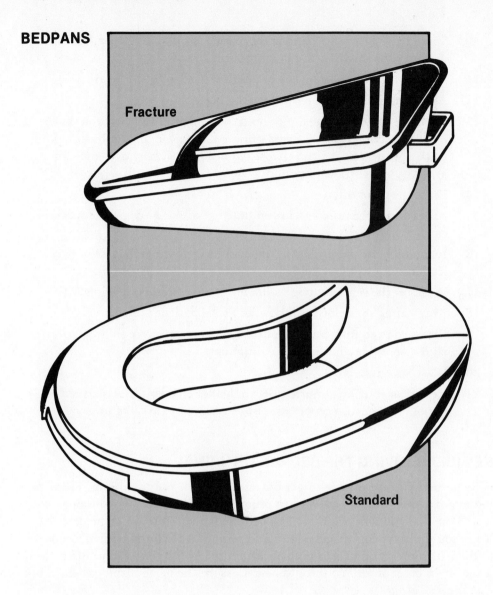

Fracture

Standard

Procedure: Giving the Bedpan

1. Assemble your equipment:
    a. Bedpan and cover, or fractional bedpan and cover
    b. Toilet tissue
    c. Wash basin with water at 115° F (46.1° C).
    d. Soap
    e. Hand towel
2. Wash your hands.
3. Identify the patient by checking the identification bracelet.
4. Ask visitors to step out of the room.
5. Ask the patient if he would like to use the bedpan.
6. Pull the curtain around the bed for privacy.
7. Take the bedpan out of the bedside table. Warm the bedpan by running warm water inside it and along the rim. Dry the outside of the bedpan.

8. Fold back the top sheets so that they are out of the way.

9. Raise the patient's gown, but keep the lower part of his body covered by the top sheets.

10. Ask the patient to bend his knees. Put his feet flat on the mattress. Raise his hips by pressing his feet on the mattress. If necessary, help the patient to raise his buttocks by slipping your hand under the lower part of his back. Place the bedpan in position under the buttocks.

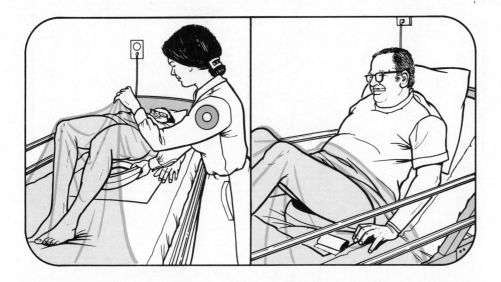

11. Sometimes the patient is unable to lift his buttocks to get on or off the bedpan. In this case turn the patient on his side with his back to you. Put the bedpan against the buttocks. Then turn the patient back onto the bedpan.

12. Replace the covers over the patient.

13. Raise the backrest and kneerest, if allowed, so the patient is in a sitting position.

14. Put toilet tissue and the signal cord where the patient can reach them easily.

15. Ask the patient to signal when he is finished.

16. Raise the side rails to the up position.

17. Wash your hands. Leave the room to give the patient privacy.

18. After a short time, or when the patient signals, return to the room. Help the patient to raise his hips so you can remove the bedpan.

19. Cover the bedpan immediately.

20. Help the patient if he is unable to clean himself. Turn the patient on his side. Clean the anal area with toilet tissue.

21. Take the bedpan to the patient's bathroom.

22. If a specimen is required, collect it at this time. Measure the urine if the patient is on intake and output.

23. Check the excreta (feces or urine) for abnormal (unusual) appearance.

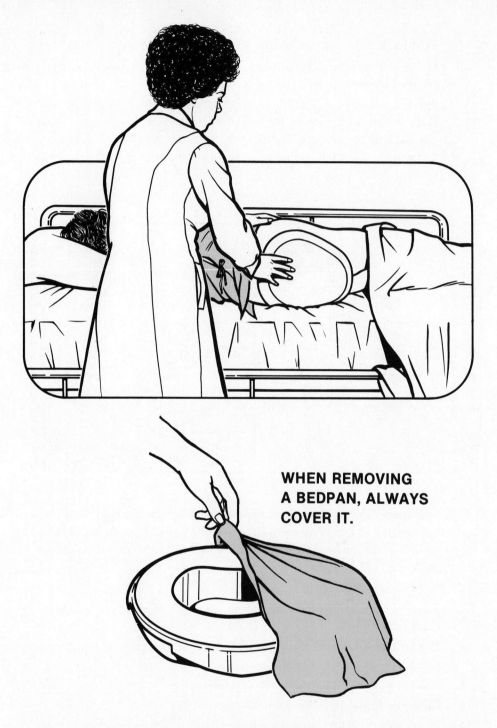

WHEN REMOVING A BEDPAN, ALWAYS COVER IT.

24.   Empty the bedpan into the patient's toilet.

25.   Every hospital has different equipment in the bathroom for cleaning the bedpan. Follow your instructions for cleaning the bedpan in your hospital. Cold water is always used to rinse the bedpan.

26.   Put the clean bedpan and cover back into the bedside table.

27.   Help the patient wash his hands in the basin of water.

28.   Make the patient comfortable. Lower the backrest as necessary. Pull back the curtains to the open position.

29.   Wash your hands.

30. Report to your head nurse or team leader your observations of anything unusual.

Procedure: Giving the Urinal

1. Assemble your equipment:
   a. Urinal and cover
   b. Basin of water at 115° F (46.1° C)
   c. Soap
   d. Towel

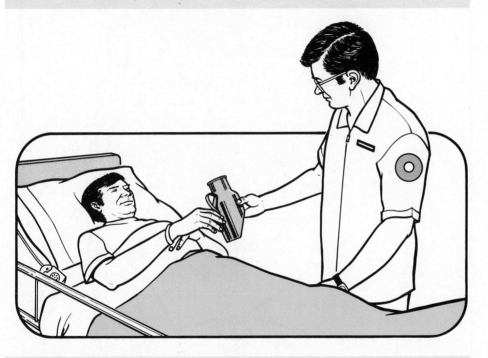

2. Wash your hands.
3. Identify the patient by checking the identification bracelet.
4. Ask visitors to step out of the room.
5. Ask the patient if he would like to use the urinal.
6. Pull the curtain around the bed for privacy.
7. Give the urinal to the patient.
8. Place signal cord within easy reach.
9. Ask the patient to signal when he is finished.
10. Wash your hands. Leave the room to give the patient privacy.
11. After a short time, or when the patient signals, return to the room.
12. Cover the urinal and take it to the patient's bathroom.
13. Check urine for abnormal (unusual) appearance.
14. Measure the urine if the patient is on intake and output. Collect a specimen if required.
15. Empty the urinal into the toilet. Rinse with cold water.
16. Put the clean urinal back in the patient's bedside table.

17. Help the patient wash his hands in the basin of water.

18. Wash your hands.

19. Report to your head nurse or team leader your observations of anything unusual.

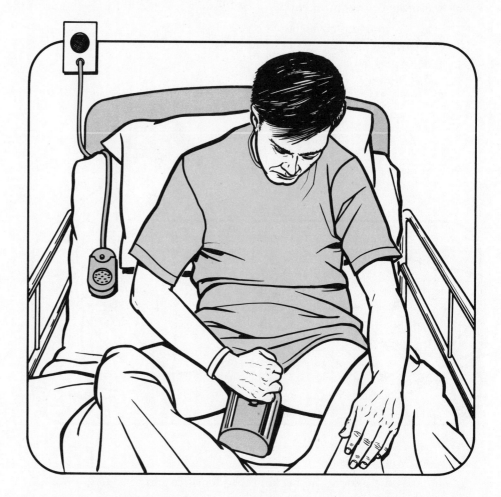

Procedure: Giving the Portable Bedside Commode

1. Assemble your equipment:
   a. Portable bedside commode
   b. Bedpan and cover
   c. Toilet tissue
   d. Basin of water at 115° F (46.1° C)
   e. Soap
   f. Towel

2. Wash your hands.

3. Identify the patient by checking the identification bracelet.

4. Ask visitors to step out of the room.

5. Tell the patient you will assist him onto the commode.

6. Pull the curtain around the bed for privacy.

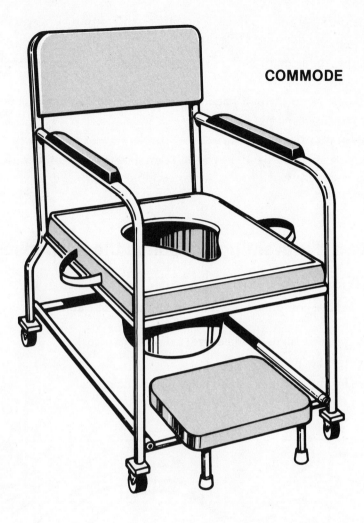

COMMODE

7. Put the commode next to the patient's bed. Open the cover and insert a bedpan under the toilet seat.

8. Help the patient out of bed and onto the commode.

9. Put toilet tissue and the signal cord where the patient can reach them easily.

10. Ask the patient to signal when he is finished.

11. Wash your hands. Leave the room to give the patient privacy.

12. After a short time, or when the patient signals, return to the room.

13. Help the patient if he is unable to clean himself.

14. Assist the patient back to bed.

15. Close the cover on the commode.

16. Help the patient to wash his hands in the basin of water.

17. Remove the bedpan from under the commode. Cover it and carry it to the patient's bathroom.

18. Check the excreta (feces or urine) for abnormal (unusual) appearance.

19. Measure output if patient is on intake and output. If a specimen is required, collect it at this time.

20. Empty the bedpan in the toilet, and clean the bedpan according to your instructions.

21. Put the clean bedpan back in the bedside table. Put the commode in its proper place.

22. Wash your hands.

23. Report to your head nurse or team leader your observations of anything unusual.

Section 2: Preventing Decubitus Ulcers (Bedsores)

OBJECTIVES: WHAT YOU WILL LEARN

When you have completed this section, you should be able:

- To recognize the signs of a bedsore (a decubitus ulcer)
- To care for the incontinent patient
- To care for the patient's skin to help prevent bedsores

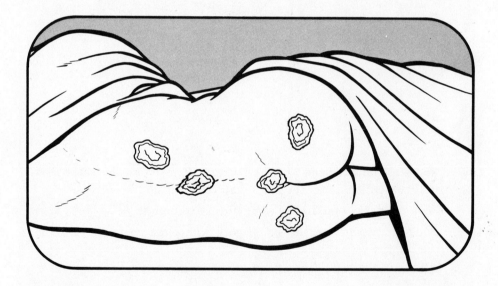

KEY IDEAS

Decubitus ulcers, called bedsores or pressure sores, are areas where the skin has broken because of prolonged pressure. Injury to the skin comes from pressure on a part of the body where there is loss of circulation (blood flow). Then the tissues are destroyed. If decubitus ulcers are not treated, they quickly get larger, become very painful, and usually become infected.

The direct cause of bedsores is interference with the circulation of blood in a part of the body. The interference is caused by pressure over the bony prominences. These are places where bones come close to the surface of the body.

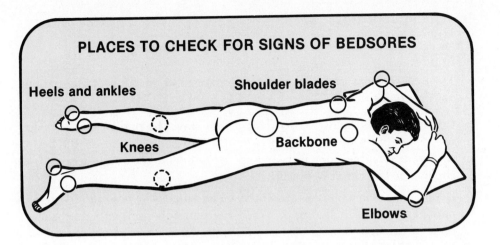

The pressure can come from the weight of the body lying in one position for too long or from splints, casts, or bandages. Even wrinkles in the bed linen can be a cause of bedsores.

Bedsores are often made worse by continued pressure, heat, moisture, and lack of cleanliness. Irritating substances on the skin such as perspiration, urine, feces, material from wound discharges, or soap that has been left on the skin after a bath—all tend to make bedsores worse.

The signs of a bedsore on the skin are heat, redness, tenderness, discomfort, and a feeling of burning. When the skin is broken, a bedsore has formed. Specific treatment for a bedsore is prescribed by a doctor. The wound, however, must be kept clean and the rules of asepsis must be followed. As you have learned, the skin is where the battle for asepsis begins.

Places to check on the body for signs of bedsores are the bony areas. These are, for example, the shoulder blades, elbows, knees, heels, ankles, and backbone. Usually these areas are covered only by a thin layer of skin. They receive a smaller supply of blood than other areas of the body. And these are the areas where bedsores are most likely to occur.

Obese patients—patients who are overly fat—develop bedsores where body parts rub against each other, causing friction. Places to check on obese patients are the folds of the body where skin touches skin, such as under the breasts, between the folds of the buttocks, and between the thighs.

Preventing bedsores is the responsibility of the entire nursing team. These sores are usually the result of carelessness or a lack of knowledge and skill in caring for patients. Once even a mild bedsore has formed, it is very hard to cure. Therefore, as a nursing aide, you have to know how to prevent bedsores and how to recognize them when they do occur. Report the first sign of a bedsore to your head nurse or team leader so that steps can be taken to prevent further damage.

The doctor may order special equipment to reduce the pressure on the skin. One way is to use an air cushion or a sponge rubber cushion under the base of the spine—that is, the sacrum or lower back. If you use an air cushion, don't fill it more than half full. More air will make it too hard.

There are special cotton rings that can be used to reduce the pressure on the heels, the elbows, and the back of the head. Also used are pillows, pads, air mattresses, alternating pressure mattresses, flotation beds or pads, booties, wheelchair pads, wheelchair flotation cushions, sheepskin pads, and commode flotation pads.

Preventing Bedsores

You can help to prevent bedsores by doing the following:

- Turn the patient often. You should change the position of the patient's body every 2 hours.

- Be careful with the use of bedpans. Don't leave the patient on the bedpan too long. And remove the pan carefully. Covering the rim of the bedpan with pads is a good idea if there appears to be danger of a bedsore. Or the rim can be powdered very well.

- Keep the patient's body as absolutely clean and dry as possible. Change the patient's gown if it is damp. Wash the patient's skin with mild soap to remove urine or feces. Use lotion on the skin to prevent contact with discharged materials from wounds, which can cause irritation.

- If a part of the patient's body shows signs of developing a bedsore, rub the area often with skin lotion. Do this at least two or three times a day. Rub with a circular motion, away from the affected part of the body. Rubbing, that is, friction, stimulates the circulation of blood in the affected area.

- Use powder where skin surfaces come together and form creases. Examples are under the breasts of women patients, between the buttocks, and in folds of skin on the abdomen. Powder helps keep these areas dry. This is especially important in caring for obese patients.

- Keep linen wrinkle-free and dry at all times.

- Remove crumbs, hair pins, and any other hard objects from the bed promptly.

- If the patient is incontinent, you may be instructed to use disposable bed protectors. These protect the linen the patient has to lie on. Be sure that plastic never touches the patient's skin.

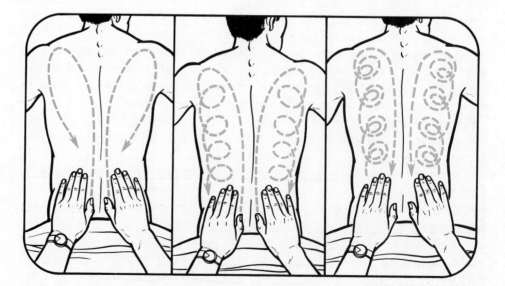

Procedure: Preventing Decubitus Ulcers (Bedsores) in the Incontinent Patient

1. Assemble your equipment:
    a. Basin of water at 115° F (46.1° C)
    b. Soap
    c. Towels
    d. Corn starch or bath powder
    e. Disposable gloves
    f. Lotion

2. Wash your hands.

3. Identify the patient by checking the identification bracelet.

4. Ask visitors to step out of the room.

5. Tell the patient you are going to wash him.

6. Pull the curtain for privacy.

7. Put on disposable gloves.

8. Wash the area that has urine or feces on it very well, removing all waste material from the skin.

9. Rinse with lots of water, changing the water frequently.

10. Dry with a circular motion to stimulate blood circulation.

11. Apply lotion to buttocks and back, massaging to stimulate blood circulation.

12. Wipe off excess lotion.

13. Powder with corn starch or bath powder.

14. Leave the top sheets loose so air can get to every part of the patient's body.

15. Turn the patient from side to side every 2 hours.

16. Keep the patient dry at all times by checking the patient every 2 hours.

17. Wash your hands.

18. Report to your head nurse or team leader any signs of decubitus ulcers (bedsores). Also report your observations of anything unusual.

WHAT YOU HAVE LEARNED

Daily personal care of patients is an essential part of your duties as a nursing aide. Patients should be allowed to help as much as possible with their daily care, if this is allowed.

You will be giving oral hygiene, bathing the patient, giving bedpans and urinals, and caring for the incontinent patient.

In giving this care, it is important to respect the patient's privacy. These tasks should be performed with tender loving care and careful, regular observations to note any pattern of change in the patient's condition.

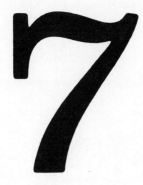

Food Service

Section 1: Therapeutic Diets

OBJECTIVES: WHAT YOU WILL LEARN

When you have completed this section, you should be able:

- To define a well-balanced diet
- To name the four basic food groups
- To list some foods included in each group
- To explain what is meant by a therapeutic diet
- To list various types of therapeutic diets
- To describe each type of therapeutic diet
- To explain the purpose of each type of therapeutic diet

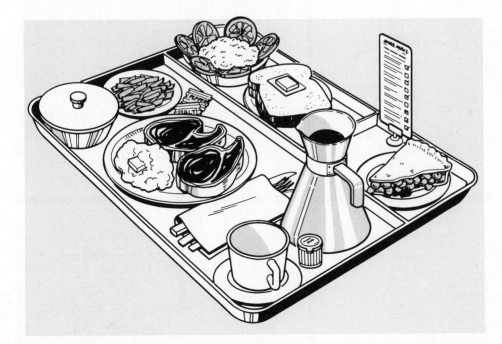

THE FOUR BASIC FOOD GROUPS

*EAT VITAL FOODS • EVERY MEAL • EVERY DAY
A SELECTED VARIETY FROM EACH GROUP*

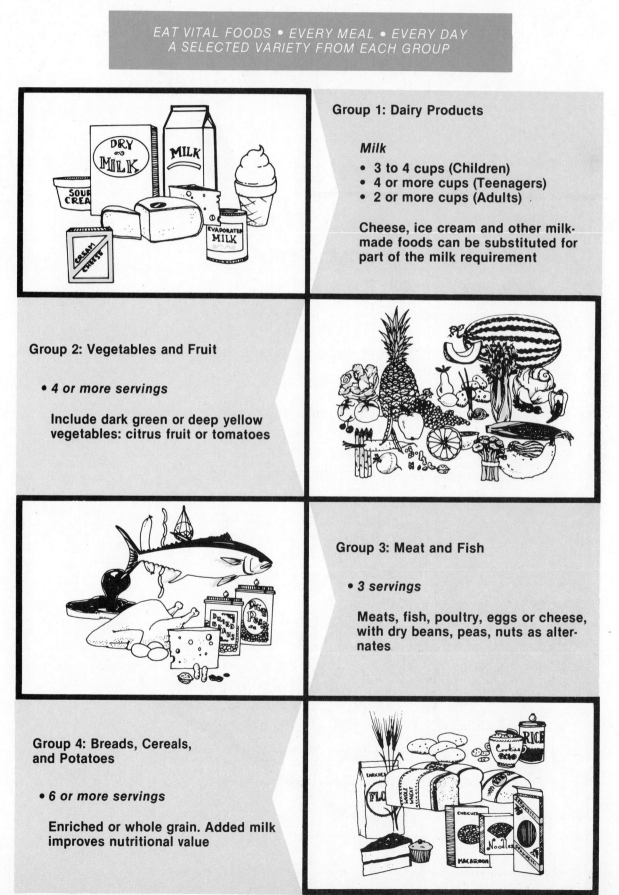

Group 1: Dairy Products

Milk

- 3 to 4 cups (Children)
- 4 or more cups (Teenagers)
- 2 or more cups (Adults)

Cheese, ice cream and other milk-made foods can be substituted for part of the milk requirement

Group 2: Vegetables and Fruit

- *4 or more servings*

Include dark green or deep yellow vegetables: citrus fruit or tomatoes

Group 3: Meat and Fish

- *3 servings*

Meats, fish, poultry, eggs or cheese, with dry beans, peas, nuts as alternates

Group 4: Breads, Cereals, and Potatoes

- *6 or more servings*

Enriched or whole grain. Added milk improves nutritional value

KEY IDEAS: REGULAR AND SPECIAL DIETS

Eating properly is very important when you are healthy and feeling well. Good nourishment is even more important when a person is ill. The food service department or dietary department in your institution will be preparing a well-balanced diet of good nourishing meals for many different patients. This basic balanced diet is often called by different names:

- Normal diet
- Regular diet
- House diet
- Full diet

A well-balanced diet is one that contains a variety of food from each of the four basic food groups at every meal.

The normal diet is sometimes changed to meet a patient's special nutritional needs. This modified diet is also known by several names:

- Therapeutic diet
- Special diet
- Restricted diet
- Modified diet

Therapeutic diets require the preparation of meals that differ from those regularly prepared for patients on the normal diet in the hospital. The special meals given to patients who cannot be on a normal diet are ordered by the doctor. They are worked out by the dietitian according to the patient's illness and what is needed for his recovery. These special meals help the doctor in treating a patient. For example, a man who has a disorder of his digestive system may be on a soft diet. A diabetic patient may be on a diet in which total calories are limited and the amounts of protein, fat, and carbohydrates are specified. A person with heart disease may be restricted to a low-salt diet or a salt-free diet. The doctor may order changes in the normal diet for several reasons. These include:

- Changing the consistency of the patient's food, as in liquid or "soft" diets
- Changing the caloric intake, as in high- or low-calorie diets
- Changing the amounts of one or more nutrients, as in a high-protein, low-fat, or low-salt diet
- Changing the amount of bulk, as in a low-residue diet
- Changing the seasonings in the patient's food, as in a bland diet
- Omitting foods that the patient is allergic to
- Changing the time and number of meals

Section 2: Nutrition for the Patient

OBJECTIVES: WHAT YOU WILL LEARN

When you have completed this section, you should be able:

- To prepare the patient before mealtime
- To serve the food tray

Types of Diets Given to Patients; What They Are and Why They Are Used

Type of diet	Description	Common purpose
Normal regular	Provides all essentials of good nourishment in normal forms	For patients who do not need special diets
Clear liquid (Hospital surgical)	Broth, tea, ginger ale, gelatin	Usually for patients who have had surgery or the very ill
Full liquid	Broth, tea, coffee, ginger ale, gelatin, strained fruit juices, liquids, custard, junket, ice cream, sherbet, soft-cooked eggs	For those unable to chew or swallow solid food.
Light or soft	Foods soft in consistency; no rich or strongly flavored foods that could cause distress	Final stage for postoperative patient before resuming regular diet
Soft (mechanical)	Same foods as on a normal diet, but chopped or strained	For patients who have difficulty in chewing or swallowing.
Bland	Foods mild in flavor and easy to digest; omits spicy foods	Avoids irritation of the digestive tract, as with ulcer and colitis patients
Low residue	Foods low in bulk; omits foods difficult to digest	Spares the lower digestive tract, as with patients having rectal diseases
High calorie	Foods high in protein, minerals, and vitamins	For underweight or malnourished patients
Low calorie	Low in cream, butter, cereals, desserts, and fats	For patients who need to lose weight
Diabetic	Precise balance of carbohydrates, protein, and fats, devised according to the needs of individual patients	For diabetic patients; matches food intake with the insulin and nutritional requirements
High protein	Meals supplemented with high protein foods, such as meat, fish, cheese, milk, and eggs	Assists in the growth and repair of tissues wasted by disease
Low fat	Limited amounts of butter, cream, fats, and eggs	For patients who have difficulty digesting fats, as in gallbladder, cardiovascular, and liver disturbances
Low cholesterol	Low in eggs, whole milk, and meats	Helps regulate the amount of cholesterol in the blood
Low sodium	Limited amount of foods containing sodium, no salt allowed on tray	For patients whose circulation would be impaired by fluid retention; patients with certain heart or kidney conditions
Salt-free	Completely without salt	

Type of diet	Description	Common purpose
Tube feeding	Milk formula or liquid forms of meat or vegetables given to the patient through a tube; follow with a glass of water	For patients who, because of a condition such as oral surgery, can't eat normally

Objectives (continued from page 165)

- To observe and record information concerning meals
- To feed the helpless patient
- To serve extra nourishment
- To distribute drinking water

KEY IDEAS: PREPARING THE PATIENT AND SERVING A MEAL

A poor appetite doesn't mean that the body's need for food is lowered. The sick person's body is in a weakened condition. The patient needs as much food as ever—if not more—to return to health. The surroundings and the food served should be as cheerful, attractive, and appetizing as possible. The sight and aroma of food often make a person hungry. You often can increase a patient's appetite by showing him what he will be eating. Also, people have a better appetite for foods they especially like. Therefore, if a patient asks for a particular food—and if he is permitted to have it—you should try to arrange for that food to be served to him. You can do this by reporting the patient's request to your team leader or head nurse.

Mealtime often is one of the highlights of the day for a convalescent patient or a patient who is not extremely sick. Mealtime is a break in the often boring routine. It gives the patient something to look forward to. Many patients also enjoy making food selections from a menu, when choices are offered. This is another time when your attitude is important. If the patient seems to want you to, look at the menu with him and make suggestions. When the food tray is delivered, do everything you can to make the patient's meal as pleasant and comfortable as possible.

As you know, eating in a pleasant, attractive place helps you enjoy your food. This is also true for the hospital patient. When a patient is going to have a meal, be sure the room is clean, quiet, free of unpleasant odors, and not too warm or cold. Take away things that might spoil the patient's appetite—items such as an emesis basin, urinal, or bedpan.

Procedure: Preparing the Patient for a Meal

1. Assemble your equipment:
   a. Bedpan or urinal
   b. Basin of warm water at 115° F (46.1° C)
   c. Washcloth
   d. Towel
   e. Robe and slippers

2.   Wash your hands.

3.   Identify the patient by checking the identification bracelet.

4.   Ask visitors to step out of the room.

5.   Tell the patient you are getting him ready for his next meal.

6.   Pull the curtain around the bed for privacy.

7.   Offer the bedpan or urinal, or assist the patient to the bathroom.

8.   Have the patient wash his hands or do this for him.

9.   Raise the backrest so the patient is in a sitting position, if this is allowed. If not, you might prop up his head by using several pillows.

10.   Clear the overbed table. Put it in a convenient position for the patient's meal.

11.   If the patient wants to sit in a chair during his meal, and if this is allowed, help him into his robe and slippers, and help him out of bed and to the chair.

12.   Wash your hands.

13.   Report to your head nurse or team leader that the patient is ready for his next meal. Also report your observations of anything unusual.

Procedure: Serving the Food

1.   Wash your hands.

2.   Check the tray before you give it to a patient. Is everything on it? All the silverware and a napkin? Does the tray look attractive? Was food spilled? Correct anything that is wrong.

3.   Be sure you are giving the tray to the right patient. Check the tray card, which will have the patient's name on it, against the identification band to be sure they match.

4.   Put the tray on the overbed table. Adjust it to a height comfortable for the patient.

5.   Arrange the dishes and silver so the patient can reach everything easily. Be sure his drinking water is handy.

6.   Help any patient who needs it. For example, if a patient seems to be weak or asks for help, you might offer to spread his napkin on his lap or tuck it under his chin. Spread butter on his bread. Cut up his meat. Pour tea or coffee. Don't give him any more help than he really needs. The more a patient can do for himself, the better.

7.   A patient may discover that he can't eat when he is served. In this case you may take his tray away and keep the hot food warm for him until he wants to eat. You will learn how to keep the food warm in your institution.

8.   When you are sure the patient can go on with his meal by himself, leave the room.

9.   Go back for the food tray when the patient has finished eating.

10.   Notice how much the patient has eaten and how much he has had to drink.

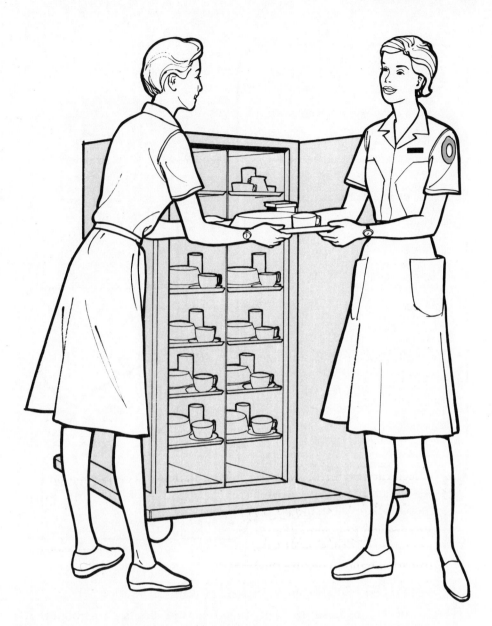

11.   Record fluid intake on the Intake and Output sheet.

12.   Record how the patient has eaten his meal on the daily activity sheet. Record this information separately for breakfast, lunch, and supper:

    a.   Did the patient eat all food served to him?

    b.   Did the patient eat about half the food served?

    c.   Did the patient eat very little food?

    d.   Did the patient refuse to accept the tray and actually ate nothing?

13.   Take the tray away and put it in its proper place.

14.   Make the patient comfortable. If he ate his meal sitting in a chair, help him back into bed.

15.   Lower the backrest, if this is what the patient wants, and if it is allowed.

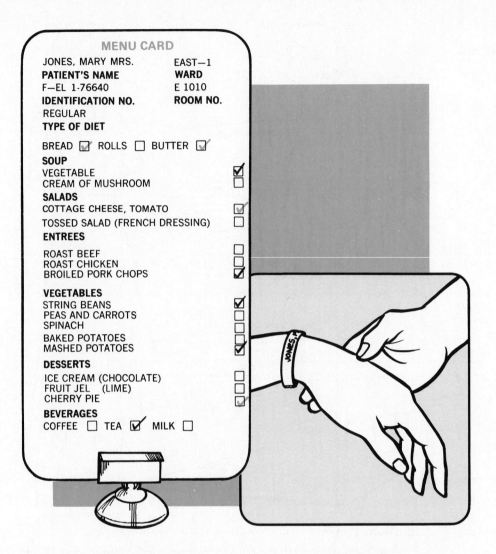

MENU CARD

JONES, MARY MRS.	EAST—1
PATIENT'S NAME	**WARD**
F—EL 1·76640	E 1010
IDENTIFICATION NO.	**ROOM NO.**
REGULAR	
TYPE OF DIET	

BREAD ☑ ROLLS ☐ BUTTER ☑

SOUP
VEGETABLE ☑
CREAM OF MUSHROOM ☐

SALADS
COTTAGE CHEESE, TOMATO ☑
TOSSED SALAD (FRENCH DRESSING) ☐

ENTREES

ROAST BEEF ☐
ROAST CHICKEN ☐
BROILED PORK CHOPS ☑

VEGETABLES
STRING BEANS ☑
PEAS AND CARROTS ☐
SPINACH ☐
BAKED POTATOES ☐
MASHED POTATOES ☑

DESSERTS

ICE CREAM (CHOCOLATE) ☐
FRUIT JEL (LIME) ☐
CHERRY PIE ☑

BEVERAGES
COFFEE ☐ TEA ☑ MILK ☐

16. Put his personal articles back where he wants them.

17. Brush crumbs from the bed. Smooth out the sheets. Straighten the bedding.

18. Wash your hands.

19. Report to your head nurse or team leader that you have served the patient his food. Also report your observations of anything unusual.

KEY IDEAS: FEEDING THE HELPLESS PATIENT

Some patients are helpless and have to be fed. The reason might be:

- They can't use their hands.
- The doctor wants them to save their strength.
- They may be too weak to feed themselves.

Usually it is hard for an adult to accept the idea of not being able to feed himself. Because a patient is helpless, he may feel resentful and depressed. Be friendly and natural. Talk pleasantly, but not too much. Help the patient overcome his resentment by encouraging him to do as much as he can. Also,

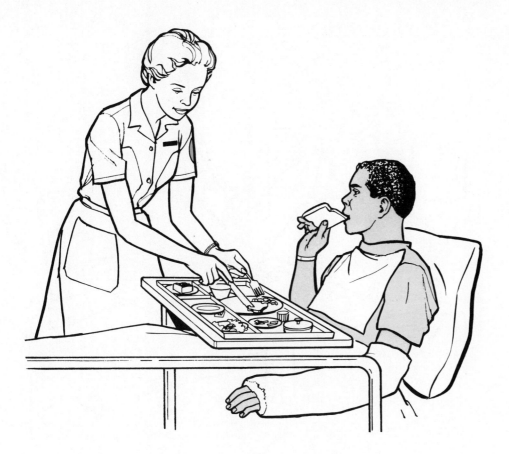

remember that because of medical reasons the patient may not always be allowed to help. You will learn how to judge the amount of help a patient can give you when he is being fed. For example, if a patient is strong enough, you might let him hold a piece of bread you have buttered for him.

When feeding a helpless patient, the most important thing is not to rush him through the meal. The time he takes to chew his food, for example, may seem long to you. But he is probably very weak; otherwise he would be feeding himself.

Remember that you should not bring the food tray or have it delivered until you have prepared the patient for his meal and are ready to feed him. Again, make sure you are serving the correct tray to the patient. Preparations before mealtime are the same for the helpless patient as for the patient who can feed himself. Be observant throughout. Watch for signs of choking.

Procedure: Feeding the Helpless Patient

1. Assemble your equipment: the patient's tray.
2. When the tray is brought into the patient's room, set it on the overbed table.
3. Wash your hands.
4. Check the name on the name card on the tray against the patient's identification bracelet.
5. Tell the patient you are going to feed him his meal.

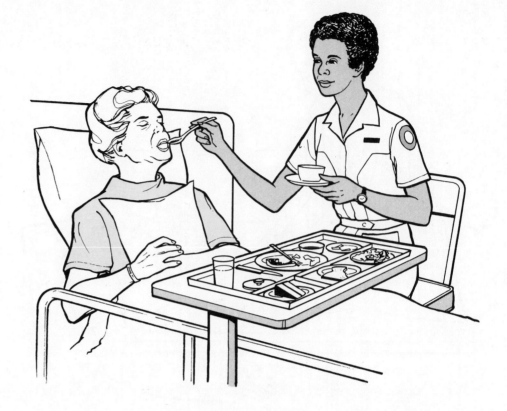

6. If you plan to be seated while you feed the patient, bring a chair to a convenient position beside the bed.

7. Check the tray to make sure everything is there. If anything is missing, have it brought in or get it yourself.

8. Tuck a napkin under the patient's chin.

9. Season the food the way the patient likes it. But do this only if his requests agree with the prescribed diet.

10. Fill the spoon only half-full. Always use a spoon when feeding a helpless patient. Give the food to the patient from the tip of the spoon, not the side. Put the food in one side of the patient's mouth so he can chew it more easily. If a patient is paralyzed on one side of his body, make sure you feed him on the side of his mouth that is not paralyzed.

11. If the patient can't see the tray, name each mouthful of food as you offer it. Offer the different foods in a logical order—soup or juice before the main course. Alternate between liquids and solid foods throughout the meal. Feed the patient as you yourself would want to eat. Or follow the patient's suggestions about how he wants to alternate between various kinds of foods and a beverage.

12. Warn the patient if you are offering something hot.

13. Use a straw for giving liquids. Hold the glass or cup in one hand and the straw in the other. Use a new straw for each beverage.

14. Feed the patient slowly. Remember that he may chew and swallow very slowly. Allow plenty of time between mouthfuls.

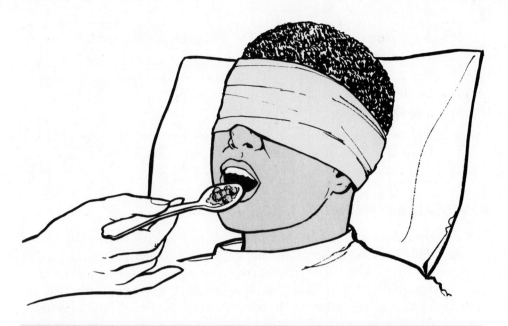

15. Encourage the patient to finish his meal, but don't force him.

16. When the patient has finished eating, help him to wipe his mouth with his napkin, or do this for him.

17. Notice how much the patient has eaten and how much he has had to drink.

18. Record fluid intake on the Intake and Output sheet.

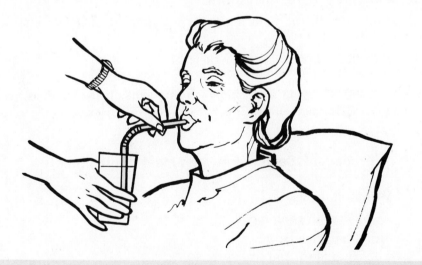

19. Record how the patient has eaten his meal on the daily activity sheet. Record this information separately for breakfast, lunch, and supper:
    a. Did the patient eat all food served to him?
    b. Did the patient eat about one-half of the food served?
    c. Did the patient eat very little food?
    d. Did the patient refuse to accept the tray and actually ate nothing?

20. As soon as you are sure the patient is finished with the tray, take it away. Put it in its proper place.

21. Adjust the backrest of the bed to make the patient comfortable, if this is allowed.
22. Brush crumbs from the bed. Smooth the sheets. Straighten the bedding.
23. Wash your hands.
24 . Report to your head nurse or team leader that you have fed the helpless patient. Also report your observations of anything unusual.

KEY IDEAS: BETWEEN-MEAL NOURISHMENTS

Extra nourishment in the form of food or drink is offered to patients during the day. This is a kind of hospital "snack" given to patients to provide quick energy or to break the routine. Patients are often given extra nourishment as part of their medical care. The snack is usually a beverage such as milk, chocolate milk, or fruit juice. Or it may be a portion of food such as gelatin, custard, crackers, or a sandwich. Some patients on special diets are allowed to have only certain kinds and amounts of extra nourishment. Other patients may not be allowed to have anything at all.

In some institutions, extra nourishment is passed out to patients by workers from the food service department. However, you may be assigned this responsibility. If you are, the head nurse or your team leader will give you a list of patients that shows:

- Those who are not to be given anything
- Those who are allowed to have certain nourishment, such as skim milk or tea
- Those who have no restrictions on their diet

A specific time for serving nourishments to patients on special diets may be given on the nourishment chart. Be sure to follow this time schedule carefully.

Procedure: Serving Between-Meal Nourishments

1. Wash your hands.
2. Assemble your equipment:
    a. Nourishment
    b. Cup, dish, and a spoon or straw
    c. Napkin
3. Identify the patient by checking the identification bracelet.
4. If a patient has a choice of items, ask him what he wants.
5. Prepare the nourishment.
6. Take the nourishment to the patient on a tray or cart.
7. Encourage the patient to take his nourishment. Help him if he needs it. Offer a straw if this is more convenient for him.
8. After the patient has finished, collect the tray. Get rid of used disposable items.

9. Record the intake for those patients who are on intake and output.

10. Wash your hands.,

11. Report to your head nurse or team leader that you have served the between-meal nourishment. Also report your observations of anything unusual.

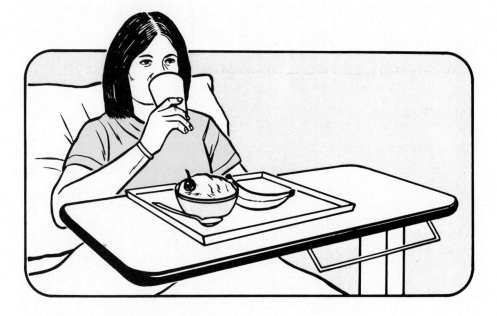

KEY IDEAS: PASSING DRINKING WATER

Part of your job as a nursing aide will be to see that the patients you are caring for have plenty of fresh water at their bedsides, unless a doctor orders otherwise. Some patients are not allowed to have more than a certain amount of water. Some, for brief periods, may not have water at all.

Fresh water is passed to patients at regular intervals during the day. Your instructor will tell you the schedule.

Disposable pitchers and cups are used in all hospitals.

Most patients like ice water. Others want water without ice, straight from the tap. You will be told which patients are allowed to have a choice. If a patient is not allowed to have ice, his water pitcher will be tagged *OMIT ICE*.

Procedure: Passing Drinking Water

NOTE: In some hospitals each pitcher is taken to the clean kitchen or utility room, filled with clean water and ice, and then returned to each individual patient. When this is done, the following procedure is not used.

1. Assemble your equipment:
    a. Moving table with small styrofoam ice chest and cover
    b. Ice cubes
    c. Scoop
    d. Paper cups

      e.   Disposable water pitchers
      f.   Straws
      g.   Paper towels

2. Wash your hands.

3. Fill the ice chest with ice cubes and cover it.

4. Put your equipment on the table.

5. Before you pass drinking water, be sure you know:
   a. Which patients are NPO (nothing by mouth)
   b. Which patients are on restricted fluids and therefore get only a measured amount of water
   c. Which patients should get only tap water (omit ice)
   d. Which patients may have ice water

6. Roll the moving table into the hall outside the patient's room.

7. Go into the room and pick up one patient's water pitcher.

8. Empty it in the sink in the room. Fill it half-full with tap water.

9. Walk to the water table in the hall. Fill the pitcher to the brim with ice cubes, being sure the scoop does not touch the water pitcher.

10. Replace the water pitcher on the same patient's table from which it was taken. If the pitcher is labeled with the patient's name, check it against the identification bracelet.

11. Throw away used paper cups.

12. Wipe the table with a clean paper towel. Discard the towel.

13. Place several clean paper cups next to the water pitcher.

14. Place several straws next to the water pitcher.

15. Be sure the patient can reach the water pitcher easily.

16. Offer to pour a fresh glass of water for the patient.

17. Wash your hands.

18. Report to your head nurse or team leader that you have passed drinking water to the patient. Also report your observations of anything unusual.

WHAT YOU HAVE LEARNED

For good health, every person needs the essential nutrients contained in all of the four basic food groups. Patients on therapeutic diets are permitted only those foods included in their strict prescribed diet. These patients must never be served any other foods. Before you serve any tray, be sure to check the identification bracelet against the name on the tray card. Observe how much the patient has eaten and record this information. Make accurate records of fluid intake on the Intake and Output sheet. Remember that you should not bring the food tray into a helpless patient's room until you are ready to feed him. When serving between-meal nourishments, check the diet list to be sure each patient is served only those foods permitted on his diet. When passing drinking water, be sure to return the patient's water pitcher to the same patient.

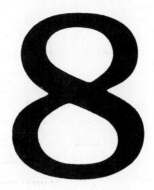

Intake and Output

Section 1: Fluid Balance

OBJECTIVES: WHAT YOU WILL LEARN

When you have completed this section, you should be able:

- To explain fluid balance and imbalance
- To give the reasons for making accurate records of fluid intake and output

KEY IDEAS

Water is essential to human life. Next to oxygen, water is the most important thing the body takes in. A person can be starving, can lose half of his body protein and almost half of his body weight, and he can still live. But losing only one-fifth of the body's fluid will result in death.

Through eating and drinking, the average healthy adult will take in about 3 1/2 quarts of fluid every day—this is his *fluid intake*. The same adult also will eliminate about 3 1/2 quarts of fluid every day—this is his *fluid output*. Fluid is discharged from the body of a healthy person in several ways:

- Most of the fluid passes through the kidneys and is discharged as urine.
- Some of it is lost from the body through perspiration.

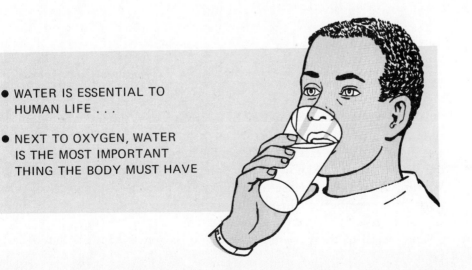

- WATER IS ESSENTIAL TO HUMAN LIFE . . .

- NEXT TO OXYGEN, WATER IS THE MOST IMPORTANT THING THE BODY MUST HAVE

- Some is evaporated from the lungs in breathing.
- The rest is absorbed and discharged through the intestinal system.

It is difficult to measure accurately the amount of fluid discharged through evaporation and breathing. Therefore, a person may seem to have a greater fluid intake than output. There is, however, a fluid balance in the normally functioning body. Fluid balance means that just about the same amount of fluid taken in by the body is also given out. The fluid taken in is called the *fluid intake.* The fluid given out, no matter how, is called the *fluid output.*

An *imbalance* of fluids in the body occurs when too much fluid is kept in the body or when too much fluid is lost. In some medical conditions, fluid may be held in the body tissues and make them swell. This is called *edema.* In other conditions, much fluid may be lost by vomiting, bleeding, severe diarrhea, or excessive sweating.

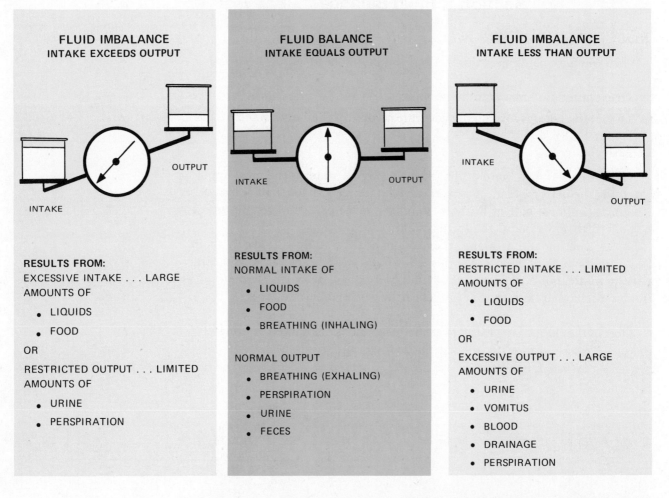

FLUID IMBALANCE
INTAKE EXCEEDS OUTPUT

OUTPUT

INTAKE

RESULTS FROM:
EXCESSIVE INTAKE . . . LARGE AMOUNTS OF

- LIQUIDS
- FOOD

OR

RESTRICTED OUTPUT . . . LIMITED AMOUNTS OF

- URINE
- PERSPIRATION

FLUID BALANCE
INTAKE EQUALS OUTPUT

INTAKE   OUTPUT

RESULTS FROM:
NORMAL INTAKE OF

- LIQUIDS
- FOOD
- BREATHING (INHALING)

NORMAL OUTPUT

- BREATHING (EXHALING)
- PERSPIRATION
- URINE
- FECES

FLUID IMBALANCE
INTAKE LESS THAN OUTPUT

INTAKE

OUTPUT

RESULTS FROM:
RESTRICTED INTAKE . . . LIMITED AMOUNTS OF

- LIQUIDS
- FOOD

OR

EXCESSIVE OUTPUT . . . LARGE AMOUNTS OF

- URINE
- VOMITUS
- BLOOD
- DRAINAGE
- PERSPIRATION

When a patient's body loses more fluid than he is taking in or retains more than he is putting out, his doctor can treat the condition in various ways. A specific method is prescribed to meet the needs of the individual patient. The only way a doctor can know when a patient's balance of fluids is not right is by knowing the patient's measurable intake and output. Therefore, it is very important for members of the nursing staff to keep accurate records of fluid intake and output.

The record of the patient's intake and output is kept for a full 24-hour period.

INTAKE AND OUTPUT SHEET

Hospital # _____   Patient Name _____

Date _____   Room # _____

	INTAKE				OUTPUT		
				URINE		GASTRIC	
Time 7-3	BY MOUTH	TUBE	PARENTERAL	VOIDED	CATHETER	EMESIS	SUCTION
TOTAL							
Time 3-11							
TOTAL							
Time 11-7							
TOTAL							
24 HOUR TOTAL							
24 Hour Grand Total ● Intake				24 Hour Grand Total ● Output			

The amounts of intake and output (I and O) are written on a special sheet of paper. It is called the Intake and Output (I&O) sheet and hangs near the patient's bed. The patient's name, room number, the hospital number, and the date are recorded at the top of the page. The Intake and Output sheet is divided into two parts—intake on the left side and output on the right side. After measuring intake or output, you will record the amount and time in the proper columns. At the end of each 8-hour shift, the amounts in each column are totaled and recorded.

Section 2: Fluid Intake

OBJECTIVES: WHAT YOU WILL LEARN

When you have completed this section, you should be able:

- To explain the meaning of fluid intake
- To accurately measure fluids, using the metric system
- To show that you can observe exact amounts of fluids consumed by the patient and record them accurately on the Intake and Output sheet

KEY IDEAS

A doctor must know exactly how much liquid is taken in every day by certain patients. Although solid foods also contain some liquid, most of the fluids in the body are taken in when a person drinks liquids. A patient's fluid intake

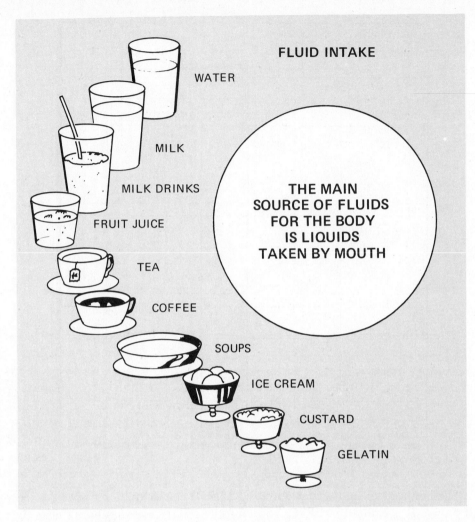

FLUID INTAKE

WATER

MILK

MILK DRINKS

FRUIT JUICE

TEA

COFFEE

SOUPS

ICE CREAM

CUSTARD

GELATIN

THE MAIN
SOURCE OF FLUIDS
FOR THE BODY
IS LIQUIDS
TAKEN BY MOUTH

ACTUAL SIZE OF
CUBIC INCH
AND
CUBIC CENTIMETER

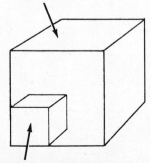

1 CUBIC INCH

1 CUBIC CENTIMETER

therefore includes everything he drinks—water, milk, milk drinks, fruit juices, soup, tea, coffee—anything liquid. Ice cream, junket, and gelatin also are usually counted as liquids.

You probably have already noticed that many quantities used in the health care field are measured in "cc." Because most hospitals use this term for measuring intake and output, you should understand what it means.

The term *cc* is an abbreviation for *cubic centimeter*, a unit of measurement in the metric system. The metric system of measurement is used in many countries of the world. In the United States, we normally use one system for measuring liquids—ounces, pints, quarts—and a different system for measuring lengths—inches, feet, yards, miles. However, scientists, engineers, and many hospital personnel use the metric system for measuring liquids, lengths, and weight, as well. The basic unit of measurement is the meter, which is a little longer than the yard. A centimeter—one one-hundredth (1/100) of a meter—is about four-tenths (4/10) of an inch long.

A cubic centimeter can be thought of as a square block with each edge of the block 1 centimeter long. If we filled this block with water, we would have 1 cubic centimeter (1 cc) of water. The list shown here includes liquid amounts that you are probably familiar with. It also gives about the same amounts in cubic centimeters.

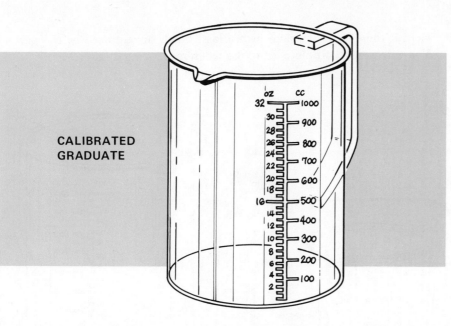

CALIBRATED
GRADUATE

The patient's liquid intake is measured in cubic centimeters (cc). A container called a graduate or a measuring cup is used to measure intake and output (I&O). The side of the graduate is marked (calibrated) with a row of short lines and numbers. These show the amount of liquid in both cubic centimeters and ounces. This graduate is like the measuring cup you use at home to measure ingredients for cooking, only larger. Another calibrated graduate used in the home is a baby's milk bottle. This, too, is marked with a row of short lines and numbers. They show the amount of milk in both ounces and cubic centimeters. When full, most baby's bottles contain 8 ounces, or 240 cubic centimeters (cc). To give the baby 4 ounces of milk, or 120 cc, you would fill it half full or to the 4-ounce line.

It is very important that you observe the exact amounts of fluids taken in by the patient and that you record them accurately. You will have to measure the amount of liquid contained in each serving container—bowl, glass, or cup—used by the patient. If your hospital does not have a list of the amounts contained in each container, bowl, glass, or cup, you will find it helpful to make such a list yourself.

Rules To Follow: Measuring the Capacity of Serving Containers

- Assemble your equipment:
  - Complete set of dishes, bowls, cups, and glasses used by the patients
  - Graduate (measuring cup)
  - Water
  - Pen and paper
- Fill the first container with water.
- Pour this water into the graduate.
- Look at the level of the water and determine the amount in cc (cubic centimeters).
- Write this information on the paper. For example: carton of milk = 240 cc.

U.S. CUSTOMARY LIQUID MEASURE WITH EQUIVALENT METRIC MEASUREMENTS

cc = cubic centemeter
cc = milliliter
ml = milliliter
oz = ounce

¼ teaspoon = 1 cc
1 teaspoon = 4 cc
30 cc = 1 oz
60 cc = 2 oz
90 cc = 3 oz
120 cc = 4 oz
150 cc = 5 oz
180 cc = 6 oz
210 cc = 7 oz
240 cc = 8 oz
270 cc = 9 oz
300 cc = 10 oz

500 cc = 1 pint
1000 cc = 1 quart
4000 cc = 1 gallon

pt = pint
qt = quart
gal = gallon

- Repeat these steps for each dish, glass, bowl, or cup used by the patients. You will have a complete list to use when measuring intake.

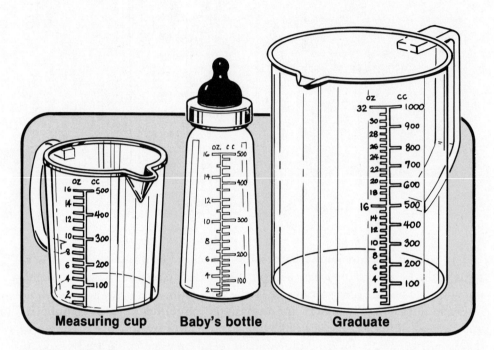

Measuring cup   Baby's bottle   Graduate

These are all containers used for measuring.

- They are all calibrated.
- They are made of metal, glass, or plastic.
- They are used for measuring liquids in cubic centimeters(cc).
- They are used for measuring liquids in ounces (oz).
- The measuring cup is used to measure liquids in the home.
- The baby's bottle is used to measure liquids in the home.
- The calibrated graduate is used to measure fluid in the hospital.

KEY IDEAS: MEASURING FLUID INTAKE

You should tell the patient that his intake is being measured. You can encourage him to help you, if he is not too ill, by asking him to keep track of how much liquid he drinks. This is not his responsibility, however. It is yours.

Fluids taken in by patients intravenously are recorded by the nurse. This record also is kept on the Intake and Output sheet, in a special column headed "Parenteral Intake." Regardless of how fluids are consumed by a patient, the important thing is that the doctor must know as accurately as possible how much fluid the patient has taken in.

The proper time for the aide to record the patient's fluids on the Intake and Output sheet is as soon as the patient has consumed the fluids. Before the end of each shift, the complete amount of intake should be added up. Your task will be to remember to record all fluid taken in each time the patient eats or drinks. Think about fluid intake every time you remove a tray, water pitcher, glass, or cup from a patient's bedside. Remember especially to check the water pitcher.

When measuring fluid intake, you will have to note the difference between the amount the patient actually drinks and the amount he leaves in the serving container. You will be required to convert (change) amounts such as 1/2 bowl of soup, 1/2 glass of orange juice, or 1/4 cup of tea into cc (cubic centimeters) when recording them.

Procedure: Determining the Amounts Consumed

1. Assemble your equipment:
    a. Graduate
    b. Pen and paper
    c. Left-over liquids
2. Pour the left-over liquid into the graduate.
3. Look at the level and determine the amount in cc.
4. Determine the amount in the full serving container.
5. Subtract the left-over amount from the full-container amount. This figure is the amount the patient actually drank.
6. Immediately record this amount on the intake side of the Intake and Output (I&O) sheet.

Section 3: Forcing and Restricting Fluids

OBJECTIVES: WHAT YOU WILL LEARN

When you have completed this section, you should be able:

*   To explain the terms *FF* and *NPO*
*   To demonstrate the nursing aide's role when a patient is on *restrict fluids*
*   To demonstrate the nursing aide's role when a patient is on *force fluids*
*   To demonstrate the nursing aide's role when a patient is on *nothing by mouth*

KEY IDEAS: FORCE FLUIDS

Patients who need to have more fluids added to their normal intake are put on *force fluids* by the doctor. *FF* is the abbreviation for force fluids. Patients on FF are required to take in extra fluids.

A patient on force fluids often needs encouragement to drink more. Some ways you can persuade the patient to drink more fluids are:

*   By showing enthusiasm and being cheerful
*   By providing different kinds of liquids

- By offering liquids without being asked
- By offering hot or cold drinks

Rules To Follow

- Check your assignment sheet or card to see if the patient is on force fluids (FF).

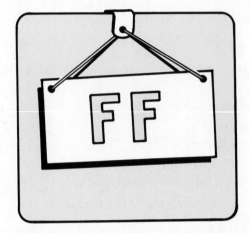

- If the patient is on force fluids, encourage him to drink the amount required. For example, 800 cc every 8 hours means that the patient would have to drink 100 cc every hour. At the end of the 8-hour shift, he would have taken in 800 cc of fluids.
- Use different kinds of fluids as permitted by the patient's therapeutic (special) diet. Examples are hot tea, gelatin, soda, ice cream, milk, juice, broth, coffee, custard, water.
- Record the amount taken in by the patient (in cc) on the intake side of the Intake and Output sheet.

KEY IDEAS: RESTRICT FLUIDS

For some patients, the doctor writes orders to *restrict fluids.* This means that fluids may be limited to certain amounts. When you are caring for a patient on **restrict fluids**, it is important to follow orders exactly and to measure accurately. Your calm and reassuring attitude can make a big difference in how the patient feels.

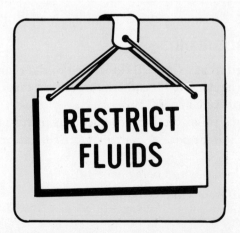

Rules To Follow

- Check your assignment sheet to see if the patient is on restrict fluids.
- If he is, the patient must stay within the limits stated by your head nurse or team leader.
- Alternate different fluids as permitted by the therapeutic diet. Be sure to limit the patient to the correct amount.
- Record the amount on the intake side of the Intake and Output sheet.

KEY IDEAS: NOTHING BY MOUTH

For some patients, the doctor writes orders that the patient is to have *nothing by mouth*. This means that the patient cannot eat or drink anything at all. You may be asked to take away the patient's water pitcher and glass at midnight. You will post a sign saying *NPO*. This is short for *nothing by mouth*. It is taken from the Latin *nils per os*, which means nothing by mouth. An NPO sign is put at the foot or the head of the bed or on the door of the patient's room. Some institutions do not allow a patient on NPO to have oral hygiene.

Patients often become very irritable and cranky when they are not allowed to have anything to eat or drink. They may, therefore, be hard for you to deal with. Calm and reassuring behavior on your part can help the patient go through a very uncomfortable period. A smile and a few kind words will go a long way here.

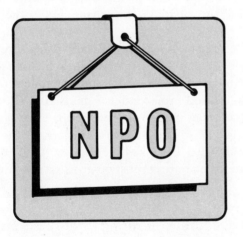

Rules To Follow

- Check the assignment sheet to see if the patient is on NPO.
- Explain to the patient that he is now on nothing by mouth.
- Remove the water pitcher and anything else by which the patient could take a drink or eat.
- Place a sign stating NPO on the bed or door.
- Do not give any liquids or food to this patient.
- Make a note on the intake side of the Intake and Output sheet that the patient is NPO.

Section 4: Fluid Output

OBJECTIVES: WHAT YOU WILL LEARN

When you have completed this section, you should be able:

- To explain fluid output
- To list the ways in which the body loses fluid
- To use the metric system accurately to measure fluid output
- To measure the exact amounts of fluid output
- To record the amounts accurately on the Intake and Output sheet

KEY IDEAS: MEASURING FLUID OUTPUT

Fluid output is the sum total of liquids that come out of the body.

To *urinate* means to discharge urine from the body. Other terms for this body function are: to void, to pass water.

The rest of the fluid that is discharged goes out of the body by a process called "insensible loss." This means that the fluid is lost without being noticed. Some of the fluid is lost through perspiration. Some is lost in the air breathed out. Also, from 100 to 200 cc of fluid is discharged from the body in feces. Output also includes emesis (vomitus), drainage from a wound or from the stomach, and loss of blood.

A patient who is on intake and output must have his output as well as his intake measured and recorded. This means that every time the patient uses the urinal, emesis basin, or bedpan, the urine and other liquids must be measured.

You should tell a patient his output is being measured and ask him to cooperate. A female patient must urinate in a bedpan or specipan. (The specipan is a disposable container that fits into the toilet bowl under the seat.) The specipan can be placed in her toilet if she is allowed out of bed. Ask the patient not to place toilet paper in the bedpan or specipan. Provide a wastepaper basket for her. Then discard tissue into the toilet or hopper. Female patients must also be asked not to let their bowels move while urinating. Male patients on output must be instructed to use a urinal.

Procedure: Measuring Urinary Output

1. Assemble your equipment:
   a. Bedpan, cover, urinal, or specipan
   b. Graduate (measuring container)
   c. Intake and Output sheet
2. Pour the urine from the bedpan or urinal into a graduate.
3. Place the graduate on a flat surface for accuracy in measurement.
4. Look carefully at the graduate to see the number reached by the level of the urine.
5. Record this amount on the output side of the Intake and Output sheet.
6. Write down the time and record the amount in cc.

7. Rinse and return the graduate.

8. Report to your head nurse or team leader your observations of anything unusual.

KEY IDEAS: PLASTIC URINE CONTAINER

Some patients have a catheter inserted into their urinary bladder by the doctor or nurse. This catheter drains all the patient's urine into a plastic urine container. The container hangs on the bed below the level of the urinary bladder. You will empty this container, measure the urine, and record the amount, always before the end of your working shift.

Procedure: Emptying a Plastic Urine Container

1. Assemble your equipment: a graduate.

2. Wash your hands.

3. Open the drain and let the urine run into the graduate.

4. Measure the amount of urinary output.

5. Record the amount immediately on the output side of the Intake and Output sheet.

CHECKING CATHETERS AND CONTAINERS

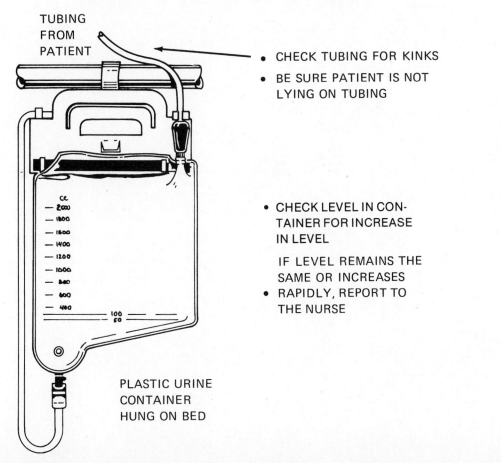

TUBING
FROM
PATIENT

- CHECK TUBING FOR KINKS
- BE SURE PATIENT IS NOT LYING ON TUBING

- CHECK LEVEL IN CONTAINER FOR INCREASE IN LEVEL

  IF LEVEL REMAINS THE SAME OR INCREASES
- RAPIDLY, REPORT TO THE NURSE

PLASTIC URINE
CONTAINER
HUNG ON BED

WHAT YOU HAVE LEARNED

It is important that you observe the exact amounts of fluids consumed by the patient and record them accurately. All fluids should be measured in cubic centimeters. Remember to record all fluids taken in each time the patient eats or drinks. Think about fluid intake whenever you remove a tray, water pitcher, glass, or cup from a patient's bedside. Be sure you know which of your patients are on force fluids, restrict fluids, nothing by mouth, and intake and output. Each time the patient who is on intake and output uses the bedpan, urinal, or specipan, measure and record the fluid output accurately on the Intake and Output sheet.

Remember to drain the urine from a urinary drainage bag into a graduate for measuring. The calibrations on the plastic urinary drainage bag are no longer accurate once the bag fills with urine.

Specimen Collection

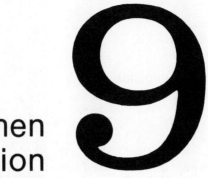

OBJECTIVES: WHAT YOU WILL LEARN

When you have completed this section, you should be able:

- To explain what specimens are
- To collect specimens correctly and exactly at the time required
- To label specimens properly
- To test urine for sugar and acetone

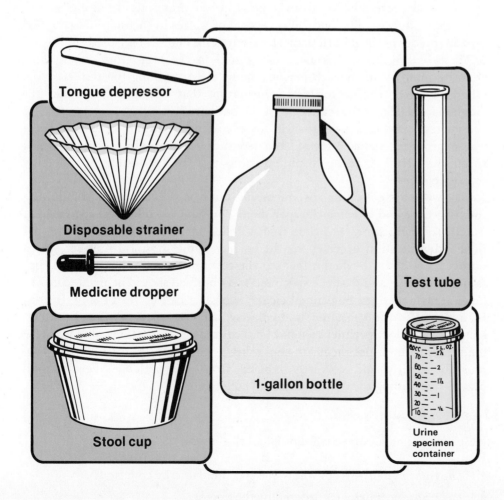

Tongue depressor

Disposable strainer

Medicine dropper

Stool cup

1-gallon bottle

Test tube

Urine specimen container

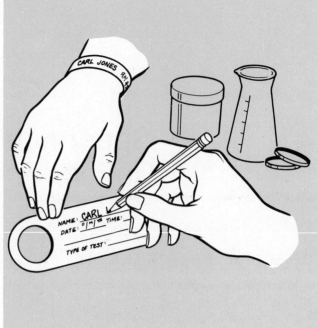

BE ACCURATE . . .

Check identification bracelet

Print clearly so the label can be easily read

Put label on specimen immediately after specimen container has been collected

Check identification bracelet

Copy the patient's name from it.

KEY IDEAS

As one of its natural living functions, the human body regularly gets rid of various waste materials. Most of the body's waste materials are discharged in the urine and feces. The body also gets rid of wastes in the material coughed up and spit out of the mouth (expectorated). This material is called *sputum*.

These body waste materials, when tested in the laboratory, often show changes going on in the sick person's body. By examining the results of the laboratory tests, the doctor gets information that can help him make his diagnosis and decide on treatment for the patient.

For these reasons, the doctor will sometimes need samples of each of these waste products—urine, feces, and sputum. These samples are called *specimens*. Members of the hospital nursing staff are responsible for collecting such specimens.

When you are collecting specimens you must be very accurate in following the procedure and labeling the specimen. You have to collect the specimen at exactly the right time—the time that is called for. You must look at the patient's identification bracelet for the correct name, hospital number, room number, and so forth when filling out the cover or label on the specimen container. The time and date the specimen was obtained should be printed on the label. The label must be printed clearly so that it can be read easily. It must be attached to the container immediately after the specimen has been collected. Unlabeled specimens should be thrown away so that mistakes won't be made. Sometimes specimens are kept until a doctor can see them. These, too, must be clearly and correctly labeled from the patient's identification bracelet, including the date and time of collection.

Need for Accuracy

Be sure you have correctly followed all the "rights" listed here:

- *The right patient*—from whom the specimen is to be collected
- *The right specimen*—as ordered by the doctor

- *The right time* — when the specimen is to be collected
- *The right amount* — exactly measured for each specimen
- *The right container* — the cup that is correct for each specimen
- *The right label* — properly filled out from the patient's identification bracelet
- *The right requisition or laboratory (lab) slip* — lists the kind of test to be done (filled out by the head nurse, team leader, or ward clerk)
- *The right method* — procedure by which you collect the specimen
- *The right asepsis* — washing your hands before and after collecting the specimen
- *The right attitude* — how you approach and speak to the patient

KEY IDEAS: ASEPSIS IN SPECIMEN COLLECTION

As you learned in Chapter 3, asepsis means "free of disease-causing organisms." When collecting specimens, it is very important to follow all the rules of medical asepsis. You must wash your hands very carefully, to prevent spreading bacteria.

ASEPSIS IN SPECIMEN COLLECTION

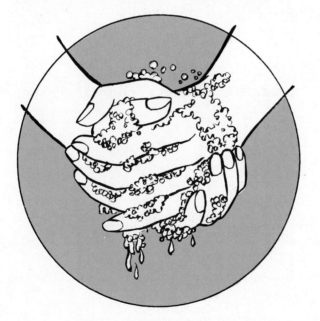

Medical asepsis means preventing the conditions that allow disease-producing bacteria to live, multiply, and spread. As a nursing aide, you will share the responsibility for preventing the spread of disease and infection by using aseptic technique.

Remember especially to wash your hands before and after collecting specimens.

KEY IDEAS: ROUTINE URINE SPECIMEN

The usual single urine specimen collected is called the *routine urine specimen.* This is the specimen that is taken routinely on admission, daily, or preoperatively by the nursing aide and sent to the laboratory.

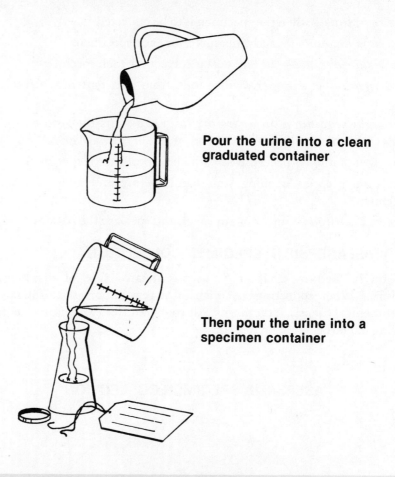

Pour the urine into a clean graduated container

Then pour the urine into a specimen container

Procedure: Collecting a Routine Urine Specimen

1. Assemble your equipment:
   a. Patient's bedpan and cover, or urinal, or specipan
   b. Graduate used for measuring output
   c. Urine specimen container and lid
   d. Label, if your hospital's procedure is not to write on the lid
   e. Laboratory request slip, which should be filled out by the head nurse, team leader, or ward clerk

2. Wash your hands.

3. Identify the patient by checking the identification bracelet.

4. Ask visitors to step out of the room.

5. Tell the patient a urine specimen is needed.

6. Pull the curtain around the bed for privacy.

7. Have the patient urinate into the bedpan, urinal, or specipan.

8. Ask the patient not to put toilet tissue into the bedpan or specipan, but to use the wastepaper basket temporarily. You will then discard the tissue in the toilet or hopper.

9. Prepare the label immediately by copying all necessary information from the patient's identification bracelet. Record the time and date.

10. Take the bedpan or urinal to the patient's bathroom or to the dirty utility room.

11. Pour the urine into a clean graduated container.

12. If the patient is on output, note the amount of the urine and record it on the Intake and Output sheet.

13. Pour urine from the graduate into a specimen container and fill it three-fourths full, if possible.

14. Put the lid on the specimen container. Put the correct label on the specimen container for the correct patient.

15. Pour the leftover urine into the toilet or hopper.

16. Clean and rinse out the graduate. Put it in its proper place.

17. Clean the bedpan or urinal and put it in its proper place.

18. Wash your hands.

19. Send or take the labeled specimen container to the laboratory with a requisition or laboratory request slip.

20. Report to your head nurse or team leader:
    - That a routine urine specimen has been obtained
    - That the specimen has been sent to the laboratory
    - The date and time of collection
    - Your observations of anything unusual

KEY IDEAS: MIDSTREAM CLEAN-CATCH URINE SPECIMEN

A special method is used to collect a patient's urine when the specimen must be free from contamination. This special kind of specimen is called a *midstream clean-catch urine specimen*. In most hospitals, a disposable midstream clean-catch package can be obtained from the CSR (Central Supply Room).

All the equipment and supplies necessary for this specimen are in the kit. Midstream means catching the urine specimen between the time the patient begins to void and the time he stops. Clean catch refers to the fact that the urine is not contaminated by anything outside the patient's body. The procedure requires careful washing of the genital area. This ensures a "clean catch" as the urine itself washes off the body opening.

Procedure: Collecting a Midstream Clean-Catch Urine Specimen

1. Assemble your equipment:
   a. Obtain a requisition slip from the ward clerk, team leader, or head nurse. Go to the CSR for a disposable kit for this specimen. If your hospital does not use disposable equipment, CSR will supply the cotton balls and solution to be used for the cleansing process according to your hospital's policy.
   b. Label, if your hospital procedure does not call for writing directly on the cover of the urine container
   c. Disposable gloves
   d. Laboratory request slip, which should be filled out by the head nurse, team leader, or ward clerk
   e. Patient's bedpan or urinal

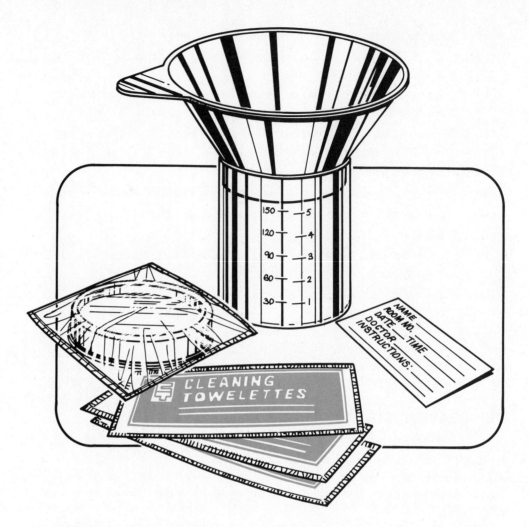

2. Wash your hands.

3. Identify the patient by checking the identification bracelet.

4. Ask visitors to step out of the room.

5. Tell the patient you need a midstream clean-catch urine specimen.

6. Pull the curtain around the bed for privacy.

7. Explain the procedure. If the patient is able, he may collect this specimen on his own, in his bathroom.

8. If the patient is not able to collect the specimen himself, help him onto the bedpan or put the urinal close by.

9. Open the disposable kit.

10. Remove towelettes from the kit.

11. For female patients:

    a. Put on the disposable gloves.

    b. Use all three towelettes to cleanse the perineal area.

    c. Separate the folds of the labia (lips) and wipe with one towelette from the front to the back (anterior to posterior) on one side. Then throw away the towelette.

      d.   Wipe the other side with a second towelette, again from front to back. Discard the towelette.

      e.   Wipe down the middle from front to back, using the third towelette, and discard it.

12.   For male patients:

      a.   If the patient is not circumcised, pull the foreskin back (retract foreskin) on the penis to clean, and hold it back during urination.

      b.   Use a circular motion to clean the head of the penis. Discard each towelette after each use.

13.   Take the urine specimen container out of the disposable kit. Ask the patient to start to urinate into either the bedpan or the urinal. After the flow of his (or her) urine has started, ask him or her to stop urinating. Place the urine specimen container under the patient and ask him or her to start urinating again. But this time catch the urine between the time the patient begins to void and the time he stops.

14.   If a funnel type of container is used, remove the funnel and discard it.

15.   Cover the urine container immediately with the cap from the kit. Be careful not to touch the inside of the container or the inside of the cap.

16.   Label right away. Copy all needed information from the patient's identification bracelet. Record the date and time of collection.

17.   Clean the bedpan or urinal. Put it in its proper place.

18.   Discard all used disposable equipment.

19.   Wash your hands.

20.   The labeled specimen container must be sent or taken to the laboratory with a requisition or laboratory request slip.

21.   Report to your head nurse or team leader:
- That a midstream clean-catch urine specimen has been obtained
- That it has been sent to the laboratory
- The date and time of collection
- Your observations of anything unusual

KEY IDEAS: 24-HOUR URINE SPECIMEN

A 24-hour urine specimen is a collection of all urine voided by a patient over a 24-hour period. All the urine is collected for 24 hours, usually from 7 a.m. on the first day to 7 a.m. the following day.

When you are to obtain a 24-hour urine specimen, it is necessary to ask the patient to void and discard the first voided urine at 7 a.m. This is because this urine has remained in the bladder an unknown length of time. The test should begin with the bladder empty. For the next 24 hours, save all the urine voided by the patient. On the following day at 7 a.m., ask the patient to void and save this specimen. In this way the doctor can be sure that all the urine for the test came into the urinary bladder during the 24 hours of the test period.

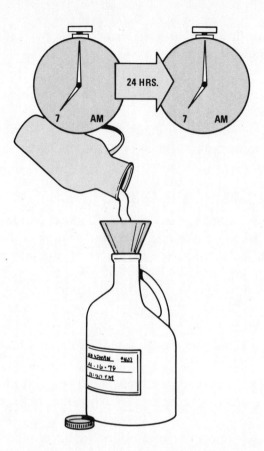

Procedure: Collecting a 24-Hour Urine Specimen

1. Assemble your equipment:
   a. Large container, usually a 1-gallon plastic disposable bottle
   b. Funnel, if the neck of the bottle is small
   c. Graduate, used for measuring output
   d. Patient's bedpan, urinal, or specipan
   e. Label for the container
   f. Laboratory request slip, which should be filled out by the head nurse, team leader, or ward clerk
   g. Tag, to be placed over or on the patient's bed, to indicate that a 24-hour urine specimen is being collected
   h. Urine specimen container and cover, if used

2. Wash your hands.

3. Identify the patient by checking the identification bracelet.

4. Ask visitors to step out of the room.

5. Tell the patient that a 24-hour urine specimen is needed.

6. Explain the procedure. Tell the patient that you will be placing the large container in his bathroom.

7. Fill in the label for the large container. Copy all needed information from the patient's identification bracelet. Record the date and time of the first collection. Attach the label to the urine specimen container. Place the container in the patient's bathroom.

8. Post the tag over or on the patient's bed. This is so all hospital personnel will be aware that a 24-hour specimen is being collected.

9. Pull the curtain around the bed for privacy each time the patient voids, if he uses a bedpan or urinal rather than a specipan or urinal in the bathroom.

10. If the patient is on intake and output, measure all the urine each time the patient voids. Write the amount on the Intake and Output sheet.

11. When the collection starts, have the patient void. Throw away (discard) this first amount of urine. This is to be sure that the bladder is completely empty. This is usually done at 7 a.m. The test will continue until the next day at 7 a.m. This first voiding should not be included in the specimen.

12. You may be instructed to refrigerate the urine. If so, fill a large bucket with ice cubes. Keep the large container in the ice, in the patient's bathroom. All nursing aides caring for this patient for the next 24 hours will be responsible for keeping the bucket filled with ice.

13. For the next 24 hours, save all urine voided by the patient. Pour the urine from each voiding into the large container.

14. At the end of the 24-hour period, have the patient void at 7 a.m. Add this to the collection of urine in the large container. This will be the last time you will collect the urine for this test.

15. The large labeled container with the entire 24-hour collection of urine is taken to the laboratory with a requisition or laboratory request slip.

16. Clean your equipment and put it in its proper place.

17. Throw away used disposable equipment.

18. Remove the 24-hour specimen tag from the patient's bed.

19. Wash your hands.

20. Report to your head nurse or team leader:
    - That a 24-hour urine specimen has been obtained
    - That the specimen has been sent to the laboratory
    - The date and time of collection
    - Your observations of anything unusual

KEY IDEAS: SPUTUM SPECIMEN

Sputum is a substance collected from a patient's mouth that contains saliva, mucus, and sometimes pus. It is thicker than ordinary saliva (spit). Most of it is coughed up from the lungs and bronchial tubes.

Procedure: Collecting a Sputum Specimen

1. Assemble your equipment:
    a. Sputum container and cover

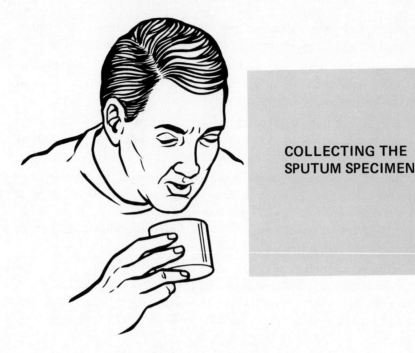

COLLECTING THE
SPUTUM SPECIMEN

b. Label, if your hospital procedure is not to write on the lid
c. Laboratory request slip, which should be filled out by the head nurse, team leader, or ward clerk

2. Wash your hands.

3. Identify the patient by checking the identification bracelet.

4. Tell the patient a sputum specimen is needed.

5. If the patient has eaten recently, have him rinse out his mouth. If he wants to have oral hygiene at this time, help him as necessary.

6. Give the patient a sputum container. Ask him to cough up (expectorate) as much sputum as he can. Tell him to cough deeply to bring up the thick material from the chest. Explain that saliva (spit) and nose secretions are not what are needed for this test.

7. The patient may have to cough several times to bring up enough sputum for the specimen. One to two tablespoons is usually the required amount.

8. Cover the container immediately. Be careful not to touch the inside of either the container or the cover to avoid contamination.

9. Label the container right away. Copy all needed information from the patient's identification bracelet. Record the time of collection and the date.

10. The labeled specimen container must be sent or taken immediately to the laboratory with a requisition or laboratory request slip. The test must be done in the laboratory before the sputum begins to dry.

11. Wash your hands.

12. Report to your head nurse or team leader:

   • That a sputum specimen has been obtained
   • That the specimen has been sent to the laboratory

- The date and time of collection
- Your observations of anything unusual

KEY IDEAS: STOOL SPECIMEN

Feces, stool, BM, bowel movement, fecal matter all can be taken to mean the same thing: the solid waste from a patient's body. The doctor sometimes orders a stool specimen to help him in the diagnosis of a patient's illness. Sometimes a warm specimen is ordered. This means that the test must be done in the laboratory while the specimen is still warm from the patient's body. You will be told whether the specimen is to be warm or cold.

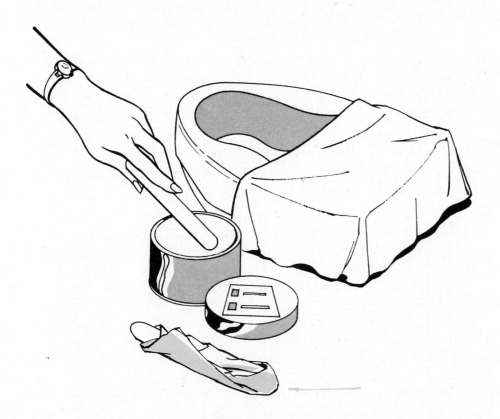

Procedure: Collecting a Stool Specimen

1. Assemble your equipment:
    a. Patient's bedpan and cover
    b. Stool specimen container
    c. Wooden tongue depressor
    d. Label, if your hospital procedure is not to write on the lid
    e. Laboratory request slip, which should be filled out by the head nurse, team leader, or ward clerk
    f. Plastic bag for warm specimen, if used by your hospital
2. Wash your hands.
3. Identify the patient by checking the identification bracelet.

4. Ask visitors to step out of the room.

5. Tell the patient that a stool specimen is needed. Explain that whenever he can move his bowels he is to call you so the specimen can be collected.

6. Pull the curtain around the bed for privacy while the patient is on the bedpan.

7. Have the patient move his bowels into the bedpan.

8. Ask the patient not to urinate into the bedpan and not to put toilet tissue in the bedpan. Provide the patient with a wastepaper basket to temporarily dispose of the toilet tissue. Then discard it in the toilet or hopper.

9. Prepare the label immediately by copying all needed information from the patient's identification bracelet. Record the time of collection and the date.

10. After the patient has had a bowel movement, take the covered bedpan to the patient's bathroom or to the dirty utility room.

11. Using the wooden tongue depressor, take about 1 to 2 tablespoons of feces from the bedpan and place them in the stool specimen container. Put the correct label on the specimen container for the correct patient.

12. Wrap the tongue depressor in a paper towel and discard it.

13. Empty the remaining feces into the toilet or hopper.

14. Clean the bedpan and return it to its proper place.

15. If your head nurse or team leader told you this is a warm specimen, it must be taken to the laboratory for examination while it is still warm from the patient's body. Place the stool specimen container, fully labeled, in the plastic bag (if used by your hospital). Attach the laboratory request slip to the bag. Carry it immediately to the laboratory.

16. Report to your head nurse or team leader:
    - That a stool specimen has been obtained
    - That the specimen has been sent to the laboratory
    - The date and time of collection
    - Your observations of anything unusual

KEY IDEAS: STRAINING THE URINE

The urine is strained to determine if a patient has passed stones (calculi) or other matter from the kidneys. The doctor may order that all urine passed by the patient is to be strained.

Procedure: Straining the Urine

1. Assemble your equipment:
   a. Paper disposable strainers or gauze squares
   b. Specimen container with cover or a small plastic bag to be used as a specimen container

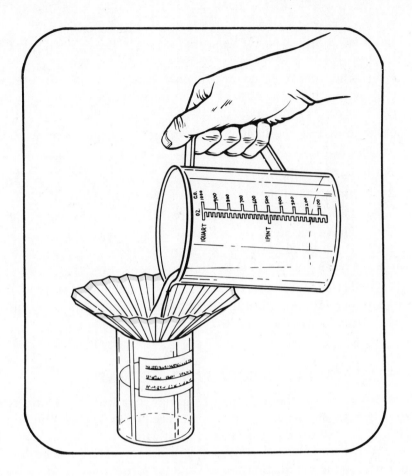

    c.   Label, if your hospital procedure is not to write on the lid

    d.   Patient's bedpan and cover, or urinal, or specipan

    e.   Laboratory request slip, which should be filled out by the head nurse, team leader, or ward clerk

    f.   Tag, to be placed over the bed indicating that all urine must be strained

2.   Wash your hands.

3.   Identify the patient by checking the identification bracelet.

4.   Ask visitors to step out of the room.

5.   Tell the patient that each time he urinates, it must be into a urinal, bedpan, or specipan. This is because it must be strained. Caution the patient not to put any tissue into the container.

6.   Pull the curtain around the bed for privacy whenever the patient voids.

7.   When the patient voids, take the bedpan or urinal to the patient's bathroom. Pour the urine through the strainer or gauze into the measuring container.

8.   Measure the amount of the voiding and record it on the Intake and Output sheet, if the patient is on intake and output.

9.   Discard the urine.

10.   If any particles show up on the gauze or the paper strainer, place the gauze or paper strainer with particles in a plastic bag or

specimen container. Do not attempt to remove the particles, because they may be lost or damaged.

11. Label the specimen container immediately. Copy all needed information from the patient's identification bracelet. Record the date and time of collection.

12. Clean and rinse the bedpan and graduate and put them in their proper places.

13. Wash your hands.

14. Report immediately to your head nurse or team leader:
    - That, in straining the urine, particles were obtained
    - That a specimen was collected
    - The date and time of collection
    - Your observations of anything unusual

15. The labeled specimen container must be sent or taken to the laboratory with a requisition or laboratory request slip at the head nurse's or team leader's request.

KEY IDEAS: TESTING FOR SUGAR AND ACETONE

When caring for a diabetic patient, you may be asked to perform certain diagnostic tests on the patient's urine. There are two basic tests: one for sugar (the Clinitest) and one for acetone (the Acetest). In your work you may collect the fresh FrU (fractional urine) specimen. But the actual test may be done in a laboratory or by the medication nurse. The term *fractional urine* is used to mean both the sugar and acetone tests, each with the collection of the fresh fractional urine specimen. The results of these tests are needed by the doctor and medication nurse for determining changes that must be made in the diabetic patient's diet and medication.

These tests are usually done four times a day: one-half hour before breakfast, lunch, supper, and bedtime.

For each test you will be using either a reagent strip or a reagent tablet. The names for these tablets or strips vary greatly according to geographical area and the pharmaceutical company from which they are purchased. When testing for sugar — doing the Clinitest — you will be using Clinitest tablets, Tes-Tape, Clinistix, or Uristix. When testing for acetone — doing the Acetest — you will be using Ketostix, Tes-Tape, acetone tablets, Uristix, or Labstix.

Some hospitals have a small individual disposable kit for these tests, which is ordered from CSR for each patient. The patient's name should be written on the still of the container. It should be kept in the patient's bathroom or a designated place in the dirty utility room.

Instructions for these tests are usually posted in every dirty utility room. You also will find instructions for these tests on the package of reagent strips or reagent tablets. All tablets and strips used for these tests are poisonous. Always put equipment in a safe place where children cannot reach them. Heat is generated during the Clinitest. Do not touch the bottom of the glass test tube while doing the tests.

A fresh specimen is needed to do both the sugar test and the acetone test. The word *fresh* is used to refer to urine that has been accumulated recently in the bladder. To obtain fresh urine, it is necessary to discard the first urine voided because this urine has remained in the bladder for an unknown length of time. One half-hour after discarding the urine, collect a fresh urine specimen for the test. This will be urine recently accumulated in the bladder. The word *fractional* is used to refer to a small portion of the urine voided. Only a very small amount of urine is needed for these tests.

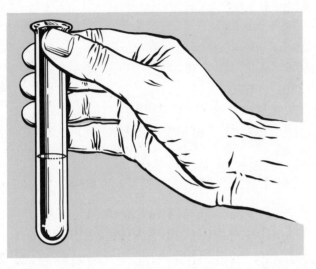

Procedure: Collecting a Fresh Fractional Urine (FrU) Specimen

1. Assemble your equipment:
   a. Patient's bedpan and cover, or urinal, or specipan
   b. Urine specimen container with lid
   c. Graduate, to measure output if the patient is on intake and output
   d. Label, if your hospital procedure is not to write on the lid

2. Wash your hands.

3. Identify the patient by checking the identification bracelet.

4. Ask visitors to step out of the room.

5. Tell the patient you need some urine for a urine test.

6. Pull the curtain around the bed for privacy.

7. Ask the patient to urinate into the bedpan or urinal or specipan a half-hour before the test is to be done, in order to empty his bladder.

8. When the patient is on intake and output, measure the urine and record the amount on the Intake and Output sheet.

9. Throw away this urine.

10. Have the patient void again at the correct time for the test so that fresh urine is used for the test.

11. Prepare a label for the container with the patient's name, copying from the patient's identification bracelet. Record the date and time of collection and the name of the specimen. Put the correct label on the specimen container for the correct patient.

12. Take the covered bedpan or urinal to the patient's bathroom or dirty utility room.

13. Measure and record the amount on the Intake and Output sheet if the patient is on intake and output.

14. Pour the urine into the urine specimen container and label it.

15. Discard the remaining urine. Wash the bedpan or urinal and put it in its proper place.

16. The labeled specimen container must be sent or taken immediately to the laboratory with a requisition or laboratory request slip.

17. Wash your hands.

18. Report to your head nurse or team leader:

   - That the fresh fractional urine specimen has been obtained
   - That the specimen has been sent to the laboratory
   - The date and time of collection
   - Your observations made of anything unusual

Procedure: The Clinitest
(2-Drop Method and 5-Drop Method)

1. Assemble your equipment:

   a. Fresh fractional urine specimen labeled with the patient's name
   b. Clean and dry test tube
   c. Color chart
   d. Medicine dropper
   e. Reagent tablet or reagent strip (Clinitest tablets, Tes-Tape, Clinistix, or Uristix)
   f. Paper cup of water for rinsing dropper
   g. Paper cup of clean water for test
   h. Paper towel

2. Wash your hands.

3. Place the paper towel on the countertop to be your work area.

4. Rinse the dropper in the paper cup that is used for rinsing only.

5. With the dropper in the upright position, place 5 drops of urine in the center of the test tube for the 5-drop method. For the 2-drop method, place 2 drops of urine in the center of the test tube. Be sure to check the package of reagent tablets to determine which method to use.

6. Rinse the dropper.

7. Place 10 drops of clean water in the center of the test tube.

8. Place 1 Clinitest tablet in the test tube. Never touch the tablet with your hands. If your hands are wet and you touch the tablet, the moisture could activate the reaction and you could be burned. Drop the tablet into the cover of the bottle. Then drop the tablet into the test tube from the cover. Then cap the bottle immediately. If the tablets are individually wrapped, open the foil carefully and drop the tablet into the test tube without touching the tablet.

9. Wait 15 seconds after the reaction (boiling) has stopped. Then gently shake the test tube.

10. Compare the test tube contents with the color chart.

11. Match the color of the liquid in the test tube to the nearest matching color on the chart. Be sure to use the color chart that goes with the tablets you have used for the test. The color chart for the 2-drop method is different from that for the 5-drop method. If the color is questionable, consult your head nurse or team leader.

12. Read the number inside the matching color box. For example: For the 5-drop method, if the color is bright orange, it will say 2% or 4+ + + + (plus) inside the orange-colored box. However, with the 2-drop method, if the color is bright orange, it will say 5% in the orange-colored box, because the 2-drop method is used to quantitate urine sugar over 2%.

13. Throw away used disposable equipment. Wash the test tube with cold water. Replace it upside down so that any remaining water will drain out. The test tube will then be ready for the next test. Rinse the medicine dropper with cold water. Put it in the rack in the upright position.

14. Wash your hands.

15. Report this amount (the number from the matching color box) to your head nurse, team leader, or medication nurse immediately. She will then enter the information on the patient's chart.

Procedure: The Clinistix Test

1. Assemble your equipment:
   a. Reagent strips
   b. Fresh fractional urine specimen, labeled with the patient's name

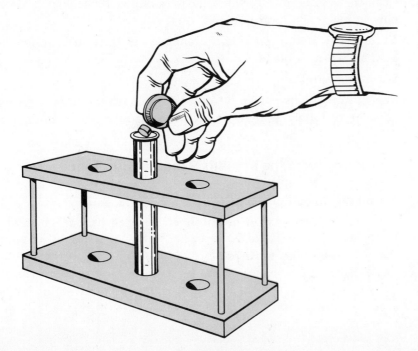

2. Wash your hands.
3. Place the reagent strip in the urine in the specimen container.
4. Wait 30 seconds and remove the strip. Compare it with the color chart. Read the results from the chart.
5. Throw away used disposable equipment.
6. Wash your hands.
7. Report your results to your head nurse, team leader, or medication nurse immediately, so that person can record the results on the patient's chart.

Procedure: Testing Urine for Acetone - The Acetest

1. Assemble your equipment:
    a. Fresh fractional urine specimen, labeled with the patient's name
    b. Color chart
    c. Medicine dropper
    d. Reagent tablet or strip (acetone tablets, Ketostix, Tes-Tape, Uristix, or Labstix)
    e. Paper cup of water for rinsing dropper
    f. Paper towel
2. Wash your hands.
3. Place 1 acetone tablet on a piece of paper towel.
4. Never touch the tablet, but drop it into the cover of its container. Then place it on the paper towel from the cover.
5. Drop 1 drop of urine to moisten the tablet. Wait 30 seconds.
6. Compare it to the color chart. Note the color of the tablet.
7. Match the color of the tablet to the color nearest matching on the chart.
8. Read the results from the chart. For example: If the color is dark purple, it will say "large quantity" on the chart.
9. Throw away used disposable equipment. Put the other equipment back in its proper place.
10. Wash your hands.
11. Report your results to your head nurse, team leader, or medication nurse immediately, so that person can record the results on the patient's chart.

Procedure: The Ketostix Reagent Strip Test

1. Assemble your equipment:
    a. Fresh fractional urine specimen, labeled with the patient's name
    b. Ketostix reagent strips
2. Wash your hands.

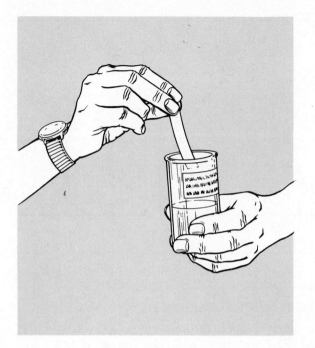

3. Place the Ketostix strip in the urine specimen.

4. Wait 30 seconds and remove the strip. Compare its color with the color chart. Read the results from the chart.

5. Throw away used disposable equipment.

6. Wash your hands.

7. Report your findings to your head nurse, team leader, or medication nurse immediately, so that person can record the results on the patient's chart.

Procedure: Collecting a Routine Urine Specimen from an Infant

1. Assemble your equipment:
   a. Urine specimen bottle
   b. Plastic disposable urine collector
   c. Label
   d. Laboratory requisition

2. Wash your hands.

3. Identify the patient by checking the identification bracelet.

4. Take off the child's diaper.

5. Make sure the child's skin is clean and dry in the genital area. This is where you are going to apply the urine collector, which is a small plastic bag.

6. Remove the outside piece that surrounds the opening of the plastic urine collector. This leaves a sticky area, which is placed around

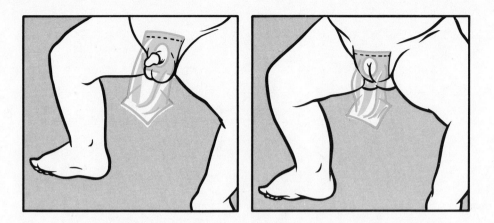

the boy baby's penis or the girl baby's vulva. Don't cover the baby's rectum.

7. Put the child's diaper on as usual.

8. Come back and check every half hour to see if the infant has voided. You can't feel the diaper to find out. You must open up the diaper and look at the urine collector.

9. When the infant has voided, remove the plastic urine collector. It comes off easily. Wash off any sticky residue.

10. Replace the child's diaper.

11. Put the specimen in the specimen container and cover it immediately.

12. Label the container properly. Check the patient's identification bracelet.

13. The labeled specimen container must be sent or taken to the laboratory with a requisition or laboratory request slip. The slip is usually filled out by the head nurse or team leader or ward clerk.

14. Wash your hands.

15. Report to your head nurse or team leader:

   • That you have collected a routine urine specimen
   • That you have sent it to the laboratory
   • The date and time of collection
   • Your observations of anything unusual

WHAT YOU HAVE LEARNED

A specimen is a sample amount of a substance taken from the patient's body. You will be collecting various specimens. A mistake in collecting or labeling a specimen may cause a mistake in the laboratory report. This might be dangerous to the patient.

Each different kind of specimen that you collect requires a different kind of container. Be sure to use the right one. All specimens must be properly labeled. Never fill the specimen container completely full.

A sputum specimen must be of coughed-up material, not saliva. Stool specimens usually must be still warm in order to be useful in the laboratory. You also will do some diagnostic testing of patients' urine. This includes straining the urine and making the sugar and acetone tests.

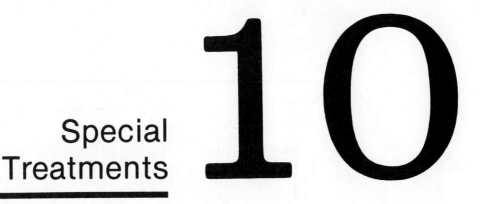

Special Treatments 10

OBJECTIVES: WHAT YOU WILL LEARN

When you have completed this chapter, you should be able:

- To administer cleansing enemas
- To administer a retention enema
- To give colostomy care
- To give daily catheter care
- To care for a patient's artificial eye

KEY IDEAS: RECTAL TREATMENTS

Cleansing enemas and oil retention enemas are given to patients by nursing aides. A cleansing enema is washing out waste materials (feces or stool) from the person's lower bowel. An oil retention enema is used to insert oil into the rectum. The reason is to soften the stool. Retention means that the patient keeps the fluid (oil) in his rectum for 20 minutes. Giving enemas has been made easier in recent years by the use of disposable, prepacked enema kits. These plastic enema kits contain an enema bag, tubing, and a clamp. The kit should be used once and then thrown away.

If the patient has any complaints, before you start giving him an enema, report this to your head nurse or team leader. Don't go ahead with the enema until you are told to do so.

Sometimes the patient says he is having a cramp-like pain after the enema has started. If this happens, stop the flow of solution until the pain goes away. If you stop the flow and then start again when the pain is gone, the full amount of solution can usually be given without causing the patient very much discomfort.

The Cleansing Enema

The cleansing enema is given only on orders from the patient's physician. This enema is used most often to promote evacuation when this doesn't happen naturally. Evacuation means discharge of the contents of the lower bowel through the rectum and anus.

Cleansing enemas may also be given in preparation for certain diagnostic tests. They are also used in preparing a patient for an operation or the delivery of a baby.

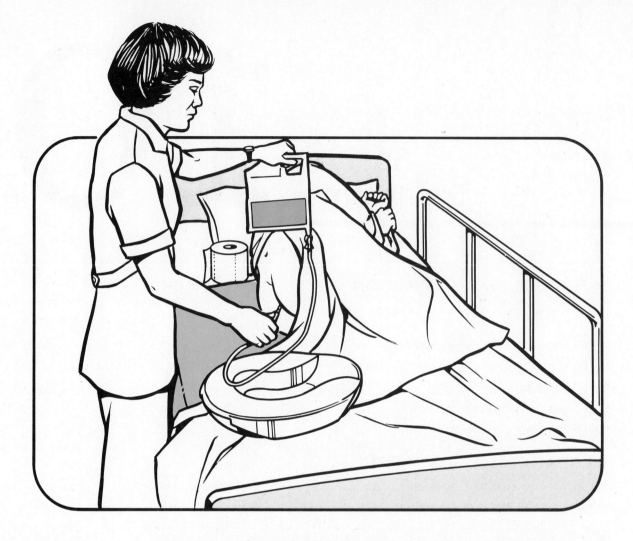

The solution used in the cleansing enema may be a commercial preparation supplied with a disposable enema kit. Or it may be a solution of salt and water, a weak mixture of soap and water, or sometimes plain tap water.

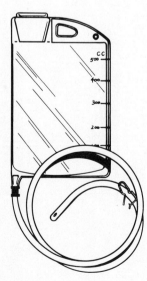

Procedure: Giving the Cleansing Enema

1. Assemble your equipment:
    a. Disposable enema kit (enema container, tubing, and clamp)
    b. Lubricating jelly
    c. Graduate
    d. Bath thermometer
    e. Solution as instructed by head nurse or team leader:
        • Soapsuds: 1 package enema soap, 1,000 cc water, 105° F (40.5° C)
        • Saline: 2 teaspoons salt, 1,000 cc water, 105° F (40.5° C)
        • Tap water only: 1,000 cc water, 105° F (40.5° C)

    f. Bedpan and cover
    g. Urinal, if necessary
    h. Emesis basin
    i. Toilet tissue

      j.   Disposable bed protector

      k.   Paper towel

      l.   Bath blanket

2. Wash your hands.

3. Identify the patient by checking the identification bracelet.

4. Ask visitors to step out of the room.

5. Tell the patient that you are going to give him an enema while he is in bed.

6. Pull the curtain around the bed for privacy.

7. Cover the patient with a bath blanket. Without exposing him, fanfold the top sheets to the foot of the bed. Have the patient covered only with the bath blanket.

8. Place the disposable bed protector under the patient's hips (buttocks).

9. Turn the patient on his left side. Bend his right knee toward his chest. (This is the left Sims' position.)

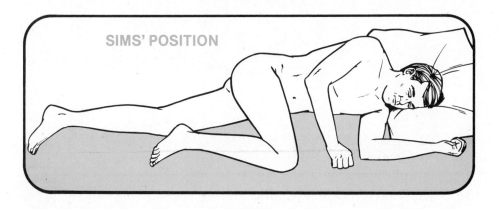

SIMS' POSITION

10. Put the bedpan at the foot of the bed within easy reach.

11. Close the clamp on the enema tubing.

12. Fill the pitcher with 1,000 cc water at 105° F (40.5° C).

13. Pour the water from the pitcher into the enema container.

14.   a.   If you are giving a soapsuds enema, add one package of enema soap to the water in the container. Use the tip of the tubing to mix the solution gently so that no suds form.

      b.   If your instructions call for a saline enema, add two teaspoons of salt to the water in the container.

      c.   If your instructions call for tap water only, do not add anything to the water.

15. Open the clamp on the enema tubing. Let the solution run through the tubing into the bedpan. This will get rid of any air in the tubing and warm the tube. Then close the clamp.

16. Put the lubricating jelly on a piece of toilet tissue. Lubricate the enema tip by rubbing the jelly on it with the tissue. Be sure the tip is well lubricated and the opening is not plugged.

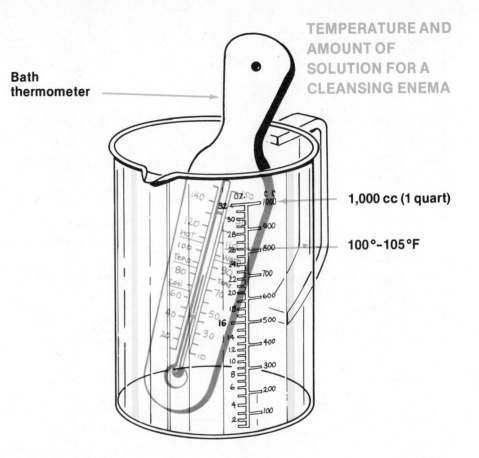

Bath thermometer

TEMPERATURE AND AMOUNT OF SOLUTION FOR A CLEANSING ENEMA

1,000 cc (1 quart)

100°–105°F

17. Expose the patient's buttocks by raising the blanket in a triangle over the anal area.

18. Raise the upper buttock so you can see the anal area.

19. Gently insert the enema tip from 2 to 4 inches through the anus into the rectum.

20. Open the clamp and hold the enema container 12 inches above the anus or 18 inches above the mattress.

21. Tell the patient to take deep breaths and to let the air out slowly. Explain that this will help relieve the cramps caused by the enema. It will also help the patient to relax.

22. When most of the solution has flowed into the patient's rectum, close the clamp. Slowly withdraw the rectal tubing. Wrap it in the paper towel to avoid contamination. Put the tubing in the enema container.

23. Help the patient onto the bedpan. Raise the back of the bed, if allowed. Put the toilet tissue where the patient can reach it easily.

24. The patient may be allowed by the nurse to go to the bathroom to expel the enema. If so, you must assist him to the bathroom. Tell the patient not to flush the toilet. This is so the results can be observed.

25. Give the patient the signal cord. Check on the patient every few minutes.

26. Dispose of the enema equipment while the patient is on the bedpan.

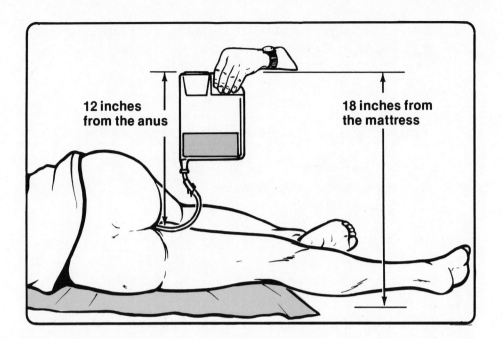

12 inches
from the anus

18 inches from
the mattress

27. When observing the results of an enema, look for anything that does not appear normal.

Report to your head nurse or team leader if the stool:
- Is very hard
- Is very soft
- Is large in amount
- Is small in amount
- Is accompanied by flatus

Collect a specimen and report to your head nurse or team leader if the stool:
- Is completely black
- Is streaked with red, white, or yellow
- Has a very bad odor
- Has little or no odor
- Looks like perked coffee grounds

28. Empty the bedpan. Clean it and put it in its proper place.

29. Remove the disposable bed protector and discard it.

30. Remove the bath blanket. At the same time, raise the top sheets to cover the patient.

31. Make the patient comfortable.

32. Wash the patient's hands.

33. Wash your own hands.

34. Report to your head nurse or team leader:
- That you have given the patient an enema
- The time and type of enema given

- The results, color of stool, consistency, flatus (gas) expelled, and unusual material noted
- Whether or not a specimen was obtained
- Your observations of anything unusual

Procedure: Giving the Ready-to-Use Cleansing Enema

1. Assemble your equipment:
   a. Disposable prepackaged enema
   b. Bedpan and cover
   c. Urinal, if necessary
   d. Disposable bed protector
2. Wash your hands.
3. Identify the patient by checking the identification bracelet.
4. Ask visitors to step out of the room.
5. Tell the patient you are going to give him a cleansing enema while he is in bed.
6. Pull the curtain around the bed for privacy.
7. Cover the patient with a bath blanket. Without exposing him, fanfold the top sheets to the foot of the bed. Have the patient covered only with the bath blanket.
8. Place the disposable bed protector under the patient's hips (buttocks).

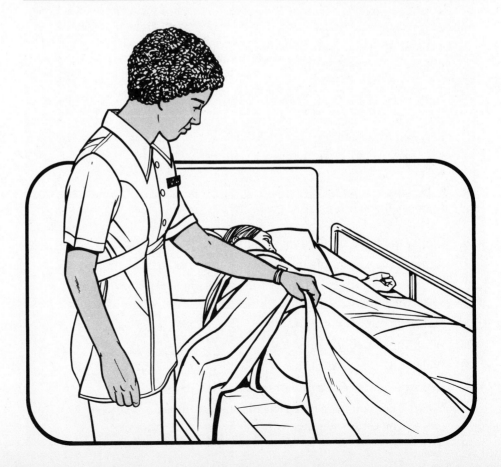

9. Turn the patient on his left side. Bend his right knee toward his chest. (This is the left Sims' position.)

10. Put the bedpan at the foot of the bed within easy reach.

11. Open the enema package. Take out the disposable enema. Remove the cap.

12. Expose the patient's buttocks by raising the blanket in a triangle over the anal area.

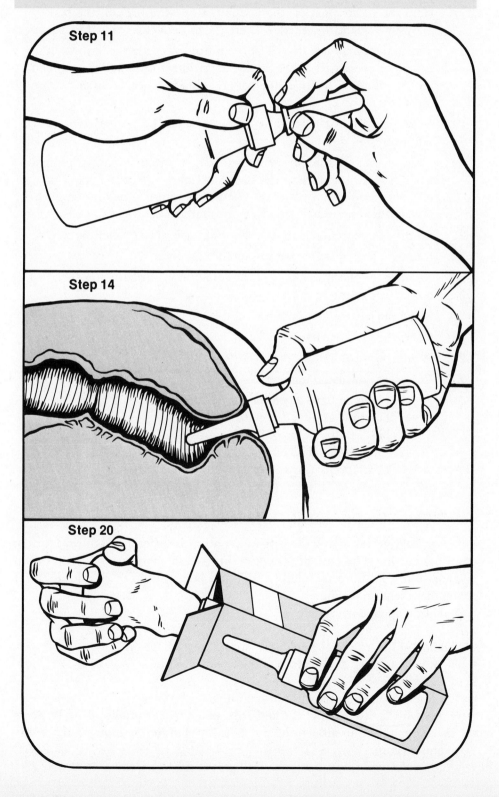

Step 11

Step 14

Step 20

13. Raise the upper buttock so you can see the anal area.

14. Gently insert the enema tip, which is already lubricated, two inches through the anus into the rectum.

15. Squeeze the plastic bottle until all the liquid goes into the patient's rectum.

16. Remove the tube from the patient's anus. Put the empty plastic bottle back in the box. You will discard it later.

17. Help the patient get on the bedpan. Raise the back of the bed, if allowed. Put the toilet tissue where the patient can reach it easily.

18. The patient may be allowed by the nurse to go into the bathroom to expel the enema. If so, you must assist him to the bathroom. Tell the patient not to flush the toilet. This is so the results can be observed.

19. Give the patient the signal cord. Check on the patient every few minutes.

20. Discard the disposable enema equipment. Return to the patient when he is finished using the bedpan. Check the contents for color of stool, consistency, amount, unusual material, or anything abnormal. If you observe anything unusual, collect a specimen.

21. Empty the bedpan, clean it, and put it back in its proper place.

22. Remove the disposable bed protector and discard it.

23. Remove the bath blanket. At the same time, raise the top sheets to cover the patient.

24. Make the patient comfortable.

25. Wash the patient's hands.

26. Wash your own hands.

27. Report to your head nurse or team leader:

   - That you have given the patient an enema
   - The time and type of enema given
   - The results, color of stool, consistency, flatus expelled, and unusual material noted
   - Your observations of anything unusual

KEY IDEAS: THE OIL RETENTION ENEMA

The procedure for giving the retention enema is different from that for the cleansing enema. The patient is expected to retain (hold in) the enema solution for 10 to 20 minutes. Usually a soapsuds enema is given 20 minutes after giving the retention enema.

Retention enemas are given:

- To help soften the feces and gently stimulate evacuation
- To lubricate the inside surface of the lower intestine
- To soften the stool, if necessary
- To ease passage of feces without straining
- To provide laxative benefits when oral laxatives are not allowed to be given
- To help the patient eliminate barium sulfate residues after x-ray examinations

- To soften fecal impaction (hard stool caught in the lower bowel) when straining might be harmful or painful

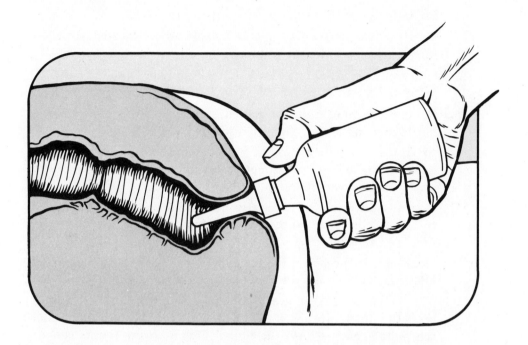

Procedure: Giving the Ready-To-Use Oil Retention Enema

1. Assemble your equipment:
   a. Disposable prepackaged ready-to-use oil enema kit
   b. Bedpan and cover
   c. Urinal, if necessary
   d. Disposable bed protector
   e. Equipment for soapsuds enema, if ordered 20 minutes after oil retention enema
2. Wash your hands.
3. Identify the patient by checking the identification bracelet.
4. Ask visitors to step out of the room.
5. Tell the patient that you are going to give him an oil retention enema while he is in bed.
6. Pull the curtain around the bed for privacy.
7. Cover the patient with a bath blanket. Without exposing him, fanfold the top sheets to the foot of the bed. Have the patient covered only with the bath blanket.
8. Place the disposable bed protector under the patient's hips (buttocks).
9. Turn the patient on his left side. Bend his right knee toward his chest. (This is the left Sims' position.)
10. Put the bedpan at the foot of the bed within easy reach.
11. Open the package. Take out the disposable prepackaged ready-to-use enema bag filled with oil. Remove the cap.

12. Expose the patient's buttocks by raising the blanket in a triangle over the anal area.

13. Raise the upper buttock so you can see the anal area.

14. Gently insert the enema tip, which is already lubricated, 2 inches through the anus into the rectum.

15. Squeeze the plastic bottle until all the liquid goes into the patient's rectum.

16. Remove the tube from the patient's anus. Put the empty plastic bottle back in the box. You will discard it later.

17. Explain to the patient that he must retain (hold in) the oil for 20 minutes. Encourage the patient to stay in the Sims' position. Check on the patient every few minutes.

18. Your instructions may require you to give a soapsuds enema after the patient has retained the oil for 20 minutes. If so, give the soapsuds enema at this time.

19. Help the patient get on the bedpan. Raise the back of the bed, if allowed. Put the toilet tissue where the patient can reach it easily.

20. The patient may be allowed by the nurse to go to the bathroom to expel the enema. If so, you must help him get to the bathroom. Tell the patient not to flush the toilet. This is so the results can be observed.

21. Give the patient the signal cord. Check on the patient every few minutes.

22. Discard the disposable enema equipment.

23. Return to the patient when he is finished using the bedpan. Check the contents for color of stool, consistency, amount, unusual material, or anything abnormal. If you observe anything unusual, collect a specimen.

24. Empty the bedpan, clean it, and put it back in its proper place.

25. Remove the disposable bed protector and discard it.

26. Remove the bath blanket. At the same time, raise the top sheets to cover the patient.

27. Make the patient comfortable.

28. Wash the patient's hands.

29. Wash your own hands.

30. Report to your head nurse or team leader:
    - That you have given the patient an enema
    - The time the oil enema was given
    - The results, color of stool, consistency, flatus expelled, and unusual material noted
    - Your observations of anything unusual

KEY IDEAS: THE HARRIS FLUSH (RETURN-FLOW ENEMA)

The Harris flush is an irrigation of the rectum. Irrigation means washing out. Clean water runs into the rectum. Gas (flatus) and water run out of the rectum. Then clean water runs into the rectum. Flatus and water run out of the rectum in the return flow. This procedure is repeated for 10 minutes until the patient is relieved of excess gas.

Procedure: Giving the Harris Flush (Return-Flow Enema)

1. Assemble your equipment:
   a. Disposable enema bag, tubing, and clamp
   b. Lubricating jelly
   c. Graduate
   d. Bath thermometer
   e. Urinal, if necessary
   f. Emesis basin
   g. Toilet tissue
   h. Disposable bed protector
   i. Paper towel
   j. Bath blanket
   k. Bedpan

2. Wash your hands.

3. Identify the patient by checking the identification bracelet.

4. Ask visitors to step out of the room.

5. Explain to the patient that you are going to give him a Harris flush.

6. Pull the curtain around the bed for privacy.

7. Cover the patient with a bath blanket. Without exposing him, fanfold the top sheets to the foot of the bed. Have the patient covered only with the bath blanket.

8. Place the disposable bed protector under the patient's hips (buttocks).

9. Turn the patient on his left side. Bend his right knee toward his chest. (This is the left Sims' position.)

10. Put the bedpan at the foot of the bed within easy reach.

11. Close the clamp on the enema tubing.

12. Fill the pitcher with 500 cc of water, 105° F (40.5° C). Measure the temperature of the water with the bath thermometer.

13. Pour the water from the pitcher into the enema container.

14. Open the clamp on the enema tubing to let water run through the tubing into the bedpan. This will get rid of any air that may be in the tubing. It also warms the tube. Then close the clamp.

15. Put the lubricating jelly on a piece of toilet tissue. Lubricate the enema tip by rubbing the jelly on it with the tissue. Be sure the tip is well lubricated and the opening is not plugged.

16. Expose the patient's buttocks by raising the blanket in a triangle over the anal area.

17. Raise the upper buttock so you can see the anal area.

18. Gently insert the enema tip from 2 to 4 inches through the anus into the rectum.

19. Open the clamp. Hold the enema container 12 inches above the anus. Allow about 200 cc of water to enter the rectum.

20. Lower the enema bag below the bed frame. Let the water run back into the enema bag without removing the tube from the patient's rectum.

21. Hold the enema bag 12 inches above the anus. Let 200 cc of water run into the patient's rectum. Then lower the bag. Allow the water to run back into the enema bag. Keep the tube in the patient's rectum.

22. Continue letting water in and out of the rectum for 10 to 20 minutes as you are instructed.

23. Tell the patient to take deep breaths. Tell him to let the breaths out slowly. Explain that this kind of breathing will help relieve the cramps caused by the enema. It will also help him to relax.

24. Observe the amount (large or small) of flatus the patient expels as the water runs out into the enema bag.

25. Remove the tubing when the treatment is finished. Wrap the enema tip in the paper towel. This is to avoid contamination. Put it in the disposable enema container.

26. Help the patient get on the bedpan. Raise the back of the bed, if allowed. Put the toilet tissue where the patient can reach it easily. Give the patient the signal cord. Check on the patient every few minutes.

27. The patient may be allowed by the nurse to go to the bathroom to expel more flatus. If so, you must help him get to the bathroom. Tell the patient to check the amount of flatus (large or small) that he expels.

28. Dispose of the enema equipment while the patient is on the bedpan.

29. Return to the patient when he is finished using the bedpan. Check the contents of the bedpan for bowel movement, color of stool, consistency, amount, unusual material, or anything abnormal. If you observe anything unusual, collect a specimen. Ask the patient if flatus was expelled.

30. Empty the bedpan, clean it, and put it back in its proper place.

31. Remove the disposable bed protector and discard it.

32. Remove the bath blanket. At the same time, raise the top sheets to cover the patient.

33. Make the patient comfortable.

34. Wash the patient's hands.

35. Wash your own hands.

36. Report to your head nurse or team leader:
    - That you have given the patient an enema
    - The time the Harris flush was given and how long it was continued
    - The results, amount of flatus expelled, and unusual material noted
    - Whether or not a specimen was obtained
    - Your observations of anything unusual

KEY IDEAS: POSITIONING THE PATIENT FOR THE ENEMA

Left Sims' Position

Most patients are given enemas in the left Sims' position.

Paraplegic Enema

Sometimes the patient can't be on his side. He may be unconscious, paralyzed, mentally confused, unable to understand, or very uncooperative. He may be unable to retain the enema fluid. In these cases, the patient lies on his back. His buttocks are raised over the bedpan with the knees separated. The patient should be draped with a small sheet so as not to be exposed. The nursing aide wears disposable gloves. The rectal tube is inserted into the patient's anus from between the legs. This is sometimes called the paraplegic method.

Rotating Enema

The patient is given one-third of the enema while he is lying on his left side. Then one-third more is given while he is lying on his abdomen (prone). The final one-third of the enema is given while the patient is lying on his right side. The reason is so the enema solution will first enter the descending colon. Then it will go to the transverse colon. Last it will enter the ascending colon. This is why it is called a rotating enema.

KEY IDEAS: DISPOSABLE RECTAL TUBE WITH CONNECTED FLATUS BAG

A rectal tube with connected bag is used to relieve the accumulation of intestinal gas (flatus) that often accumulates in the patient's lower bowel. You will use the rectal tube only once a day for 20 minutes, unless otherwise instructed. The whole kit—tube and bag—is discarded after one use.

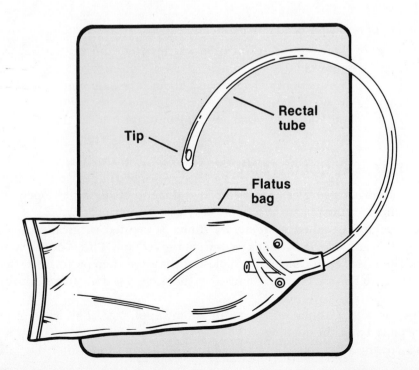

Procedure: Using the Disposable Rectal Tube with Connected Flatus Bag

1. Assemble your equipment:
    b. Disposable rectal tube with connected flatus bag
    b. Small piece of adhesive tape
    c. Tissue
    d. Lubricating jelly
2. Wash your hands.
3. Identify the patient by checking the identification bracelet.
4. Ask visitors to step out of the room.
5. Explain to the patient that you are going to insert a rectal tube.
6. Pull the curtain around the bed for privacy.
7. Turn the patient on his left side. Bend his right knee toward his chest. (This is the left Sims' position.)
8. Expose the patient's buttocks by raising the top sheets in a triangle over the anal area.
9. Lubricate the tip of the rectal tube. Do this by squeezing lubricating jelly onto the tissue and rubbing the jelly on the tip. (If the rectal tube is already lubricated, this step is not necessary.)
10. Raise the patient's upper buttock so you can see the anal area.
11. Gently insert the rectal tube 2 to 4 inches through the anus into the rectum.
12. Use a small piece of adhesive tape to attach the tube to the patient's buttocks in order to hold the tube in place.
13. Let the tube remain in place for 20 minutes. Then remove and discard the equipment. (Usually this procedure is done once in a 24-hour period.)
14. Wash your hands.
15. Report to your head nurse or team leader:
    - The time the rectal tube was inserted and the time it was removed
    - The patient's comments about the amount—small or large—of flatus that he expelled through the tube
    - Your observations of anything unusual

KEY IDEAS: THE COLOSTOMY

A colostomy is a surgical operation. It is done to create a new opening on the abdomen for the release of solid wastes (feces) from the body.

The opening is called a *stoma*. A stoma is created surgically to divert (change the path of) the patient's feces from the rectum. This is done when his colon is diseased, as in cancer. The colostomy is most often performed when it is necessary to remove tumors. Sometimes the surgery is done to permit repair of bowel injuries.

A person with a stoma must wear an ostomy appliance. This is a collecting device placed over the opening.

As a nursing aide, you will be taking care of the colostomy after the patient

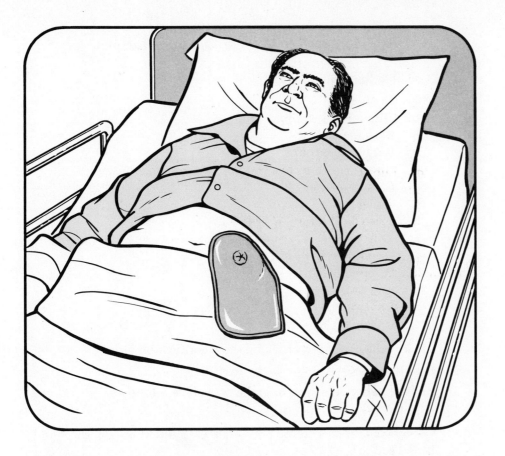

has been fitted with an ostomy appliance. This is usually called an old colostomy.

Sometimes the patient is able and wants to care for his colostomy himself. In this case, get permission from the nurse for him to do this.

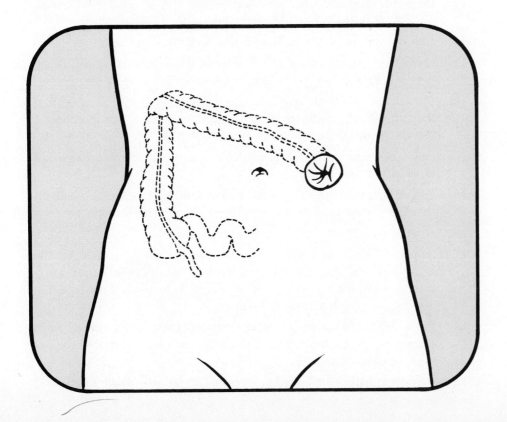

Procedure: Caring for an Old Colostomy

1. Assemble your equipment:
    a. Bedpan
    b. Disposable bed protectors
    c. Bath blanket
    d. Large emesis basin
    e. Clean colostomy belt (ostomy appliance), adjustable
    f. Clean stoma bag
    g. Toilet tissue
    h. Basin of water at 115°F (46.1°C)
    i. Soap
    j. Disposable washcloths
    k. Disposable gloves
    l. Towels
    m. Lubricant

2. Wash your hands.

3. Identify the patient by checking the identification bracelet.

4. Ask visitors to step out of the room.

5. Tell the patient that you will take care of his colostomy.

6. Pull the curtain around the bed for privacy.

7. Cover the patient with the bath blanket. Fanfold the top sheet and bedspread to the foot of the bed.

8. Put the disposable bed protector under the patient's hips. This is to keep the bed from getting dirty.

9. Place the bedpan and emesis basin within easy reach.

10. Have the wash basin (with water at 115° F (46.1° C), soap, disposable washcloth, and bath towels on the bedside table.

11. Remove the soiled plastic bag (stoma bag) from the belt.

12. Open the belt. Protect it if it is clean and can be used again. If the belt is dirty, remove it. It will have to be replaced with a clean belt.

13. Put the soiled plastic bag into the bedpan. Wipe the area around the colostomy with toilet tissue. This is to remove any loose feces. Put the tissue in the bedpan or emesis basin.

14. Soap the washcloth. Gently wash the entire colostomy area with a circular motion.

15. Rinse the entire area very well. Be careful not to leave any soap on the skin. (Soap has a drying effect and may irritate the skin.)

16. Dry the area gently with a bath towel.

17. Apply a small amount of lubricant around the area of the colostomy. Put it on the skin nearby. The lubricant is to prevent irritation to the skin. Wipe off all excess lubricant. This is so the ostomy device will stick to the skin.

18. Put a clean adjustable belt on the patient. Use a clean stoma bag in place through the loop. This is to catch any other excretions the patient may have later.

19. Remove the disposable bed protector. Change any damp linen.

20. Replace the top sheet and bedspread on the patient. Remove the bath blanket.

21. Make the patient comfortable. Ask him how he wants his bed raised, if allowed.

22. Remove all used equipment. Dispose of waste material in large garbage containers with covers in the dirty utility room.

23. Clean the bedpan and replace it where it belongs.

24. Empty the wash basin. Wash it throughly with soap. Rinse it. Dry it and return it to its proper place.

25. Wash your hands.

26. Report to your head nurse or team leader:
    - That the colostomy was cleaned
    - The amount of drainage
    - The consistency of the excretions
    - Your observations of anything unusual

KEY IDEAS: PERINEAL CARE

Perineal care is always given before catheter care. It provides cleanliness and comfort for the patient. It helps to prevent irritation and infection.

Procedure: Giving Perineal Care

1. Assemble your equipment:
    a. Disposable bed protector
    b. Bedpan and cover
    c. Graduated container
    d. Cotton balls

2. Wash your hands.

3. Identify the patient by checking the identification bracelet.

4. Ask visitors to step out of the room.

5. Tell the patient that you are going to give perineal care—that you are going to clean the genital area.

6. Pull the curtains around the bed for privacy.

7. Be sure there is plenty of light.

8. Cover the patient with a bath blanket. Without exposing him, fanfold the top sheets to the foot of the bed. Have the patient covered only with the blanket.

9. Fill the graduated container with warm water at 100° F (37.7° C), or use the solution provided in your hospital.

10. Place the disposable bed protector under the patient's buttocks.

11. Help the patient to get on the bedpan.

12. Pour the warm water or warm solution over the perineal (genital) area.

13. Dry the patient gently with the cotton balls.

14. Remove the bedpan and disposable bed protector. Place them at the foot of the bed or on a chair.

15. Cover the patient with the top sheets. Remove the bath blanket. Make the patient comfortable.

16. Empty, rinse, and put the equipment back where it belongs.

17. Discard disposable equipment.

18. Wash your hands.

19. Report to your head nurse or team leader:
    - That you have given the patient perineal care
    - The time and date it was given
    - Your observations of anything unusual

KEY IDEAS: DAILY CATHETER CARE

A catheter is a tube inserted through the patient's urethra into the bladder to allow for drainage. The catheter is specially made so that it will stay in place within the patient's bladder.

Daily catheter care is very important to prevent infection. Medical aseptic technique should be used at all times when you are handling and caring for the equipment.

The catheter is attached to tubing that should be taped loosely to the inner side of the patient's thigh. This is so it does not pull. This tubing leads to a plastic urine container. The container is attached to the bed frame. It is lower than the level of the urinary bladder so there is a constant downhill flow from the patient. The urine collects in a plastic container.

This is a closed drainage system. The system must never be opened. If the patient is allowed to get out of bed, the container is carried at a lower level than the patient's bladder. A careful record of urinary output is kept for all patients who have catheters in place.

Procedure: Giving Daily Catheter Care

1. Assemble your equipment:
    a. Disposable catheter care kit
    b. Disposable gloves

2. Wash your hands.

3. Identify the patient by checking the identification bracelet.

4. Ask visitors to step out of the room.

5. Tell the patient you are going to give him catheter care on the tube he has in place. Make sure the patient's genital area has already been washed.

6. Pull the curtains around the bed for privacy.

7. Make sure there is plenty of light. You will be watching for crusting, lesions, or anything else abnormal.

8. Cover the patient with a bath blanket. Without exposing him, fan fold the top sheets to the foot of the bed. Have the patient covered with only the blanket.

9. Open the catheter kit.

10. Put on the disposable gloves.

11. Take the applicators from the kit. The applicators are covered with antiseptic solution. Apply antiseptic solution on the entire area where the catheter enters the patient's body. Gently separate the labia on female patients. If the male patient has a foreskin, gently pull it back to apply antiseptic solution to the entire area.

12. Apply antiseptic solution to the four inches of the tube closest to the patient.

13. Apply the antiseptic ointment where the tube is inserted.

14. Cover the patient with the top sheets. Remove the bath blanket. Make the patient comfortable.

15. Remove the disposable bed protector.

16. Discard the disposable equipment.

17. Wash your hands.

18. Report to your head nurse or team leader:
    - That catheter care has been given
    - The time it was given
    - Your observations of anything unusual

THE URINARY CATHETER

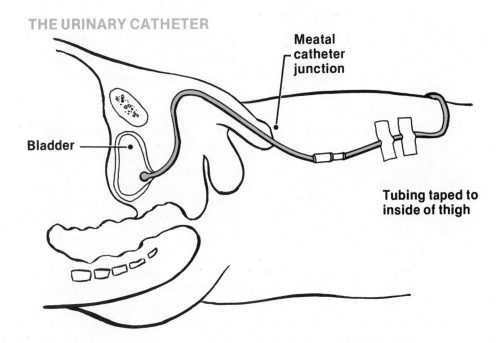

Meatal catheter junction

Bladder

Tubing taped to inside of thigh

KEY IDEAS: CARE OF THE PATIENT'S ARTIFICIAL EYE

Cleaning the patient's artificial eye is part of daily personal hygiene. Often a patient can't care for it himself. If he has an artificial eye, it must be cared for properly to prevent infection and encrustation. (Encrustation means formation of dried mucus material in the eye socket and around the artificial eye.)

Procedure: Caring for the Artificial Eye

1. Assemble your equipment:
    a. An eyecup half-filled with lukewarm water (98° F–100° F, 36.6° C–37.7° C) and labeled with the patient's name and room number
    b. Gauze, 4 x 4 (2 pieces), for the bottom of the cup
    c. Small basin with lukewarm water
    d. Cotton balls (4)
    e. Optional: any special cleansing solution the doctor may order

2. Wash your hands.

3. Ask visitors to step out of the room.

4. Identify the patient by checking the identification bracelet.

5. Tell the patient you are going to take care of his eye.

6. Pull the curtains around the bed for privacy.

7. Help the patient to lie down on the bed. This is to prevent accidental dropping of the artificial eye.

8. Clean any external secretions from the patient's upper eyelid. Use cotton balls and warm water from the basin. Clean from the nose to the outside of the eye. Use gentle strokes.

9. Remove the artificial eye. To do this, carefully depress the lower eyelid with your thumb. Lift the upper lid gently with your forefinger. The eye should slide out and down.

10. Place the eye in the cup on the 4 x 4 gauze. Let it soak in the water.

11. Clean the eye socket. Wash off external matter and encrustations with cotton balls and water. Using gentle strokes, work from the inner canthus to the outer. This means that you move from the nose to the outside of the eye area.

12. Take the eyecup to the patient's bathroom. Close the drain in the sink. Fill the sink one-half full with water to prevent breakage if the eye is dropped.

13. Wash the eye with running water. Use plain water unless the doctor ordered a special solution. Leave the eye in the gauze and rub gently between your thumb and forefinger. Do not use alcohol, ether, or acetone. These dissolve the plastic of the artificial eye and also may dull the luster.

14. Rinse the eye under running lukewarm water (98° F–100° F, 36.6° C–37.7° C). Then dry it. Use the second 4 x 4 gauze. Discard the water from the eyecup. Place the slightly moistened eye on dry gauze in the eyecup. A slightly moistened eye is easier to insert. Return to the patient's bedside.

15. If the patient cannot wear the eye, store it in the eyecup with water.

16. Wash your hands thoroughly a second time before inserting the artificial eye.

17. Insert the eye in the patient's eye socket. Have the notched edge toward the nose. Raise the upper lid with your forefinger. With your other hand, insert the eye. Place the eye under the upper lid. Then depress the lower lid. The eye should settle in place.

18. Discard your used supplies. Leave the patient's area neat.

19. Report to your head nurse or team leader that you have completed care of the artificial eye. Also, report your observations of anything unusual.

WHAT YOU HAVE LEARNED

The guiding principles for all forms of special treatments are effectiveness, safety, good aseptic technique, and consideration for the patient's comfort. The disposable, ready-to-use equipment and the correct technique help you meet all these requirements conveniently and efficiently.

Observing and Recording Vital Signs

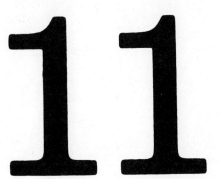

Section 1: Vital Signs

OBJECTIVES: WHAT YOU WILL LEARN

When you have completed this section, you should be able:

- To explain vital signs
- To state the average adult normal rates

KEY IDEAS

When the body is not functioning normally, changes happen in the measurable rates of the vital signs. Everyone who is taking and recording information about patients' vital signs must be very careful and accurate. When you record the readings, write carefully. Make sure your handwriting is clear and easy to read. If you are not sure of your readings, tell your head nurse or team leader. All hospitals use these abbreviations for the vital signs:

- Temperature = T
- Pulse = P
- Respiration = R
- Blood Pressure = BP
- Vital Signs = TPR & BP

When your head nurse or team leader says:

- "Take temps," she means take the patient's temperature, pulse, and respiration.
- "Take vital signs," she means take the patient's temperature, pulse, respiration, and blood pressure.
- "Take blood pressure," she means take the patient's blood pressure, pulse, and respiration.

Write down the numbers for the patient's temperature, pulse, respiration, and blood pressure right away. If you are using a TPR book, check to find the right column. The columns have certain hours of the day written at the top—for example, 8 a.m., 12 noon.

VITAL SIGNS

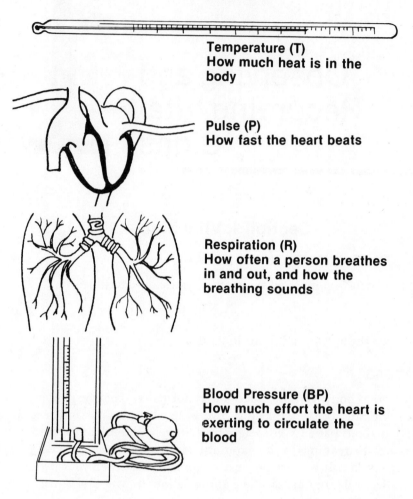

Temperature (T)
How much heat is in the body

Pulse (P)
How fast the heart beats

Respiration (R)
How often a person breathes in and out, and how the breathing sounds

Blood Pressure (BP)
How much effort the heart is exerting to circulate the blood

Check the patient's name. Be sure you are writing the vital signs opposite the right name and at the right time. Report to the nurse if there are changes in the patient's temperature, pulse, respiration, or blood pressure. In most hospitals this is done by drawing a red circle around the number on the "temp" board or in the TPR book.

Average Normal Adult Rates

Temperature: 98.6°F or 37°C

Pulse: 72–80 beats per minute

Respiration: 16–20 per minute

Section 2: Measuring the Patient's Temperature

OBJECTIVES: WHAT YOU WILL LEARN

When you have completed this section, you should be able:

- To read a thermometer accurately
- To demonstrate the procedure for taking oral temperatures
- To demonstrate the procedure for taking rectal temperatures
- To demonstrate the procedure for taking axillary temperatures

KEY IDEAS: BODY TEMPERATURE

Body temperature is a measurement of the amount of heat in the body. The body creates heat in the process of changing food into energy. The body also loses heat—through perspiration, respiration (breathing), and excretion. The balance between the heat produced and the heat lost is the body temperature. The normal adult body temperature is 98.6° Fahrenheit, or 37° Centigrade.

The body temperature is measured with an instrument called a thermometer. This is a delicate, hollow glass tube with mercury sealed inside it. Mercury is an element that is very sensitive to temperature. It expands (gets larger) when the temperature goes up. Mercury contracts (gets smaller) when the temperature goes down. Even if the temperature rises only a little, the mercury will expand and travel up the tube. The outside of the thermometer is marked with lines, or *calibrations*, and numbers. These markings help us measure exactly the readings given by the level of the mercury.

There are two kinds of glass thermometers:

* An oral thermometer is used to take a patient's temperature by mouth or by axilla (in the patient's armpit).

* A rectal thermometer is used to take a patient's temperature by inserting the thermometer into the patient's rectum.

Many hospitals now also use a battery-operated electronic thermometer. This instrument has both a rectal (red) and an oral (blue) attachment called a probe. A disposable plastic cover is used over the *probe* for each patient. Many hospitals now also use chemically treated single-use paper and plastic thermometers.

Care of Glass Thermometers

* Glass thermometers break easily. Handle them with care. Be especially careful to avoid breaking a thermometer while it is in a patient's mouth or rectum.

* When a thermometer breaks, it shatters. Mercury is a poison.

TYPES OF THERMOMETERS

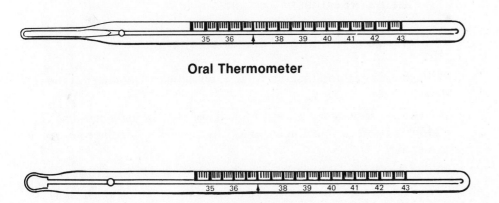

Oral Thermometer

Rectal Thermometer

• Check the containers in which the thermometers are kept. Follow your instructions for cleaning these containers. You are expected to see that the containers are filled with the proper disinfectant solution.

Procedure: Shaking Down the Thermometer

1. Before using the thermometer, check to make sure it is not cracked or the bulb is not chipped.

2. Stand away from hard objects. When you shake the thermometer, avoid striking it against something hard and breaking it. While you are practicing, you might stand with your arm over a mattress or pillow in case you drop the thermometer.

3. Hold the thermometer tightly between your fingers and your thumb at the stem end farthest from the bulb. That is the end that doesn't go into the patient's mouth.

4. When you are sure that you have a good hold on the thermometer, shake your hand loosely from the wrist. Do it as if you were shaking water from your fingers.

5. Snap your wrist again and again. This will shake down the mercury to the lowest possible point. This should be below the numbers and lines.

6. Do this always before and after using a thermometer.

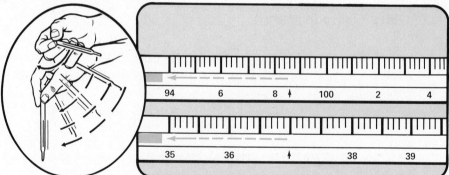

SHAKE THE MERCURY DOWN TO THE LOWEST POINT BELOW THE NUMBERS AND LINES

Procedure: Reading a Fahrenheit Thermometer

1. With your thumb and first two fingers, hold the thermometer at the stem.

2. Hold the thermometer at eye level. Turn the thermometer back and forth between your fingers until you can clearly see the column of mercury.

3. Notice the scale or calibrations. Each long line stands for 1 degree.

4. There are 4 short lines between each of the long lines. Each short line stands for 2 tenths (or .2) of a degree.

5. Between the long lines that represent 98° and 99°, look for a longer line with an arrow directly beneath it. This special line stands for normal body temperature.

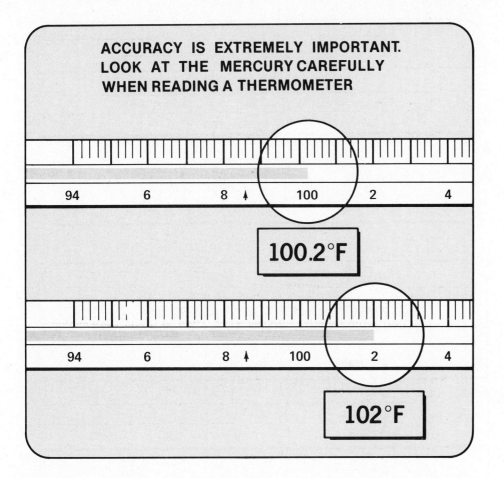

**ACCURACY IS EXTREMELY IMPORTANT.
LOOK AT THE MERCURY CAREFULLY
WHEN READING A THERMOMETER**

100.2°F

102°F

6. Look at the end of the mercury. Check the line or number where the mercury ends. If it is one of the short lines, notice the next longer line toward the silver tip that goes into the patient's mouth. The temperature reading is the degree marked by that long line plus 2, 4, 6, or 8 tenths of a degree. Example: If the mercury ends after the 99 line, but on the second short line, the temperature is 99.4° F.

7. Write down the patient's temperature right away. If you are using a TPR book, check to find the right column next to the patient's name and the right time of day. Write the patient's temperature using the figure you read on the thermometer. Some hospitals will write 99.4° F. Others will write 99⁴. Follow the method used in your hospital.

Procedure: Reading a Centigrade (Celsius) Thermometer

1. With your thumb and first two fingers, hold the thermometer at the stem.

2. Hold it at eye level. Turn the thermometer back and forth between your fingers until you can clearly see the column of mercury.

3. Notice the scale or calibrations. Each long line shows one degree.

4. There are 9 short lines between each number. These short lines are 1, 2, 3, 4, 5, 6, 7, 8, and 9 tenths of a degree. If the mercury ended

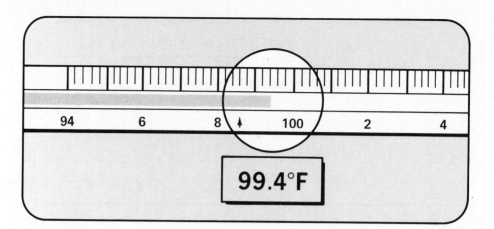

99.4°F

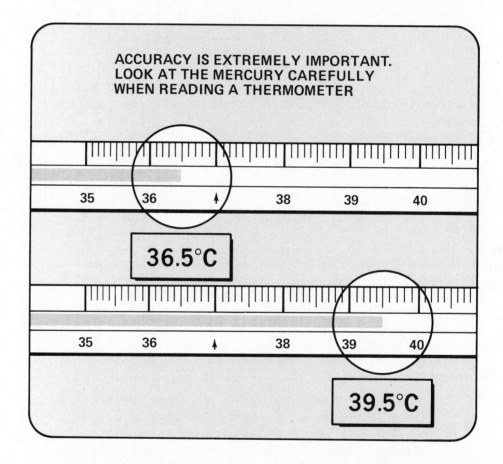

ACCURACY IS EXTREMELY IMPORTANT.
LOOK AT THE MERCURY CAREFULLY
WHEN READING A THERMOMETER

36.5°C

39.5°C

after the 36 and on the third short line, the temperature would read 36.3° C. If the mercury ended after long line 37 and on the eighth short line, the temperature would read 37.8° C. If the mercury ends after line 37 on the fifth short line, the temperature would be referred to as 37.5° C.

5.   Write down the patient's temperature right away. If you are using a TPR book, check to find the correct column next to the patient's name and the right time of day. Write the patient's temperature using the figure you read off the thermometer. Some hospitals will write 37° C. Others will write 37. Follow the method used in your hospital.

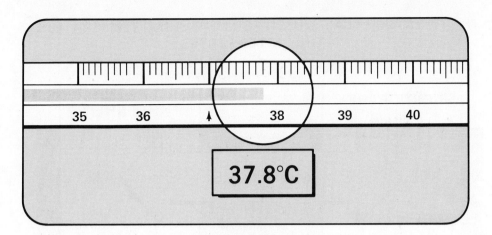

For recording the patient's temperature, three symbols are needed:

° = degrees

F = Fahrenheit

C = Centigrade

You will record the patients' temperatures according to the style used in your hospital.

Fahrenheit temperature can be written in two ways:

$$98.6° \text{ F or } 98^{\underline{6}}° \text{ F}$$

If you are using a centigrade (Celsius) thermometer, the temperature would be written:

$$37° \text{ C or } 37.3° \text{ C or } 37^{\underline{3}}° \text{ C}$$

You would write R with the temperature reading if a rectal temperature was taken. You would write A beside the temperature reading if an axillary temperature was taken.

USING AN ORAL THERMOMETER

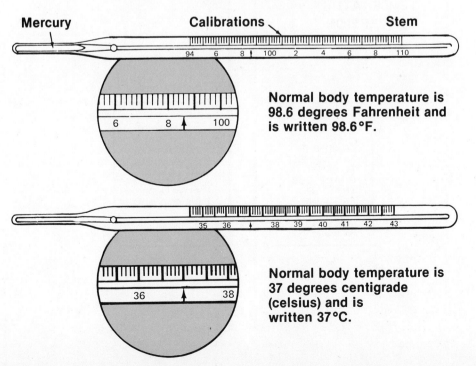

Normal body temperature is 98.6 degrees Fahrenheit and is written 98.6°F.

Normal body temperature is 37 degrees centigrade (celsius) and is written 37°C.

THE TWO MAJOR SCALES USED FOR MEASURING TEMPERATURE IN THE UNITED STATES

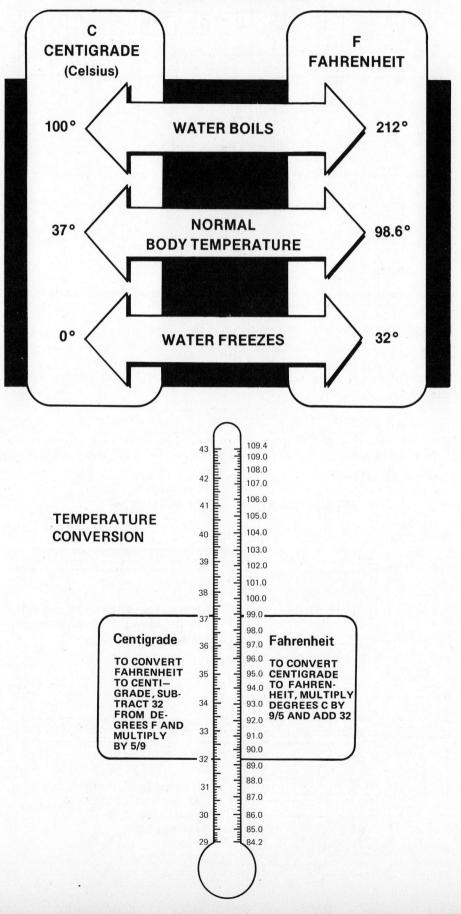

INSERTING THE ORAL THERMOMETER

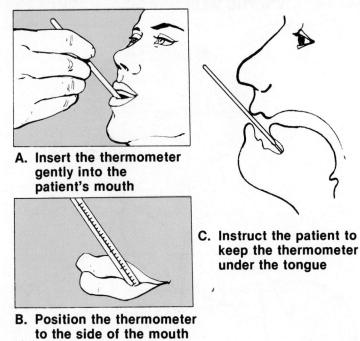

A. Insert the thermometer gently into the patient's mouth

B. Position the thermometer to the side of the mouth

C. Instruct the patient to keep the thermometer under the tongue

Procedure: Taking an Oral Temperature

1. Assemble your equipment:
   a. Oral thermometer
   b. Tissue
   c. Temp. board, a TPR book, or the form used in your hospital
2. Wash your hands.
3. Identify the patient by checking the identification bracelet.
4. Tell the patient that you are going to take his temperature.
5. Ask the patient if he has recently had hot or cold fluids or if he has been smoking. If the answer is yes, wait 10 minutes before taking an oral temperature.
6. Ask visitors to step out of the room.
7. Pull the curtain around the bed for privacy.
8. The patient should be in bed or sitting in a chair.
9. Take the thermometer out of its container. Rinse with cold water. (This will remove the taste of the disinfectant solution it is kept in.)
10. Shake the mercury down.
11. Put the bulb end in the patient's mouth under the tongue. Ask him to keep his mouth and lips closed.
12. Leave the thermometer in the patient's mouth for eight minutes, to get the most accurate reading.
13. Take the thermometer out of the patient's mouth. Hold the stem end and wipe the thermometer with the tissue. Wipe from the stem end of the thermometer toward the bulb end.
14. Read the thermometer.

SHAKING DOWN THE MERCURY OF A THERMOMETER

15. Record the temperature in the TPR book, or on the temp. board or the form used in your hospital.

16. Shake the mercury down. Replace the thermometer in its container.

17. Make the patient comfortable.

18. Wash your hands.

19. Report to your head nurse or team leader if the oral temperature was above 100° F or 37.8° C. (Many hospitals report an oral temperature above 100° F or 37.8° C by circling the figure in red on the temp. board.) Also, report your observations of anything unusual.

KEY IDEAS: TAKING A RECTAL TEMPERATURE

Remember that you will always use a rectal thermometer for taking rectal temperatures. Notice that the rectal thermometer has a small round bulb on one end. This bulb prevents the thermometer from injuring the sensitive lining of the patient's rectum. You will not have to wait for a doctor to write an order to take the temperature by rectum under the following conditions:

- When the patient is an infant or a child under 12 years old
- When the patient is having warm or cold applications on his face or neck
- When the patient cannot keep his mouth closed on the thermometer
- When the patient finds it hard to breathe through his nose
- When the patient has sneezing or coughing spells
- When the patient's mouth is dry or inflamed (red)
- When the patient is restless, delirious, unconscious, or confused
- When the patient has had major surgery in the area of his face or neck
- When the patient is getting oxygen by cannula, catheter, face mask, or oxygen tent
- When the patient has a nasogastric tube (Levin's tube, NG tube) in place
- When the patient's face is partially paralyzed as from a stroke

Procedure: Taking a Rectal Temperature

1. Assemble your equipment:
   a. Rectal thermometer
   b. Tissue
   c. Lubricating jelly
   d. Temp. board, TPR book, or the form used in your hospital
2. Wash your hands.
3. Identify the patient by checking the identification bracelet.
4. Ask visitors to step out of the room.
5. Tell the patient that you are going to take his temperature by rectum.
6. Pull the curtain around the bed for privacy. Lower the backrest on the bed, if allowed.
7. Take the thermometer out of its container. Rinse it off with cold water. Handle only the stem.
8. Carefully inspect the bulb of the thermometer for cracks or chipped places. A broken thermometer could seriously injure the patient's rectum.
9. Hold the thermometer at the stem end. Shake it down until the mercury is below the numbers and lines.
10. Put a small amount of lubricating jelly on a piece of tissue. Then lubricate the bulb of the thermometer with the lubricated tissue. This makes it easier to insert the thermometer.

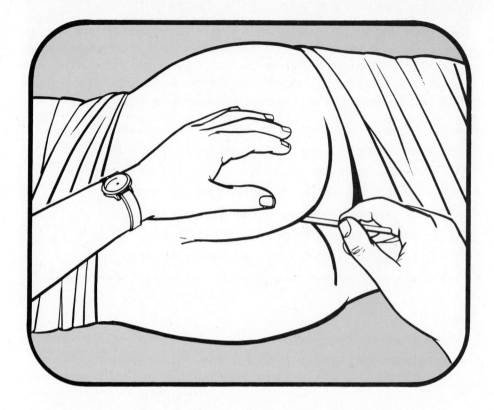

11. Ask the patient to turn on his side. Or turn him yourself, if necessary. Turn back the top covers just enough so that you can see the patient's buttocks. Avoid overexposing him.

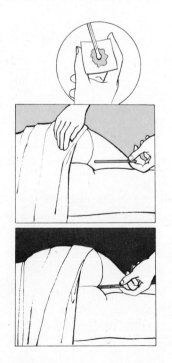

12. With one hand, raise the upper buttock until you can see the anus, the opening to the rectum. With the other hand, slip the bulb one inch through the anus into the rectum.

13. If the patient is an infant, remove the diaper. Lay the baby on his back. Raise his legs with one hand. Insert the thermometer with the other hand one-half inch into the rectum. Always hold the thermometer while it is in the child's rectum.

14. Hold the thermometer in place. If the patient is able, he may hold it. However, do not leave a patient with a rectal thermometer in the rectum.

15. Leave the thermometer in place for three minutes.

16. Remove the thermometer from the patient's rectum. Holding the stem end of the thermometer, wipe it with a tissue from stem to bulb.

17. Read the thermometer.

18. Record the temperature right away in the TPR book or on the temp. board or hospital form. Note that this is a rectal temperature by writing an R in front of the figure. This is necessary because an average rectal temperature is slightly higher than an oral one.

19. Shake the mercury down until it is below the numbers and lines.

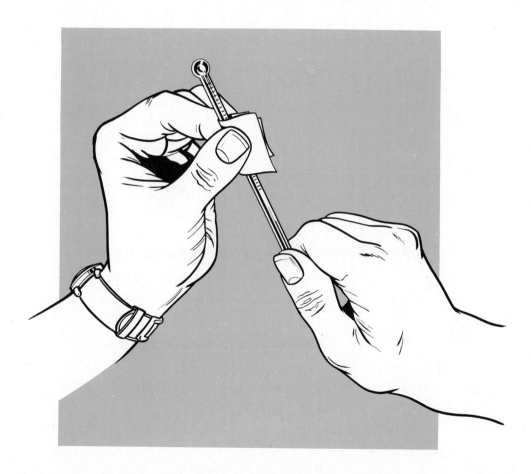

20. Replace the thermometer in its container.

21. Make the patient comfortable.

22. Wash your hands.

23. Report to your head nurse or team leader if the rectal temperature is higher than 101° F or 38.3° C. (Many hospitals report the rectal temperature over 101° F or 38.3° C by circling the figure in red on the temp. board, in the TRP book, or on the form used in your hospital.) Also report your observations of anything unusual.

Procedure: Taking an Axillary Temperature

1. Assemble your equipment:
    a. Oral thermometer
    b. Tissue
    c. Temp. board, TPR book, or the form used in your hospital

2. Wash your hands.

3. Identify the patient by checking the identification bracelet.

4. Ask visitors to step out of the room.

5. Tell the patient that you have to take his temperature.

6. Pull the curtain around the bed for privacy.

7. Holding the stem end, remove the oral thermometer from its container.

8. Rinse the thermometer with cold water and dry it with tissue. Shake the mercury down.

9. Carefully inspect the bulb of the thermometer for scratches or chipped places. A broken thermometer could seriously injure the patient.

10. Remove the patient's arm from the sleeve of his gown. If the axillary region is moist with perspiration, pat it dry with a towel.

11. Place the bulb of the oral thermometer in the center of the armpit (axilla). The thermometer then should be held upright by the arm and the chest.

12. Put the patient's arm across his chest or abdomen.

13. If the patient is unconscious or is too weak to help, you will have to hold the thermometer in place.

14. Leave the thermometer in place 10 minutes. Stay with the patient.

15. Remove the thermometer. Wipe it off with tissue from the stem to the bulb.

16. Read the thermometer.

17. Shake the mercury down until it is below the numbers and lines.

18. Replace the thermometer in its container.

19. Record the patient's temperature on the temp. board, in the TPR book, or hospital form. Note that this is an axillary temperature by writing A in front of the figure.

20. Put the patient's arm back in the sleeve of his gown.

21. Make the patient comfortable.

22. Wash your hands.

23. Report to your head nurse or team leader if the axillary temperature was over 99° F (37.2° C). (Many hospitals report an axillary temperature over 99° F by circling the figure in red on the temp. board, in the TPR book, or on the form used in your hospital.) Also, report your observations of anything unusual.

Procedure: Using a Battery-Operated Electronic Oral Thermometer

1. Assemble your equipment:
   a. Disposable plastic probe cover
   b. Battery-operated electronic thermometer
   c. Oral (blue) attachment
   d. Temp. board, TPR book, or the form used in your hospital

2. Wash your hands.

3. Identify the patient by checking the identification bracelet.

4. Ask visitors to step out of the room.

Battery-Operated Electronic Thermometer

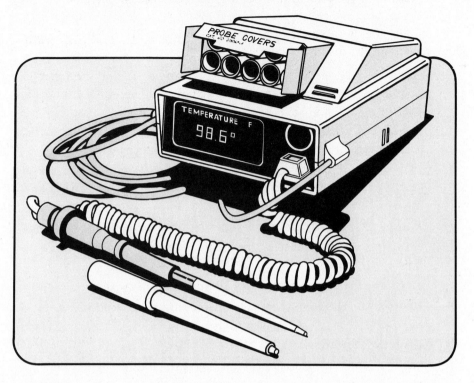

5. Tell the patient that you are going to take his temperature.

6. Pull the curtain around the bed for privacy.

7. Check to be sure that the oral (blue top) probe connector is properly seated in its receptacle on the base of the unit.

8. Remove the probe from its stored position. Insert it into a probe cover.

9. Slowly insert the covered probe into the patient's mouth until the metal tip is at the base under the tongue to the back of the patient's mouth.

10. Hold the probe in the patient's mouth. It is much heavier than a glass thermometer and some patients are unable to hold it.

11. Wait about 15 seconds for the buzzer to ring for a computed temperature reading. Then remove the probe from the patient's mouth.

12. Record the temperature on the temp. board, in the TPR book or hospital form. This is very important because when you return the probe to its stored position, the reading automatically returns to zero.

13. Discard the used probe cover immediately without touching it.

14. Return the probe to its stored position in the face of the thermometer.

15. Store the thermometer in its charging stand whenever it is not in use.

16. Make the patient comfortable.

17. Wash your hands.

18. Report to your head nurse or team leader if the oral temperature was over 100° F (37.8° C). Also, report your observations of anything unusual.

Procedure: Using a Battery-Operated Electronic Rectal Thermometer

1. Assemble your equipment:
   a. Plastic disposable probe cover
   b. Battery-operated electronic thermometer
   c. Rectal (red) attachment
   d. Temp. board, TPR book, or the form used in your hospital

2. Wash your hands.

3. Identify the patient by checking the identification bracelet.

4. Ask visitors to step out of the room.

5. Tell the patient that you are going to take his temperature. Remember that the average normal rectal temperature is 99.6° F (37.5° C).

6. Pull the curtain around the bed for privacy.

7. Check to be sure the rectal (red top) probe connector is properly seated in its receptacle on the base of the thermometer.

8. Remove the probe from its stored position and insert it into a probe cover.

9. Slowly insert the covered probe through the patient's anus into the rectum one-half inch.

10. Hold the probe in the patient's rectum.

11. Wait for the buzzer to ring for a computed temperature reading. Then remove the probe from the rectum.

12. Record the temperature on the temp. board, in the TPR book, or hospital form. This is very important because when you return the probe to its stored position, the reading automatically returns to zero.

13. Discard the used probe cover immediately without touching it.

14. Return the probe to its stored position in the face of the thermometer.

15. Store the thermometer in its charging stand whenever it is not in use.

16. Make the patient comfortable.

17. Wash your hands.

18. Report to your head nurse or team leader if the rectal temperature was over 101° F (38.3° C). Also, report your observation of anything unusual.

Procedure: Using a Battery-Operated Electronic Oral Thermometer To Take An Axillary Temperature

1. Assemble your equipment:
   a. Plastic disposable probe cover
   b. Battery-operated electronic thermometer
   c. Oral (blue) attachment
   d. Temp. board, TPR book, or the form used in your hospital

2. Wash your hands.

3. Identify the patient by checking the identification bracelet.

4. Ask visitors to step out of the room.

5. Tell the patient that you are going to take his temperature.

6. Pull the curtain around the bed for privacy.

7. Check to be sure the oral (blue top) probe connector is properly seated in its receptacle on the base of the unit.

8. Remove the probe from its stored position and insert it into a probe cover.

9. Place the covered probe in the center of the patient's armpit (axilla).

10. Put the patient's arm across his chest. Hold the probe in place.

11. Wait (about 15 seconds) for the buzzer to ring for a computed temperature reading. Then remove the probe from the patient's axilla.

12. Record the temperature in the TPR book or on the temp. board or hospital form. This is very important because when you return the probe to its stored position, the reading automatically returns to zero.

13. Discard the used probe cover immediately without touching it.

14. Return the probe to its stored position in the face of the thermometer.

15. Store the thermometer in its charging stand whenever it is not in use.

Normal Readings for Each Type of Thermometer

Types of thermometers	Normals		Time left in place
	°C	°F	
ORAL	37°	98.6°	8 minutes
AXILLARY (Oral)	36.4°	97.6°	10 minutes
RECTAL	37.5°	99.6°	3 minutes

Report any change in temperature to your head nurse or team leader.

16. Make the patient comfortable.

17. Wash your hands.

18. Report to your head nurse or team leader if the axillary temperature was over 99° F (37.2° C). Also report your observations of anything unusual.

Section 3: Taking a Pulse

OBJECTIVES: WHAT YOU WILL LEARN

When you have completed this section, you should be able:

- To count the pulse
- To accurately report the rate and rhythm of the pulse

KEY IDEAS

Each time the heart beats, it pumps a certain amount of blood into the arteries. This causes the arteries to expand (get bigger). Between heartbeats, the arteries contract and return to their normal size. The heart pumps the blood in a steady rhythm. The rhythmic expansion and contraction of the arteries, which can be measured to show how fast the heart is beating, is called the *pulse*. Measuring the pulse is a simple method of learning something about how the circulatory system is functioning.

The pulse measures how fast the heart is beating. At certain places on the body, the pulse easily can be felt under a person's fingers. One of the easiest places to feel the pulse is at the wrist. This is called a *radial pulse* because you

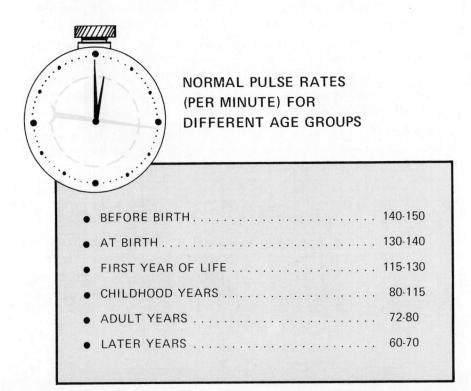

NORMAL PULSE RATES
(PER MINUTE) FOR
DIFFERENT AGE GROUPS

- BEFORE BIRTH 140-150
- AT BIRTH 130-140
- FIRST YEAR OF LIFE 115-130
- CHILDHOOD YEARS 80-115
- ADULT YEARS 72-80
- LATER YEARS 60-70

are feeling the radial artery. When taking the pulse, you must be able to report accurately the following:

- <u>Rate</u>—the number of pulse beats per minute
- <u>Rhythm</u>—the regularity of the pulse beats, that is, whether or not the length of time between the beats is steady and regular
- <u>Force of the beat</u>

The normal average rate of pulse for adults is 72 beats per minute. The range of normal rates for adults is from 72 to 80 beats per minute.

Procedure: Taking a Radial Pulse

1. Assemble your equipment:
   a. Watch with a second hand
   b. TPR book, temp. board, or form used in your hospital
2. Wash your hands.
3. Identify the patient by checking the identification bracelet.
4. Ask visitors to step out of the room.
5. Tell the patient that you are going to take his pulse.
6. If the patient is standing, ask him to sit down. Or have him lying in a comfortable position in bed.
7. The patient's hand and arm should be well supported and resting comfortably.
8. Find the pulse by putting the tips of your middle three fingers on the palm side of the patient's wrist in a line with his thumb directly next to the bone. Press lightly until you feel the beat. If you press too hard, you may stop the flow of blood and obliterate the pulse. Then you would not be able to feel the pulse. Never use your thumb. Your thumb has a pulse beat and you would be counting your own pulse instead of the patient's. When you have found the pulse, notice the rhythm. Notice if the beat is steady or irregular. Notice the force of the beat.
9. Look at the position of the second hand on the watch. Then start counting the pulse beats (what you feel) until the second hand comes back to the same number on the clock.
   - *Method A:* Count the pulse beats for 1 full minute and report the full minute count. This is always done if the patient has an irregular beat.
   - *Method B:* Count for 30 seconds, until the second hand on the watch is opposite its position when you started. Then multiply the number of beats by 2. This is the number you record. For example, if you count 35 for 30 seconds, the count for 1 full minute is 70.
10. Record the pulse count on the temp. board, in the TPR book or on the form used in your hospital right away. Be sure you write in the correct column and next to the patient's name.

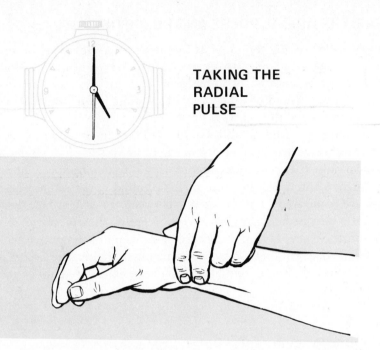

TAKING THE RADIAL PULSE

11. Make the patient comfortable.

12. Wash your hands.

13. Report to your head nurse or team leader if the pulse rate was under 60 or over 100, or if the pulse was irregular by circling in red the number on the temp. board, in the TPR book, or on the hospital form. In some hospitals, *irregular* (IRR) is written near the pulse number to report an irregular pulse. Also, report your observations of anything unusual.

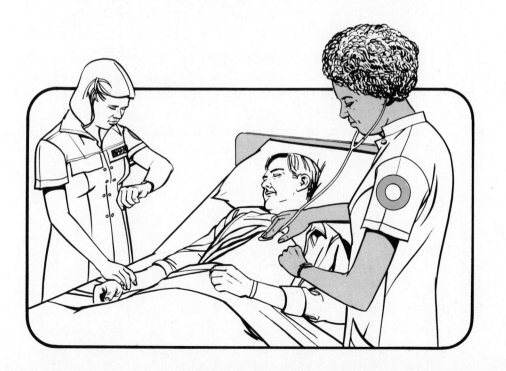

KEY IDEAS: THE APICAL PULSE AND PULSE DEFICIT

The pulse rate is usually the same as the heart rate. However, in some patients the heartbeats are not strong enough to be transmitted along the arteries. This may be because of some forms of heart disease. For these patients an apical pulse would be taken. An apical pulse is a measurement of the heartbeats at the apex of the heart.

Sometimes the patient has a "pulse deficit." This means that there is a difference between the apical heartbeat and the radial pulse rate. To determine this, the apical pulse (heart rate) is counted with a stethoscope over the apex of the heart. At the same time, the pulse rate is counted at the radial pulse. The two figures are compared. The difference between the apical heartbeat and the radial pulse beat is the *pulse deficit*. This is called the *apical pulse deficit*. For maximum accuracy, both pulses should be taken at the same time by two nursing aides. A different method calls for one nursing aide who first takes the apical pulse and then takes the radial pulse. This is considered not as accurate as the first method.

Procedure: Taking an Apical Pulse

1. Assemble your equipment:
   a. Stethoscope and antiseptic swabs
   b. Watch with a second hand
   c. Temp. board, TPR book, or the form used in your hospital. In most hospitals, this reading is always reported directly to the head nurse or team leader.
   d. Note paper

2. Wash your hands.

3. Identify the patient by checking the identification bracelet.

4. Ask visitors to step out of the room.

5. Explain to the patient that you are going to take his apical pulse.

6. Pull the curtain around the bed for privacy.

7. Uncover the left side of the patient's chest. Avoid overexposing his body.

8. Clean the earplugs of the stethoscope with antiseptic solution. Put the earplugs in your ears.

9. Locate the apex of the patient's heart by placing the bell (or diaphragm) of the stethoscope under the patient's left breast. Listen for the heart sounds.

10. Count the heart sounds for a full minute.

11. Write the full minute count on the note paper.

12. Cover the patient and make him comfortable.

13. Clean the earplugs of the stethoscope. Return the equipment to its proper place.

14. Make the patient comfortable.

15. Wash your hands.

16. Report to your head nurse or team leader that you have taken the patient's apical pulse and what the apical pulse rate was. Also, report your observations of anything unusual.

Procedure: Measuring the Apical Pulse Deficit

1. Assemble your equipment:
   a. Stethoscope and antiseptic swabs
   b. Watch with a second hand
   c. TPR book or temp. board, if this is where this pulse reading is recorded in your hospital. However, in most hospitals this reading would always be reported directly to the head nurse or team leader.
   d. Note paper
2. Wash your hands.
3. Identify the patient by checking the identification bracelet.
4. Ask visitors to step out of the room.
5. Explain to the patient that you are going to take his pulse deficit.
6. Pull the curtain around the bed for privacy.
7. There are two methods of taking the apical pulse deficit.
   - *Method One:* Two nursing aides do this procedure together at the same time. One counts the radial pulse. The other counts the apical pulse. The difference between the two pulses is known as the apical pulse deficit. This method is used for maximum accuracy.
   - *Method Two:* The nursing aide first takes the apical pulse, then the radial pulse. The difference between the two pulses is known as the pulse deficit. However, since they are not taken at the same time, it is not considered as accurate as the first method.
8. Count the apical pulse and the radial pulse for a full minute.
9. Write the figure for the pulse deficit on note paper.
10. Make the patient comfortable.
11. Clean the equipment and return it to its proper place.
12. Wash your hands.
13. Report to your head nurse or team leader:
    - That you have taken the patient's pulse
    - The apical pulse rate
    - The radial pulse rate
    - The pulse deficit
    - Your observations of anything unusual

Section 4: Counting Respirations

OBJECTIVES: WHAT YOU WILL LEARN

When you have completed this section, you should be able:

- To count a patient's respirations accurately
- To determine if the patient's breathing is labored or noisy

KEY IDEAS: COUNTING RESPIRATIONS

The human body must have a steady supply of air. The body needs the oxygen in the air in order to change food into heat and energy. When you breathe in, air is sucked into the lungs. There—in the lungs—oxygen is taken out of the air. The oxygen is absorbed into the blood. The blood then carries the oxygen to the body cells. In the body cells it is burned up (oxidized) to produce energy for the body.

Respiration is the process of inhaling and exhaling. One respiration includes breathing in once and breathing out once. When a person breathes in, his chest gets larger (expands). When he breathes out, his chest gets smaller (contracts). When you count respirations, the patient should be lying on his back. You watch his chest rise and fall as he breathes. Or you feel his chest rise and fall with your hand. Either way, you should count respirations without the patient knowing it. If he thinks his breathing is being counted, he will not breathe naturally. What you want to count is his natural breathing. Besides counting the respirations, you will be noticing whether the patient seems to breathe easily or seems to be working hard to get his breath. When a person is working hard to get his breath, it is called *labored* respiration. You must also notice whether his breathing is noisy.

Normal adults breathe at a rate of from 16 to 20 times a minute. Children breathe more rapidly. Old persons breathe more slowly. Exercise, digestion, emotional stress, disease conditions, drugs, stimulants, heat, and cold all can affect the number of times per minute that a person breathes.

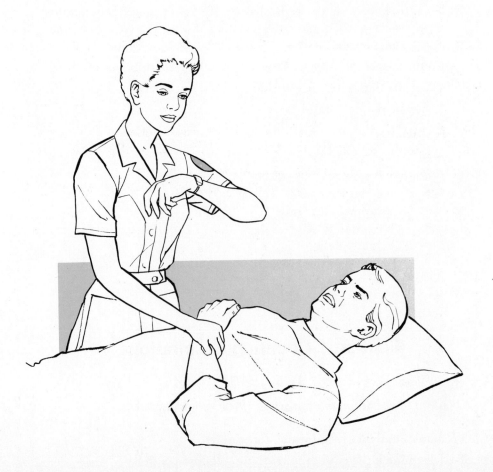

Procedure: Counting Respirations

1. Assemble your equipment:
   a. Watch with a second hand
   b. TPR book, temp. board, or form used by your hospital
2. Wash your hands.
3. Identify the patient by checking the identification bracelet.
4. Ask visitors to step out of the room.
5. Hold the patient's wrist just as if you were taking his pulse. This way he won't know you are watching his breathing. Count the patient's respirations, without his knowing it, immediately after counting his pulse.
6. If the patient is a child who has been crying or is restless, wait until he is quiet before counting respirations. If a child is asleep, count his respirations before he wakes up. Always take a child's pulse and respiration before you measure his temperature.
7. One rise and one fall of the patient's chest counts as one respiration.
8. If you can't clearly see the chest rise and fall, fold the patient's arms across his chest. Then you can feel his breathing as you hold his wrist.
9. Check the position of the second hand on the watch. Count "one" when you see the patient's chest rising as he breathes in. The next time his chest rises, count "two." Keep doing this for a full minute. Report the number of respirations you count.
10. You may be permitted to count for 30 seconds. Count the respirations for one-half minute and then multiply the number you counted by two. For example, if you count 8 respirations in 30 seconds, your number for a full minute is 16.
11. If the patient's breathing rhythm is irregular, always count for a whole minute. Observe the depth of the breathing while counting the respirations.
12. Write down the number you counted immediately on the temp. board, in the TPR book, or on the form used in your hospital. Be sure you are in the proper column, opposite the correct patient's name.
13. Note whether the respirations were noisy or labored.
14. Make the patient comfortable.
15. Wash your hands.
16. Report to your head nurse or team leader the time, regularity, whether the respirations were noisy or labored, and if the respirations were less than 14 or more than 28 a minute. Also, report your observations of anything unusual.

Section 5: Taking Blood Pressures

OBJECTIVES: WHAT YOU WILL LEARN

When you have completed this section, you should be able:

- To explain systolic pressure
- To explain diastolic pressure
- To use aneroid and mercury types of blood pressure equipment accurately and efficiently
- To take a patient's blood pressure accurately

KEY IDEAS

Blood pressure is the force of the blood pushing against the walls of the blood vessels. When you take a patient's blood pressure, you are measuring this force of the blood flowing through the blood vessels.

There is always a certain amount of pressure in the arteries. This is because the heart, by pumping, is constantly forcing blood to circulate. The blood goes first into the arteries. It then circulates through the whole body.

The amount of pressure in the arteries depends on two things:

- The rate of heartbeat
- How easily the blood flows through the blood vessels

The heart contracts as it pumps the blood into the arteries. When the heart is contracting, the pressure is highest. This pressure is called the *systolic* pressure. As the heart relaxes between each contraction, the pressure goes down. When the heart is most relaxed, the pressure is lowest. This pressure is called the *diastolic* pressure. When you take a patient's blood pressure, you are measuring these two rates—the systolic pressure and the diastolic pressure.

In young healthy adults, the normal blood pressure range is between 100 and 140 millimeters (mm) mercury (Hg) systolic pressure. It is between 60 and 90 millimeters (mm) mercury (Hg) diastolic pressure.

The way these figures are written is:

$$120/80 \text{ or } \frac{120 = \text{systolic}}{80 = \text{diastolic}}$$

When a patient's blood pressure is higher than the normal range for his age and condition, it is referred to as *high blood pressure* or *hypertension*. When a patient's blood pressure is lower than the normal range for his age or condition, it is referred to as *low blood pressure* or *hypotension*.

Instruments for Measuring Blood Pressure

When you take a patient's blood pressure, you will be using an instrument called a *sphygmomanometer*. Sphygmomanometer is a combination of three Greek words:

- Sphygmo, meaning pulse
- Mano, meaning pressure
- Meter, meaning measure

This instrument, however, is usually called simply the *blood pressure cuff*. The four main parts of this instrument are: manometer, valve, cuff, and bulb.

Two kinds of instruments are used for taking blood pressure. One is called the mercury type. The other is called the aneroid (dial) type. Both kinds have an inflatable cloth-covered rubber bag, or cuff. The cuff is wrapped around the patient's arm. Both kinds also have a rubber bulb for pumping air into the

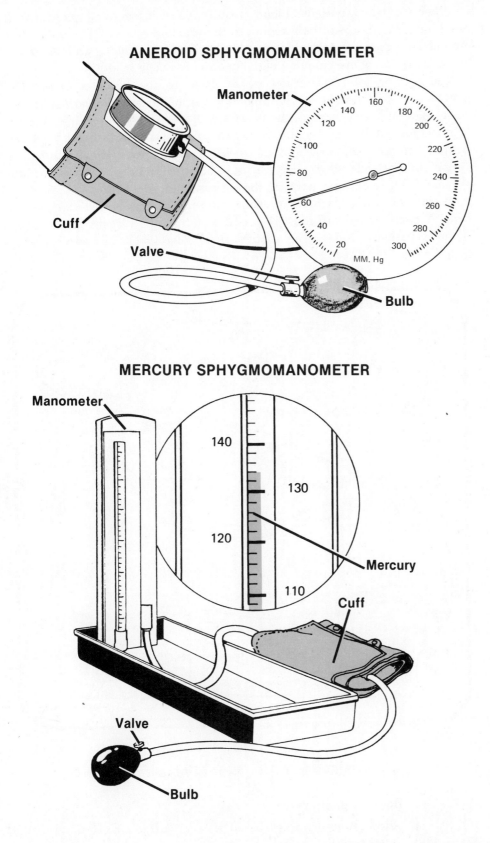

ANEROID SPHYGMOMANOMETER

Manometer

Cuff

Valve

Bulb

MERCURY SPHYGMOMANOMETER

Manometer

Mercury

Cuff

Valve

Bulb

cuff. The procedure for measuring blood pressure is the same, except for taking the reading. When you use the mercury type, you will be watching the level of a column of mercury on a measuring scale. When you use the dial (aneroid) type, you will be watching a pointer on a dial.

When you take a patient's blood pressure, you will be doing two things at the same time. You will be listening to the brachial pulse as it sounds in the brachial artery in the patient's arm. You also will be watching an indicator—either a column of mercury or a dial—in order to take a reading.

You will be using a stethoscope to listen to the brachial pulse. The stethoscope is an instrument that makes it possible to listen to various sounds in the patient's body, such as the heartbeat or breathing sounds in the chest. The stethoscope is a tube with one end that picks up sound when it is placed against a part of the body. This end is either bell-shaped and called a *bell* or round and flat and called a *diaphragm*. The other end of the tube splits into two parts. These parts have tips on the ends and fit into the listener's ears.

In many hospitals, the blood pressure equipment hangs on the wall over the bed. A smaller-sized cuff must be used for children or a larger size for obese (very fat) patients. Don't use a patient's arm that has an IV (intravenous) setup in it.

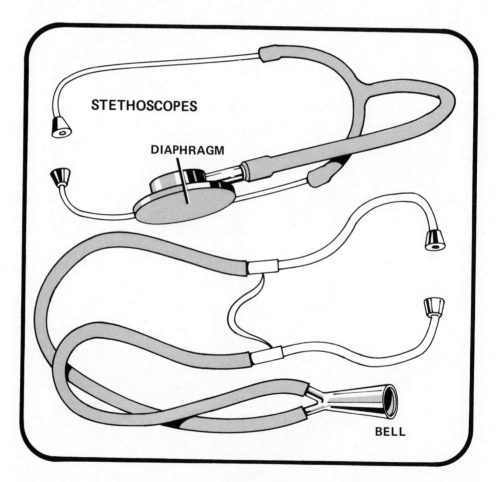

STETHOSCOPES

DIAPHRAGM

BELL

Procedure: Taking Blood Pressure

1. Assemble your equipment:
   a. Sphygmomanometer (blood pressure cuff)
   b. Stethoscope
   c. Antiseptic pad
   d. BP board, blood pressure book, or form used in your hospital

2. Wash your hands.

3. Identify the patient by checking the identification bracelet.

4. Ask visitors to step out of the room.

5. Tell the patient that you are going to take his blood pressure.

6. Act calm. You want to prevent extra apprehension and excitement in the patient.

7. Have the patient resting quietly. He should be either lying down or sitting in a chair.

8. If you are using the mercury apparatus, the measuring scale should be level with your eyes.

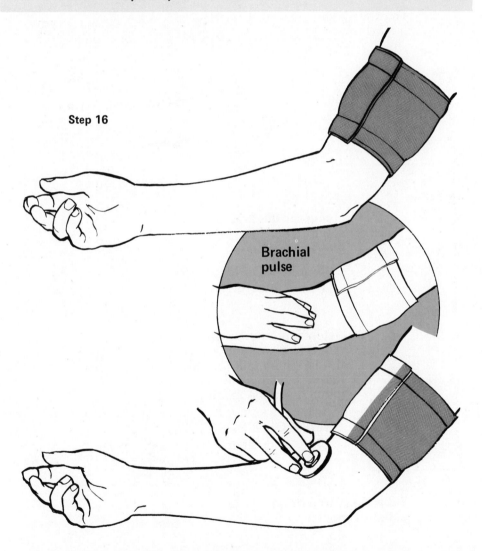

Step 16

Brachial pulse

9. The patient's arm should be bare up to the shoulder, or the patient's sleeve should be well above the elbow.

10. The patient's arm from the elbow down should be resting fully extended on the bed. Or it might be resting on the arm of the chair, well supported, with the palm upward.

11. Unroll the cuff and loosen the valve on the bulb. Then squeeze the compression bag to deflate it completely.

12. Wrap the cuff around the patient's arm above the elbow snugly and smoothly. But don't wrap it so tightly that the patient is uncomfortable from the pressure.

13. Leave the area clear where you will place the bell or diaphragm of the stethoscope.

14. Be sure the manometer is in position so you can read the numbers easily.

15. Wipe the earplugs of the stethoscope with the antiseptic pads. Put the plugs in your ears.

16. With your fingertips, find the patient's brachial pulse at the inner side of the arm above the elbow (brachial artery). This is where you will place the diaphragm or bell of the stethoscope. The diaphragm should be held tightly against the patient's skin, but it should not touch the cuff of the apparatus.

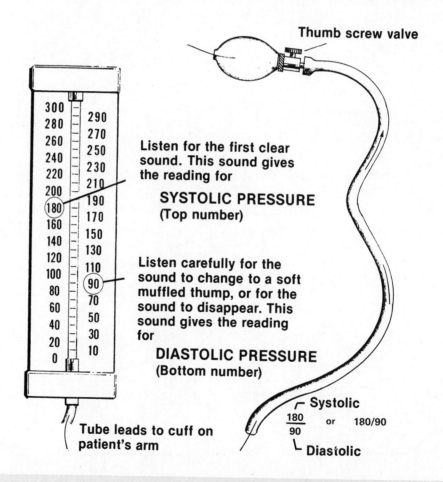

Thumb screw valve

Listen for the first clear sound. This sound gives the reading for

SYSTOLIC PRESSURE
(Top number)

Listen carefully for the sound to change to a soft muffled thump, or for the sound to disappear. This sound gives the reading for

DIASTOLIC PRESSURE
(Bottom number)

Tube leads to cuff on patient's arm

Systolic
$\frac{180}{90}$ or   180/90
Diastolic

17. Tighten the thumbscrew of the valve to close it. Turn it clockwise. Be careful not to turn it too tightly. If you do, you will have trouble opening it.

18. Hold the stethoscope in place. Inflate the cuff until the dial points to 170.

19. Open the valve counter clockwise. This allows the air to escape. Let it out very slowly until the sound of the pulse comes back. A few

seconds must go by without sounds. If you do hear pulse sounds immediately, you must stop the procedure. Then completely deflate the cuff. Wait a few seconds. Then inflate the cuff to a much higher calibration—above 200. Again, loosen the thumbscrew to let the air out. Listen for a repeated pulse sound. At the same time, watch the indicator.

20. Note the calibration that the pointer passes as you hear the first sound. This point indicates the systolic pressure (or the top number).

21. Continue releasing the air from the cuff. When the sounds change to a softer and faster thud or disappear, note the calibration. This is the diastolic pressure (or bottom number).

22. Deflate the cuff completely. Remove it from the patient's arm.

23. Record your reading on the BP board, in the BP book, or on the form used in your hospital.

24. After using the blood pressure cuff, roll it up over the manometer and replace it in the case.

25. Wipe the earplugs of the stethoscope again with antiseptic swab. Put the stethoscope back where it belongs.

26. Make the patient comfortable.

27. Wash your hands.

28. Report to your head nurse or team leader:
    - That you have taken the patient's blood pressure reading
    - The time that you took the reading
    - Your observations of anything unusual

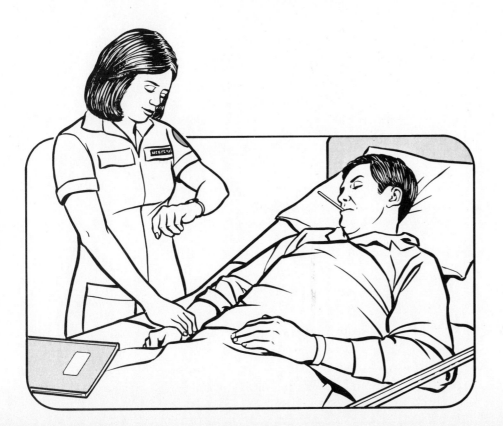

WHAT YOU HAVE LEARNED

The vital signs are temperature, pulse, respiration, and blood pressure. Temperature, pulse, and respirations (TPRs) are measured at the same time, as one procedure. Careful, accurate recording of this information is very important. The procedures for measuring the vital signs must be practiced many times for you to be able to carry them out skillfully and accurately.

Patient Admission, Transfer, and Discharge

12

Section 1: Admitting the Patient

OBJECTIVES: WHAT YOU WILL LEARN

When you have completed this section, you should be able:

- To admit a patient to your nursing unit by following the correct procedure
- To welcome the patient and his visitors in a pleasant and courteous manner
- To observe the patient carefully and record all the information needed
- To make the patient feel comfortable and help him to adjust to the hospital environment

KEY IDEAS

A patient coming into a hospital is usually frightened and uncomfortable. Maybe he is not seriously ill or in pain. Even so, he probably does not like being there. This is a time when you, as a member of the nursing team, are very important to the patient. Being pleasant and courteous will make the patient's arrival easier for him. A nice welcome will create a favorable first impression.

Introduce yourself. Learn the patient's name and use it often. Remember that the way you speak and behave will have a lot to do with the patient's impression of the hospital. Smile, be friendly. Don't appear to be rushed or busy with other things. Do your work quietly and efficiently.

Procedure: Admitting the Patient

1. Assemble your equipment:
    a. Admission checklist
    b. Urine specimen container and laboratory requisition slip, to be filled out by the head nurse or ward clerk
    c. Hospital gown or pajamas
    d. Clothing list
    e. Envelope for valuables
    f. Portable scale
    g. Blood pressure cuff and stethoscope

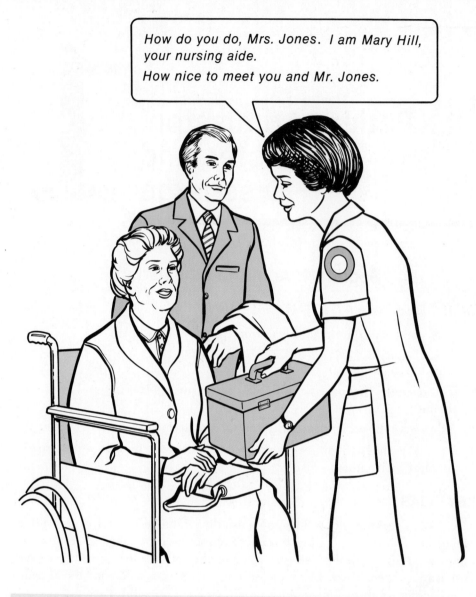

> *How do you do, Mrs. Jones. I am Mary Hill, your nursing aide.*
>
> *How nice to meet you and Mr. Jones.*

     h.   Admission pack
     i.   Thermometer
     j.   Bedpan, urinal, emesis basin, and wash basin

2. Wash your hands.

3. Fanfold the bed covers down to open the bed.

4. Place the hospital gown or pajamas at the foot of the bed.

5. Put the bedpan, urinal, emesis basin, wash basin, and admission pack in their proper place in the bedside table.

6. When the patient comes up to the floor, introduce yourself to the patient and to his visitors. Smile, be friendly. Call the patient by his name. Shake hands and tell the patient your name and job title.

7. Escort the patient to his room. Introduce him to his roommates, if he has any.

8. Ask the relatives and visitors to leave the room while you finish admitting the patient.

9. Close the door in a private room. Or draw the curtain or put a screen in place around the bed so the patient has privacy.

10. Ask the patient to change into the hospital gown or pajamas. If necessary, help the patient get undressed and into the gown.

11. Help the patient to get into the bed.

12. Raise the side rails on the bed, if necessary.

13. Complete the admission checklist that follows the admitting procedure. Cover each detail of the admission procedure. Be sure to fill out the list accurately and completely. Write carefully so your writing can be read easily.

14. Make the patient comfortable. Fix the lights the way he wants them. Be sure the sheets and blankets are arranged properly.

15. Have the patient put his toilet articles and small belongings in or on the bedside table.

16. Find out whether the patient is allowed to have drinking water. If so, fill the water pitcher.

17. Make the patient familiar with his new surroundings. Remember to show the patient where the signal cord is. Attach the signal cord to the bed where the patient can reach it easily. Explain how the intercom system works. Show him how to operate the remote-control TV.

18. Explain the hospital policy on radios, television, newspapers, and mail. Tell the patient when meals will be served.

19. Find out whether the patient is allowed to have the head of his bed elevated and the knee gatch on his bed as high or low as he

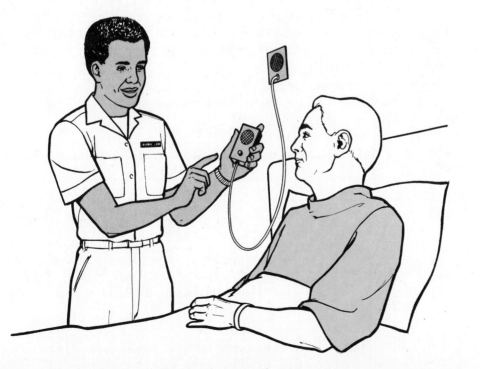

A SAMPLE ADMISSION CHECKLIST
(Fill in every statement and check every appropriate item)

Patient's name _____ Room number____

Time of admission _____a.m./p.m.   Date of admission _____

Unit ready to receive patient? Yes☐No☐ Equipment ready? Yes☐No☐

Admitted by stretcher_____ wheelchair_____ walking_____

Check identification bracelet? Yes☐No☐ Bed tag in place? Yes☐No☐

Did the patient need help to get undressed? Yes☐No☐

Is the patient in bed at this time? Yes☐No☐ Time_____a.m./p.m.

Side rails up? Yes☐No☐

Bruises, marks, rashes, or broken skin noted? Yes☐No☐
   If yes, describe _____

Weight_____ Height_____ Scale used? Yes☐No☐

Temperature____ Pulse____ Respirations____ BloodPressure____

Admission urine specimen collected? Yes☐No☐ Sent to lab? Yes☐No☐

Unusual behavior noted? Yes☐No☐ Unusual appearance noted? Yes☐No☐
   If yes, describe _____

Does the patient have any difficulty with the English language? Yes☐No☐

Is the patient allergic to food? Yes☐No☐ Allergic to drugs? Yes☐ No☐

Reason for admission _____

Complaints _____

Dentures? Yes☐No☐ Partial? Yes☐No☐ Full? Yes☐No☐ Denture cup?
   Yes☐No☐

Vision problems? Yes☐No☐ Does the patient wear glasses? Yes☐No☐

Valuables: Money? Yes☐No☐ Describe _____
   Jewelry? Yes☐ No☐ Describe _____

Is the patient hard of hearing? Yes☐No☐ Hearing aid? Yes☐No☐
   Artificial limb? Yes☐No☐ Brace? Yes☐No☐

Is the patient calm? Yes☐No☐ Is the patient very anxious? Yes☐No☐
   Angry? Yes☐No☐ Is the patient agitated or very excited? Yes☐No☐

Has the patient ever had X rays taken in this hospital before? Yes☐No☐

Has the patient been admitted to this hospital before? Yes☐No☐

Is the clothing list completed? Yes☐No☐ Signed by_____

Is the signal cord attached to the bed? Yes☐No☐

Have drugs brought into the hospital by the patient been given to the charge
   nurse? Yes☐No☐

Name of the nurse drugs were given to _____

Was the patient told not to eat or drink anything until the doctor's visit?
   Yes☐No☐

Admitted by _____

wants it. If so, adjust these to suit him. Usually, it is more comfortable for the patient to have his knees raised a little when the head of the bed is elevated. Explain how the bed works and show him how to do it himself.

20. Take your completed checklist to your head nurse or team leader. Report your observations of anything unusual. Then tell the visitors they may go back into the room.

Procedure: Weighing and Measuring the Patient

1. Assemble your equipment:
   a. Portable balance scale
   b. Paper towel

2. Wash your hands.

3. Identify the patient by checking the identification bracelet.

4. Ask visitors to step out of the room.

5. Tell the patient that you are going to weigh him.

6. Pull the curtain around the bed for privacy.

7. Balance the scale. To do this, make sure the scale is standing level. Both weights (poises) must point to zero (0). Turn the balance screw until the pointer of the balance beam stays steadily in the middle of the balance area. The scale is now balanced.

8. Place a paper towel on the stand of the scale to protect the patient's feet.

9. Have the patient remove his robe and slippers. Assist him if necessary.

10. Help the patient to stand with both feet firmly on the scale.

11. Have the patient place both his hands at his side.

12. Adjust the weights (poises) until the balance pointer is again in the middle of the balance area.

13. Note the patient's weight. Write it down.

14. Raise the measuring rod above the patient's head.

15. Have the patient turn so that his back is against the measuring rod. Be sure he is standing very straight, with his heels touching the measuring bar.

16. Bring the measuring rod down so that it rests on the patient's head.

17. Note the patient's height. Write it down.

18. Raise the measuring rod. Help the patient to step off the scale.

19. Assist the patient back into bed, or help him to put on his robe and slippers.

20. Make the patient as comfortable as possible.

21. Wipe the entire scale with disinfectant solution.

22. Put the scale back where it belongs.

23. Wash your hands.

24. Report to your head nurse or team leader the patient's weight and height. Also report your observations of anything unusual. If the patient has dressings (bandages), this should be reported.

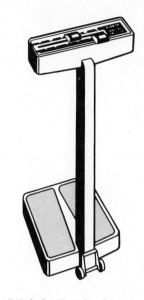

Weight Equivalents

Kilograms (kg)	Ounces (oz)	Pounds (lb)
	4	¼
	8	½
	12	¾
.50	16	1
22.68		50
45.36		100

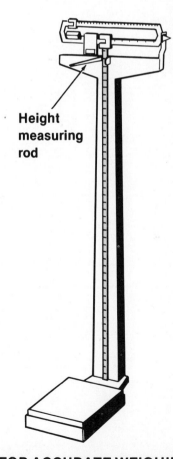

Height measuring rod

Rules To Follow: Taking Care of the Patient's Valuables

You may be responsible for taking care of the patient's jewelry, money, or other valuables at the time of admission.

- Itemize the valuables on the admission checklist.

FOR ACCURATE WEIGHING, SCALE MUST STAND LEVEL

- Ask the patient to place his valuables in the envelope.
- Close the envelope while you are with the patient. Make sure he sees you do this.
- Have the patient or relative sign the itemized list.
- Give the envelope to your head nurse or team leader. She will dispose of it in the proper way:
  a. The security officer picks it up and takes it to the hospital vault.
  b. A relative takes it home.
  c. A bonded admission clerk comes to the floor to take valuables to the safe. This clerk then gives the patient a receipt for his valuables.
- Being careful in describing these valuables on the itemized list is very important. It is not your job to decide how much any article is worth. A good description might be: "gold-colored metal earrings," rather than "gold earrings"; a "silver-colored ring with a clear stone," rather than a "diamond white gold ring"; a "silver-colored metal bracelet," rather than a "silver bracelet"; a "white stone necklace," rather than a "pearl necklace"; a "fur coat," rather than a "mink coat." Never touch the patient's money. Let the patient count it. Then you record the amount on the admission checklist.

Section 2: Transferring the Patient

OBJECTIVES: WHAT YOU WILL LEARN

When you have completed this section, you should be able:

- To transfer a patient to another unit within the hospital, following the correct procedure
- To help the patient to stay calm and feel comfortable

KEY IDEAS

During his stay, a patient may be transferred from one unit to another. This may be done for several reasons:

- He may have asked for a private room but none was available when he was admitted.
- He may ask to be transferred from a private room to a semiprivate room.
- He may be moved to another unit because of a change in his medical condition.

A patient may become alarmed if a doctor orders his transfer. In this case, try to calm the patient. Explain that the change is being made only for his benefit. Before you help in transferring a patient, be sure his new unit is ready to receive him.

Procedure: Transferring the Patient

1. Assemble your equipment, according to the needs of the patient:
   a. Wheelchair
   b. Stretcher
   c. Cart

- **Be sure the new unit is ready to receive the patient**
- **Help the patient remain calm**
- **Speak to him in a way that shows you care about him as a person**

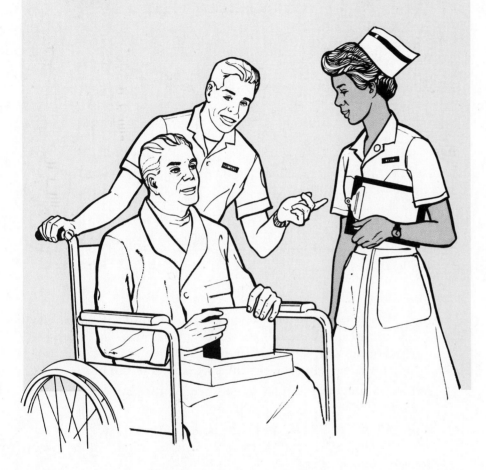

2. Wash your hands.

3. Identify the patient by checking the identification bracelet.

4. Ask visitors to leave the room.

5. Tell the patient you are going to transfer him to his new room.

6. Check to be sure the new unit is ready to receive the patient.

7. Collect the patient's personal belongings and equipment that is to be moved with him.

8. Transport the patient to this new unit:

   a. The patient can be moved in his own bed from one room to another. Personal belongings can be placed on the bed and moved with the patient. Or, if he has many personal articles, you may need a cart to move them.

   b. You may have to transport the patient by stretcher or

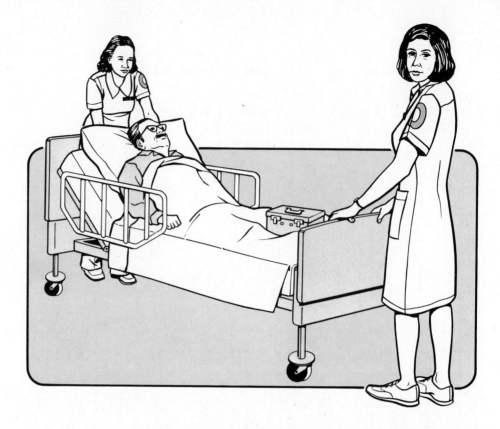

wheelchair to his new room. Here you will help the patient from the stretcher or wheelchair into his new bed. In these cases, put the patient's belongings and equipment on a cart. Move them after the patient is settled in the new unit.

9. Follow all safety precautions when wheeling the patient to his new room.

10. Give the patient both physical and emotional support. For example, he may need to be reassured that his visitors will be given his new room number.

11. Introduce the patient to his new roommate if there is one.

12. Make the patient comfortable in his new room.

13. Introduce him to the nursing staff who will be taking care of him now.

14. Arrange the unit. Help the patient to put away his personal possessions.

15. Report to the head nurse or team leader in the new nursing unit. Tell her that the patient is now in the new unit. Describe how the patient reacted to the transfer.

16. Return to your own floor. Strip the old bed. Take equipment that is not being used to the dirty utility room.

17. Wash your hands.

18. Report to your head nurse or team leader that the patient has been transferred to the new unit. Report the time and date and your observations of anything unusual.

Section 3: Discharging the Patient

OBJECTIVES: WHAT YOU WILL LEARN

When you have completed this section, you should be able:

- To discharge a patient from the hospital, following the correct procedure
- To keep the patient from becoming too tired before he leaves
- To assist the patient graciously and safely as he leaves the hospital

KEY IDEAS

The patient being discharged is often still weak and may tire easily. Your task at this time is a pleasant one. The patient is usually happy to know he can go home. The main things to remember are:

- The patient must not get too tired
- He must be sure to take with him everything that belongs to him

Written permission from a doctor is required for the patient to be discharged. Your head nurse or team leader will tell you when the doctor has

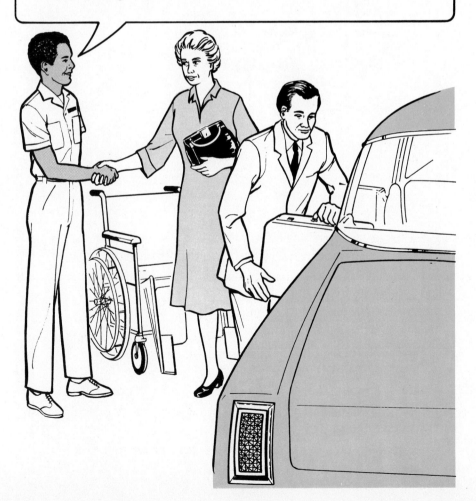

ordered that the patient is to be discharged. If the patient tries to leave, and you have not been told that the discharge order has been written by the doctor, tell your head nurse or team leader immediately. Also, every patient must be taken in a wheelchair to the business office, cashier, or discharge desk before leaving the hospital.

Patients are sometimes discharged from a hospital to another health care institution, such as a nursing home. These patients may leave the hospital in an ambulance. Your head nurse may give you special instructions for the care of these patients.

Normally, there is a certain hour—usually just before or after lunch—when most patients are discharged. This is so their rooms can be cleaned and made ready for new patients, who are often admitted early in the afternoon.

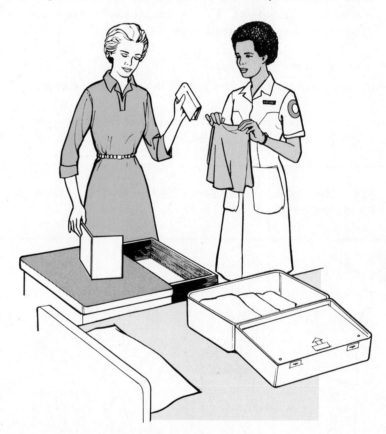

Procedure: Discharging the Patient

1. Assemble your equipment:
   a. Wheelchair
   b. Discharge slip
   c. Cart
2. Wash your hands.
3. Identify the patient by checking his identification bracelet.
4. Collect all of the patient's personal possessions for him. Help him to pack everything that belongs to him.
5. Be sure all valuables and medications are returned to the patient.
6. Help the patient get dressed, if necessary.

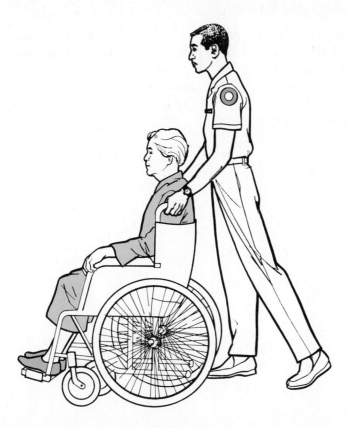

7. Make sure the patient has his written instructions from the head nurse, such as:

    a. Doctor's orders to follow at home
    b. Prescriptions
    c. Follow-up schedule of appointments with the doctor or the clinic

8. Bring the wheelchair to the patient's bedside. Help the patient get into it. Remember: All patients being discharged must leave the hospital in a wheelchair.

9. Before wheeling the patient off the floor, get the discharge slip from the head nurse or ward clerk.

10. Take the patient in the wheelchair to the discharge desk or cashier or business office. Give the clerk the discharge slip. Get a release form in return.

11. Wheel the patient to the front door. Help him out of the wheelchair and into his car or bus.

12. Take the wheelchair and release form back to your floor.

13. Report to your head nurse or team leader that the patient has been discharged. Report the time of discharge, the type of transportation used, and who it was that accompanied the patient—husband, daughter, friend. Also report your observations of anything unusual. Give the release form to your head nurse or team leader.

14. Wipe the entire wheelchair with an antiseptic solution.

15. Strip the linen from the bed. Put it in the dirty linen hamper.

16. Wash your hands.

WHAT YOU HAVE LEARNED

When you admit a new patient to your unit, you will make him comfortable, ease his fears, and help him adjust to his new surroundings. You will be taking care of your patient's personal possessions and valuables.

You will be helping in the procedure for transferring a patient from one hospital area or unit to another. Most important is relieving the patient of anxiety and making him comfortable.

You will have the usually pleasant task of helping your patients to get ready for discharge from the hospital, making sure they have all their possessions and that everything goes smoothly.

Physical Examinations, Body Positions, and Tubes and Tubing

13

Section 1: Your Role in the Physical Examination

OBJECTIVES: WHAT YOU WILL LEARN

When you have completed this section, you should be able:

- To assemble the equipment necessary for a routine physical examination
- To prepare the patient for the examination

KEY IDEAS

One of your important tasks during a patient's physical examination is to make him as relaxed, comfortable, and reassured as you can. Another impor-

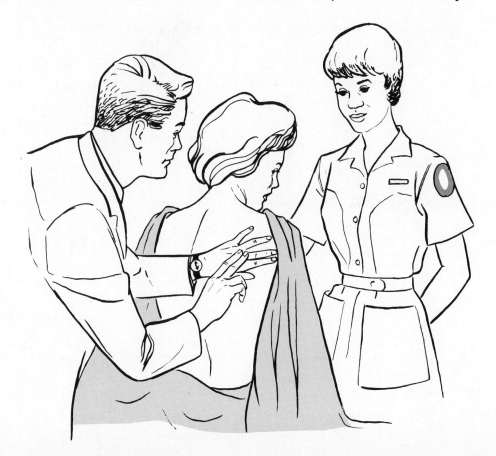

tant task is to prepare the patient and assemble the equipment for the examination. During the examination, you may help the doctor in several ways.

In preparing for an examination, you will be getting the patient ready, putting his unit in order, and collecting the equipment needed for the examination.

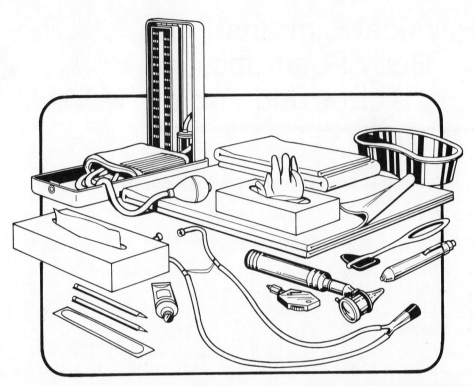

Procedure: Preparing the Patient for a Physical Examination

1. Assemble your equipment:
    a. Examination cart or box
    b. Extra lighting, if necessary
2. Wash your hands.
3. Identify the patient by checking the identification bracelet.
4. Ask visitors to step out of the room.
5. Explain to the patient that you are going to get him ready for a physical examination by the doctor (using the name of the doctor).
6. Pull the curtain around the bed for privacy.
7. Check the lighting in the room. If necessary, arrange for good lighting.
8. Bring the examination cart or box into the unit and put it in its proper place.
9. If the patient is wearing a hospital gown, untie the gown at the back and neck.
10. If the patient is wearing his or her own nightclothes, have the patient change into a hospital gown.
11. Offer the bedpan or urinal to the patient before the examination. There are several reasons for this:
    a. The patient will be less uncomfortable.

> b. Examination of the abdomen and pelvic regions will be easier for the doctor.
>
> c. You can collect a specimen and be ready for the doctor's request.

12. Cover the patient with a bath blanket or large sheet. Remove the top sheet and bedspread from the bed without exposing the patient.

13. The top sheet, blanket, or bedspread can be used during the examination for draping the patient. Draping a patient keeps him from being exposed during the examination. The sheet, blanket, or bedspread may be called the *drape*.

14. Wash your hands.

15. Report to your head nurse or team leader that you have prepared the patient for the physical examination. Also report the time and your observations of anything unusual.

Rules To Follow: During the Examination

1. Wash your hands before and after assisting with the examination.

2. When you hand a tongue depressor to the doctor, first tear the paper disposable covering halfway down. Never touch the tongue depressor with your fingers.

3. As the doctor takes it, pull the paper covering completely off. This way the doctor can take it by one end and put the clean end in the patient's mouth. When the doctor is finished with the tongue depressor, hold out an emesis basin so the doctor can drop it into the basin. The tongue depressor is discarded after the examination.

4. When the doctor asks for a flashlight, turn it on before you hand it to him.

5. The doctor may ask you to shine the flashlight into the patient's mouth. Follow his instructions.

6. When the doctor is ready to examine the patient's body, he will ask you to remove the patient's gown. Have a towel ready to cover the part of the patient's body the doctor is not examining.

7. When the doctor is ready to examine the patient's abdomen, fold the drape down to the patient's hips. Place a gown or towel across his chest.

8. When the doctor has finished this part of the examination, pull the drape back over the patient's chest.

9. When the doctor examines the patient's legs and feet, expose both legs so the doctor can compare them. He may use a percussion hammer to test the patient's reflexes.

10. Sometimes the doctor will ask the patient to stand up while he is examining the patient's feet and body alignment. Put a paper towel on the floor for the patient to stand on. Be sure the patient is properly draped.

11. When the examination is finished, make the patient comfortable.

12. Remove all of the equipment. Discard the disposable supplies. Put everything else back in its proper place.

EXAMINATION OF PATIENT'S ABDOMEN

- Place towel or gown over patient's chest
- Fold bedding down to patient's hips

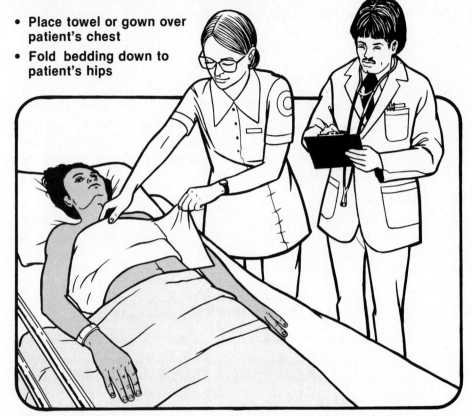

EXAMINATION OF PATIENT'S LEGS

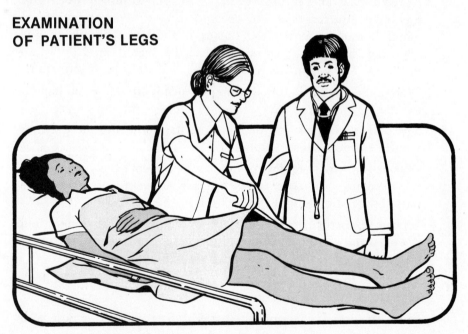

Section 2: Draping and Positioning the Patient

OBJECTIVES: WHAT YOU WILL LEARN

When you have completed this section, you should be able:

- To describe the positions used for physical examinations

- To help the patient get into these positions
- To arrange the patient's drape

KEY IDEAS

A patient will be standing or lying in different positions for certain kinds of examinations. Learn the names of these positions so you can accurately follow your instructions when positioning the patient for a certain kind of examination.

REVERSE TRENDELENBURG

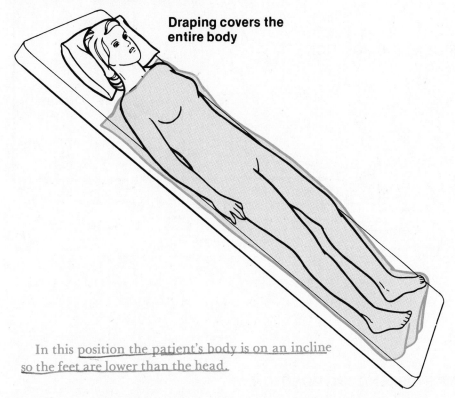

Draping covers the entire body

In this position the patient's body is on an incline so the feet are lower than the head.

HORIZONTAL RECUMBENT POSITION (SUPINE POSITION)
Draping covers the entire body

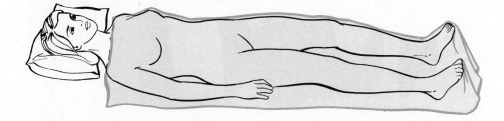

The patient lies on her back with her legs together and extended, or with her knees bent slightly to relax the muscles of the abdomen. A pillow is placed under the patient's head. The drape is spread loosely over the patient's body.

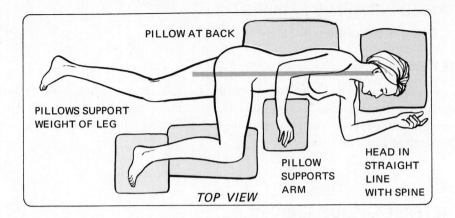

PILLOW AT BACK

PILLOWS SUPPORT
WEIGHT OF LEG

PILLOW
SUPPORTS
ARM

HEAD IN
STRAIGHT
LINE
WITH SPINE

TOP VIEW

SIDE-LYING POSITION

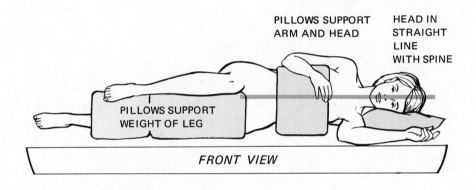

PILLOWS SUPPORT
ARM AND HEAD

HEAD IN
STRAIGHT
LINE
WITH SPINE

PILLOWS SUPPORT
WEIGHT OF LEG

FRONT VIEW

TRENDELENBURG POSITION
Draping covers the entire body

The position is used for surgery on the pelvic organs. The patient's head is low; her body is on an incline, carefully supported to prevent her from slipping out of position or being injured.

DORSAL LITHOTOMY POSITION

- Drape a folded sheet across the patient's chest
- Place a second sheet over the patient's legs

This is the same as the dorsal recumbent position, except that the patient's legs are well separated and the knees are bent more. This position is used often for examination of the bladder, vagina, rectum, and perineum. Sometimes with this position the patient's feet are placed in stirrups if an examination table is being used.

SEMI-FOWLER POSITION

Draping covers the entire body

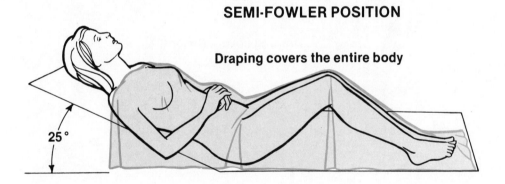

25°

This is similar to Fowler's position except that the back rest is at a lower angle (25°). The patient's knees are slightly bent.

PRONE POSITION

Draping covers the entire body

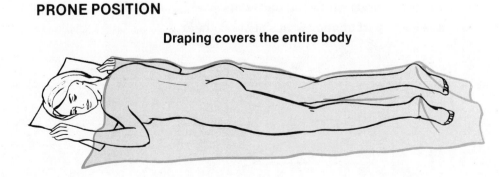

The patient lies on her abdomen with her arms at her sides, or bent at the elbows. Her head is turned to the side.

DORSAL RECUMBENT POSITION
Draping covers the entire body

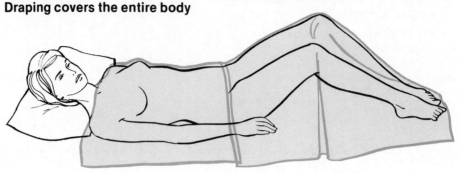

The position is similar to the horizontal recumbent position, except that the patient's legs are parted, the knees are bent, and the soles of the feet are flat on the bed. Drape the female patient by putting a sheet, folded once, across her chest. Put a second sheet crosswise over her legs loosely, so that the perineal region (the area of the body between the thighs) can be exposed for examination.

FOWLER'S POSITION
Draping covers the entire body

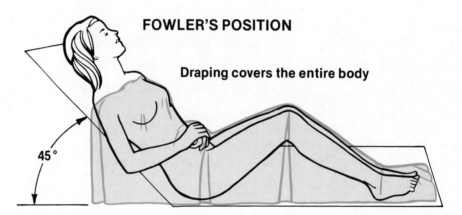

45°

This position is also called the high Fowler's position. The patient is partly sitting, with the back rest of the bed at a 45° angle. The knees are slightly bent and are supported, perhaps by a pillow.

LEFT LATERAL POSITION
- Drape top of body with a folded sheet
- Drape lower part of body with a second sheet

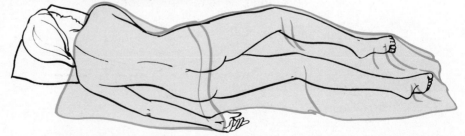

The patient lies on her left side. The hips are closer to the edge of the bed than the shoulders. The knees are bent, one more than the other.

KNEE-CHEST POSITION
Draping covers the entire body

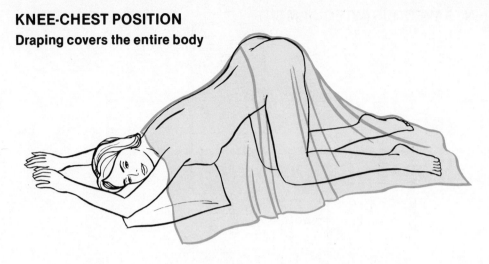

The patient rests on her knees and chest. The head is turned to one side with the cheek on a pillow. The patient's arms are extended slightly, bent at the elbows. Although the arms help support the patient, the main body weight is supported by the knees and chest. The knees are bent so that they are at right angles to the thighs. Draping is done with two sheets, one for the upper part of the body and one for the lower part. This position is used for examining the rectum and vagina.

LEFT SIMS' POSITION
Draping covers the entire body

The Sims' position is also called the "semiprone position." The patient lies on her left side. The patient's cheek is resting on a small pillow that is placed under the head. The right knee is bent against the patient's abdomen. The left knee is also bent, but not so much. The left arm is placed behind the body; the right arm rests in a way that is comfortable for the patient. This position is used for rectal examinations.

Section 3: Catheters, Tubes, and Tubing

OBJECTIVES: WHAT YOU WILL LEARN

When you have completed this section, you should be able:

- To change the patient's gown with an intravenous (IV) tube running into his body

INTRAVENOUS (IV) EQUIPMENT

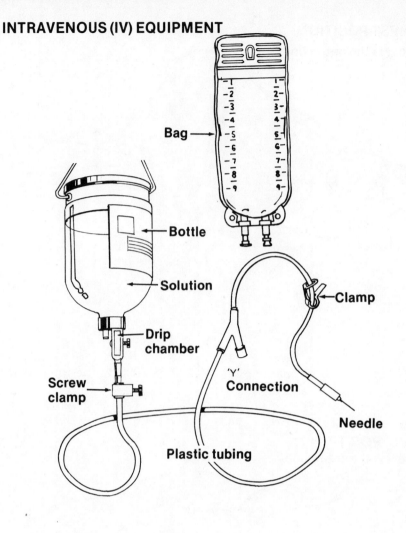

- To check the intravenous bottle, drip chamber, tubing, and the patient's arm, so that you can promptly report anything unusual to your head nurse or team leader
- To describe two methods of giving oxygen to patients

KEY IDEAS: INTRAVENOUS (IV) EQUIPMENT

Intravenous tubing is used often in the hospital to put fluids into the patient's body. The tube is connected to a bottle or plastic container. The container holds a fluid such as a clear sterile solution, usually a form of sugar or salt. The other end of the tube is connected to a needle. The needle is inserted by the doctor or the nurse into the patient's vein, usually in the arm. The purpose is to give fluids and nourishment to the body. It may be used to change the balance of certain chemicals in the patient's body. The solution flows from the bottle into the patient's vein and is circulated through his body.

The amount of fluid that can flow into the patient's body is controlled by a clamp on the tube. This clamp allows only a certain number of drops per minute to flow from the bottle. You should never touch this clamp. Only a doctor or a nurse may change or regulate the amount of flow of a solution. You may have to move the patient in bed or change his postion without stopping the flow of the solution.

Rules To Follow

1. If the needle has been inserted in the patient's hand or arm, tell him and help him to keep his arm straight. He may cut off the flow of solution if he bends his wrist or elbow.

2. Make sure the patient is never lying on top of the tubing. Watch for and straighten out any kinks that may form in the tubing. This may happen when the patient changes his position. Pressure or kinks might stop the flow of the solution.

3. To remove a patient's soiled gown:
    a. Untie the gown
    b. Remove the arm without the IV from the sleeve.
    c. Carefully remove the gown from the arm with the IV, considering the tube and the container as part of the arm. Move the sleeve down the arm, over the tubing, and up to the bottle.
    d. Remove the bottle from the hook, being careful not to lower the bottle below the area on the patient's arm where the needle is inserted.
    e. Slip the gown over the bottle, and return the bottle to its hook.

4. To put a clean gown on the patient, consider the bottle and tube as part of the patient's arm.
    a. Carefully lift the bottle from the hook. Don't let the bottle be lower than the area on the patient's arm where the needle has been inserted.
    b. Then quickly slip the sleeve of the gown over the bottle.
    c. Replace the bottle on the hook.
    d. Slip the gown down the tube and then over the patient's arm. (You can do this only if the bottle is not wider than the sleeve of the gown.)

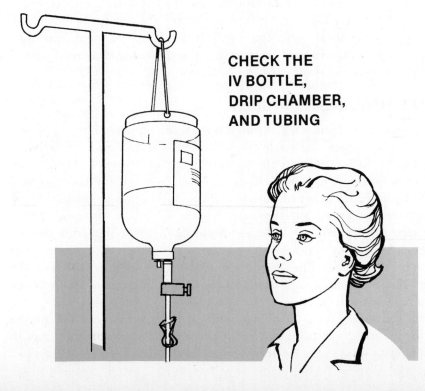

**CHECK THE
IV BOTTLE,
DRIP CHAMBER,
AND TUBING**

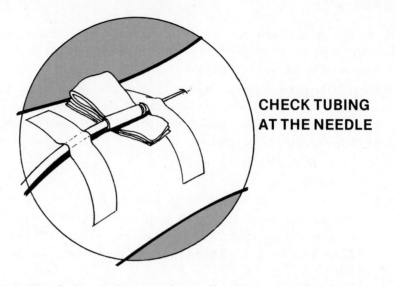

**CHECK TUBING
AT THE NEEDLE**

5.   Watch for and report immediately to your head nurse or team leader:

   a.   When you can't see drops of solution passing from the bottle into the tubing, but there is still some solution in the bottle.
   b.   When the plastic drip chamber is completely filled with the solution.
   c.   When you see blood in the tubing at the needle end.
   d.   When all the solution has run out of the bottle or the bottle is almost empty.
   e.   When the patient has deliberately or accidentally removed the needle.
   f.   When the tubing has been disconnected and is saturating the bed while the patient is bleeding freely from the connection.
   g.   When the patient complains of pain or tenderness at the site (place) where the needle is inserted.
   h.   When you notice a lumpy, raised, or inflamed area on the patient's skin near the place where the needle is inserted. This might mean that the solution is not running into the vein but, instead, is running into the tissue nearby. This is called *infiltration* of an IV solution.

KEY IDEAS: NASOGASTRIC TUBES

A nasogastric tube is inserted through one of the patient's nostrils *(naso)*. Then it is passed down the back of the patient's throat and through the esophagus until the end reaches the patient's stomach *(gastric)*. These tubes are used for nasogastric, or tube, feedings. In such feedings, fluids or liquified (blenderized) foods are given to a patient through the tube at regular times. Nasogastric feeding is also called *gavage.*

Nasogastric tubes may also be used to drain fluids by suction from the patient's stomach. Also, sometimes a doctor wants a specimen of the contents of the stomach to be tested. Then the nasogastric tube is used to withdraw the specimen. This is called *lavage.* It refers to the washing out of the stomach through a nasogastric tube.

When a nasogastric tube is being used to drain substances out of the stomach or to collect a specimen, the patient is given nothing by mouth (NPO). The food would only be drawn back out through the tube. When you

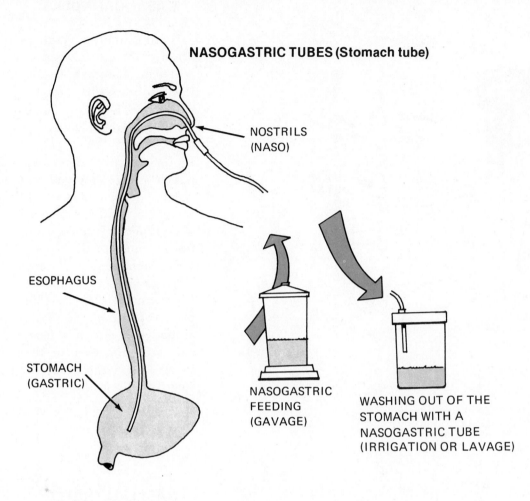

NASOGASTRIC TUBES (Stomach tube)

NOSTRILS
(NASO)

ESOPHAGUS

STOMACH
(GASTRIC)

NASOGASTRIC
FEEDING
(GAVAGE)

WASHING OUT OF THE
STOMACH WITH A
NASOGASTRIC TUBE
(IRRIGATION OR LAVAGE)

are caring for patients with nasogastric tubes in place, you should follow these rules:

- Never pull on the tube when moving the patient or changing his position.
- Keep the tube clean and free from mucus deposits at the entrance to the nostril.
- Remember to refasten the connecting tubing to the patient's clean gown after you have finished bathing him. This eases the strain on the tube and prevents an accidental withdrawal.
- If the patient begins to gag or vomit while the tube is in place, report this immediately to the head nurse.

KEY IDEAS: SUCTION

Fluids are removed from the patient's body through tubes by gravity or suction. When fluids are removed by gravity, the collecting container is placed near the patient at a level that is lower than his body. The fluid drips into the container. Suction is also used to remove thick secretions that cannot be drawn out easily by gravity.

Sometimes suction is used in emergency situations. This may happen when a patient cannot breathe because his respiratory passages are blocked by mucous secretions.

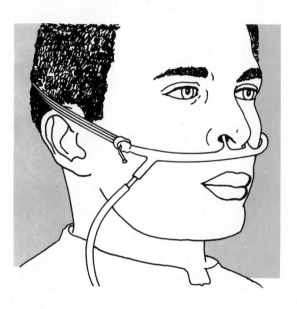

NASAL CANNULAS

Nasal cannulas, or tubes, are used to give oxygen to a patient. The cannulas are inserted into the patient's nostrils. They are used when the patient needs extra oxygen, not when equipment must provide a patient's total supply of oxygen. The cannula, which is made of plastic, is a half-circle length of tubing with two openings in the center. It fits about one-half inch into the patient's nostrils. Nasal cannulas are held in place by an elastic band around the patient's head and are connected to the source of oxygen by a length of plastic tubing.

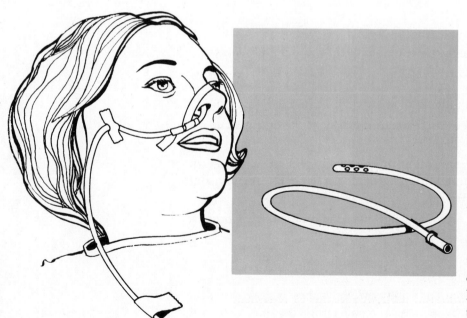

NASAL CATHETER

This catheter is a piece of tubing that is longer than a cannula. It is inserted through the patient's nostril into the back of his mouth. The nasal catheter is a more effective way to give oxygen to the patient than the nasal cannula. The nasal catheter is used when the patient must have additional oxygen at all times. It is more effective than an oxygen tent or an oxygen mask and is less likely to frighten the patient. The nasal catheter is fastened to the patient's forehead or cheek with a piece of adhesive tape that holds it steady.

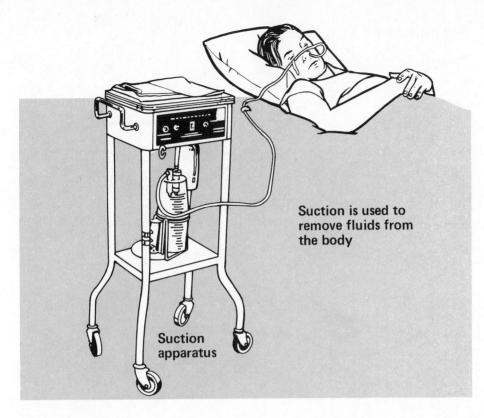

Suction is used to remove fluids from the body

Suction apparatus

Rules To Follow

1. Report immediately to the head nurse or team leader if you see what looks like leakage in the tube and suction system.

2. Never open the collecting containers to empty the drainage without instructions from your head nurse or team leader.

3. Never raise the drainage bottle.

4. Never disconnect the tubing.

5. Never remove the clamp that is kept at the bedside of a patient who has closed-chest drainage.

6. Tell your head nurse or team leader if the level of fluid in the container stops rising. The tubing may be blocked or drainage may be complete.

7. The drainage collected through the tubes is measured at regular times. The color and kind of material being drained may have to be noted. You may be asked to take these measurements and record them on the output side of the Intake and Output sheet.

8. If a specimen of the drainage is needed, collect the amount specified by the head nurse or team leader.

9. If there is a rapid increase in the amount of material being drained, or any change in the material itself, report this to your head nurse or team leader right away.

KEY IDEAS: URINARY CATHETERS

The urinary catheter is the most common kind of catheter used for taking fluids out of the body. This catheter is made of plastic. The catheter is in-

THE URINARY CATHETER

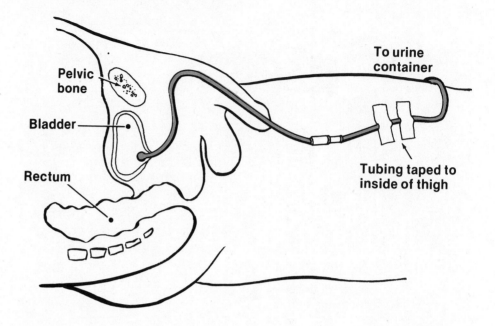

serted through a patient's urethra into his bladder. The urinary catheter may be used to take a sterile specimen. This catheter also may be used when a patient is unable to urinate naturally. Or it may be used to measure the amount of urine left in the bladder after a patient has voided naturally.

Sometimes a urinary catheter is used for only one withdrawal of urine. Sometimes, however, it is kept in place in the bladder for a number of days or even weeks. In most hospitals only a doctor or a nurse can insert or withdraw a catheter.

Sometimes the bladder-drainage catheter is used to help keep an incontinent patient dry. An incontinent patient is one who cannot contain his urine or feces. The catheter is specially made so that it will stay in place within the bladder. It really is two tubes, one inside the other. The inside tube is connected at one end to a kind of balloon. After the catheter has been inserted, the balloon is filled with water or air so the catheter won't pass out through the urethra. Urine drains out of the bladder through the outer tube. The urine collects in a container. The container is attached to the bed frame lower than the patient's urinary bladder. This is always a closed system, which means it is never opened.

Rules To Follow

1. Check from time to time to make sure the level of urine has gone up. If the level stays the same, report this to your head nurse or team leader.

2. If the patient says he feels that his bladder is full, or that he needs to urinate, report this to your head nurse or team leader.

3. If the patient is allowed to get out of bed for short periods, the bag goes with the patient. It must be lower than the patient's urinary bladder at all times.

PLASTIC URINE CONTAINER
HUNG ON BED FRAME

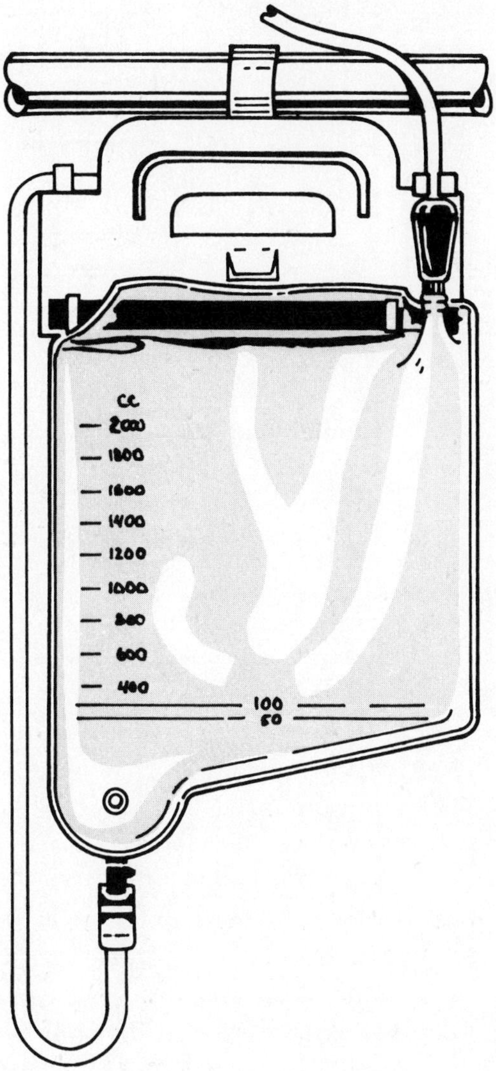

Tubing from patient
- **Check tubing for kinks**
- **Be sure patient is
  not lying on tubing**

4. Check to make sure there are no kinks in the catheter and tubing. Be sure the patient is not lying on either one. This would stop the flow of urine.

5. The catheter should be taped at all times to the patient's inner thigh. This keeps it from being pulled out of the bladder.

6. All patients with urinary drainage through a catheter are on output. You must keep a careful record of urinary output.

7. Catheter care should be done daily for these patients.

8. Report to your head nurse or team leader any complaints of burning, tenderness, or pain in the patient's urethral area.

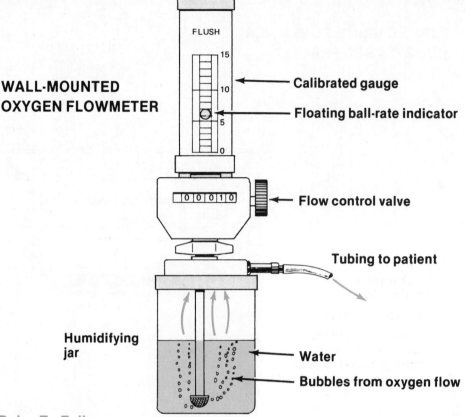

FLUSH

15

**WALL-MOUNTED
OXYGEN FLOWMETER**

10

— **Calibrated gauge**

— **Floating ball-rate indicator**

5

0

|0|0|0|1|0|

— **Flow control valve**

Tubing to patient

**Humidifying
jar**

— **Water**

— **Bubbles from oxygen flow**

Rules To Follow

1. Because oxygen is being used, be sure to observe all fire regulations in effect in your hospital.

2. Check the flowmeter, a piece of equipment that shows the rate at which oxygen is being given to the patient.

3. The tubing connected to the source of oxygen should be taped to the patient's gown or bedclothes. This helps to keep it in place and will prevent injury to the patient's nostrils if the tubing is accidentally pulled.

4. Make sure the tubing is not kinked. Also, it should not be under any part of the patient's body. This might slow down or stop the flow of oxygen.

5. A humidifying jar should be used with both the nasal oxygen cannula and the nasal oxygen catheter. The water level in the humidifying jar should be kept high enough so that it bubbles as the oxygen goes through it.

6. Inhalation therapy or respiratory therapy departments are responsible in most hospitals for the inhalation therapy treatments the patient might be receiving. Such departments take care of the oxygen equipment and make adjustments in the treatments by checking with the doctor, head nurse, or team leader.

WHAT YOU HAVE LEARNED

As a nursing aide you will be called upon to prepare the patient for a physical examination by the doctor. Your role in assisting the doctor includes positioning and draping the patient.

Part of your work will be observing and checking to make sure that intravenous tubes and other tubes and catheters attached to the patient's body are functioning properly.

All of the tubes and catheters used in modern hospitals today are disposable. This means that these tubes and catheters are discarded in the proper place after one use.

Warm and Cold Applications

14

OBJECTIVES: WHAT YOU WILL LEARN

When you have completed this chapter, you will be able:

- To explain why warm or cold applications are used
- To keep the application at the right temperature
- To explain what generalized and localized mean
- To explain the difference between moist and dry applications
- To begin applications at the right time
- To keep applications in place for the right length of time
- To check applications at the right times
- To keep the patient safe
- To keep the patient comfortable
- To follow the correct procedures

KEY IDEAS: REASONS FOR WARM AND COLD APPLICATIONS

Heat may be applied to an area of the body to speed up the healing process. This is done in the following way: Heat dilates (expands) the blood vessels in the body area. This causes more blood to circulate to the injured tissues nearby. More blood can bring more food and oxygen. These are needed for the repair (healing) of tissue. Warm tub baths, sometimes with medication in the water, are often prescribed for this reason. A sitz bath is an example. Warm water is applied to the patient's perineal or rectal area to speed up healing after childbirth or surgery.

Heat may also be applied to an area of the body to ease the pain caused by inflammation and congestion. When the blood vessels become dilated, the increased supply of blood may absorb and carry away the fluids that are causing the inflammation and pain. For example, people with certain bone and joint conditions often get relief from pain and can increase the movement of their body parts because of exercises in warm water.

Cold may be applied to a small (localized) body area or to the whole body. When cold is applied to a small area, the blood vessels contract (become smaller). This contraction may help to prevent or reduce swelling. The application helps in the case of a sprained ankle or the beginnings of a black eye.

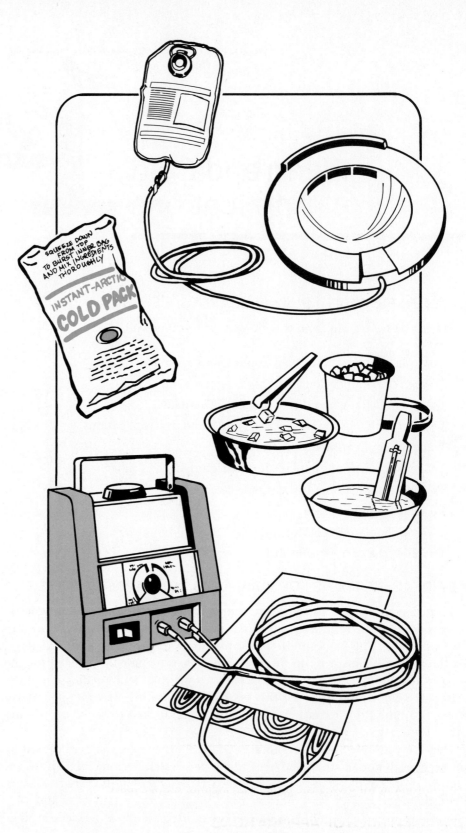

The contraction slows down the flow of blood. Therefore it reduces the amount of body fluids that are carried into the injured area. This also prevents or reduces the pain that usually goes along with the swelling.

Cold may be applied to control bleeding. When cold is applied, the blood vessels contract. The blood flow becomes slower. Less blood is able to seep out

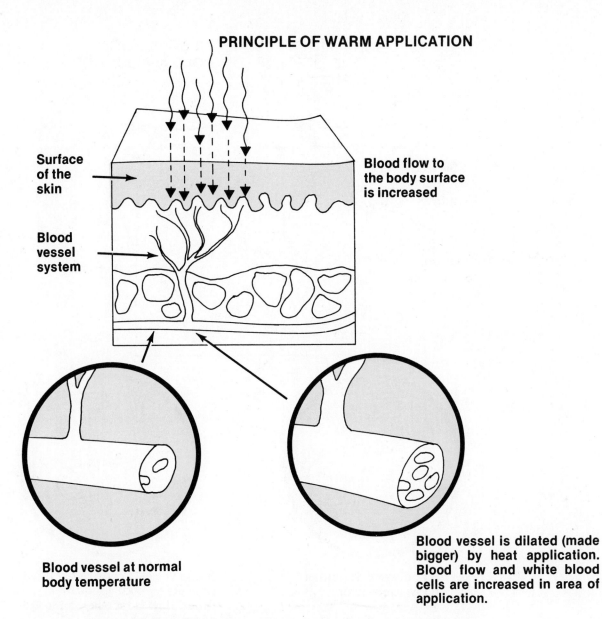

PRINCIPLE OF WARM APPLICATION

Surface of the skin

Blood vessel system

Blood flow to the body surface is increased

Blood vessel at normal body temperature

Blood vessel is dilated (made bigger) by heat application. Blood flow and white blood cells are increased in area of application.

through a cut or other wound. For example, when a patient has had a tonsillectomy, an ice collar or ice pack may be applied to the neck region.

Cold may be applied to a patient's entire body. This is usually done to lower a patient's body temperature when he has a fever. Special equipment is used to lower the body temperature. The equipment may include:

- An oxygen tent with a temperature regulator
- Applications of cold wet packs
- Equipment for giving the patient an alcohol sponge bath

TEMPERATURES OF APPLICATIONS

For a warm application, always use a bath thermometer first to test the temperature of the water. Temperatures for different kinds of heat applications are:

- Warm soak . . . . 100°F (37.8°C)
- Warm compress . . . . 115°F (46.1°C)

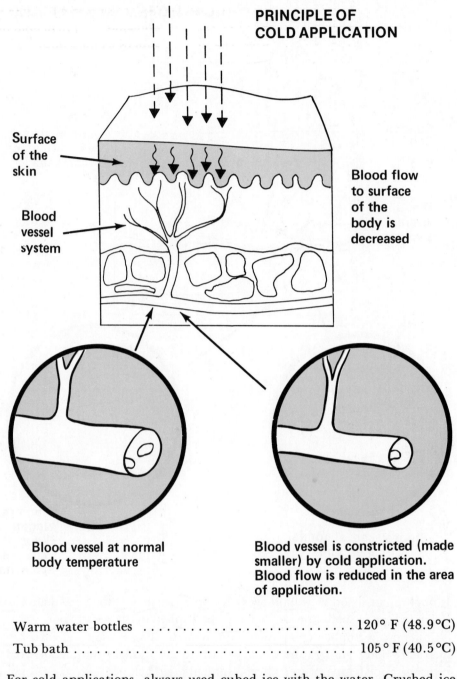

PRINCIPLE OF COLD APPLICATION

Surface of the skin

Blood vessel system

Blood flow to surface of the body is decreased

Blood vessel at normal body temperature

Blood vessel is constricted (made smaller) by cold application. Blood flow is reduced in the area of application.

- Warm water bottles .... 120° F (48.9°C)
- Tub bath .... 105° F (40.5°C)

For <u>cold applications, always used cubed ice with the water. Crushed ice melts too fast. Also it may stick to the cloths and be too cold for the patient's skin.</u> Keep the application cold by adding ice as necessary. <u>Never cover the cold application with linen or any other material after it has been applied to the patient's body. If you cover it, <u>heat will be trapped beneath the cover.</u> Then the application will become warm and will have to be changed sooner than usual.</u>

KEY IDEAS: LOCALIZED AND GENERALIZED APPLICATIONS

Be sure you know exactly where on the patient's body the warmth or cold is to be applied. A <u>generalized application is one in which a warm or cold application is applied to a patient's whole body. A <u>localized application is one that is applied to a specific part or area of a patient's body.</u></u>

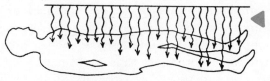

GENERALIZED APPLICATIONS
Applying warmth or cold to the
patient's entire body

**LOCALIZED
APPLICATIONS**
Applying warmth or cold to a
specific part or area of the body

Moist and Dry Applications

All applications are either <u>moist</u> or <u>dry</u>. <u>A moist application is one in which water touches the skin</u>. A <u>dry application is one in which no water touches the skin</u>. There are several types of both moist and dry applications.

Moist	Dry
Soak—warm or cold	Ice cap and ice collar
Compress—warm or cold	Warm water bottle
Tub	Heat lamp
Alcohol sponge bath	Aquamatic K pad
Sitz bath	Thermal blankets
Cool wet packs	Electric heat cradle
Commercial unit warm pack	Commercial unit cold pack

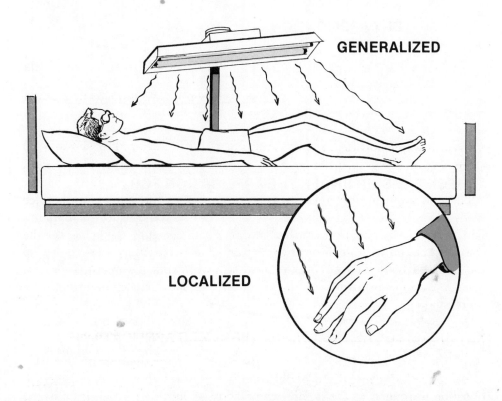

GENERALIZED

LOCALIZED

Compresses and soaks are both moist applications. They can be either warm or cold. A compress is a localized application. A soak can be either localized or generalized. In applying a compress, a cloth is dipped into water, wrung out, and applied to the skin. To apply a soak, you immerse the body or body part completely in the water. Warm water bottles, ice caps, and aquamatic K pads are considered dry applications because they have a dry surface. Water is used only inside the equipment and never touches the skin. Dry applications are sometimes used to keep moist applications at the correct temperature.

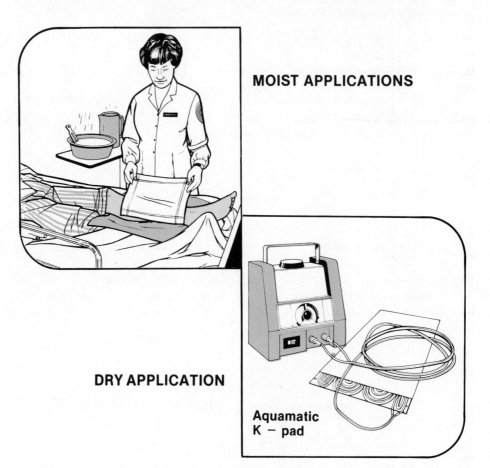

MOIST APPLICATIONS

DRY APPLICATION

Aquamatic K – pad

CHECK THE SKIN UNDER THE APPLICATION FOR

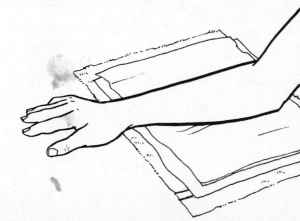

- **Discoloration of the skin: red or white**
- **If you think the patient is being burned discontinue treatment**
- **Report to your head nurse or team leader immediately**

Length of Applications

Follow the instructions given to you by the head nurse or team leader for the exact time to begin the applications. Also follow her instructions about how long the application is to stay in place.

In some hospitals an ice cap is applied for 10 minutes, removed for 10 minutes, and then reapplied. Following orthopedic surgery, however, ice caps are often ordered continuously on the cast.

Do not put an ice cap or warm water bottle on an area of the body for more than 1 to 2 hours at a time. After 2 hours, remove the cap or bottle for one-half hour before continuing the applications. Soaks and compresses may be kept on the body part for a certain period of time (continuous). Or they may be used for 15 or 20 minutes and then taken off at intervals during the day (intermittent).

Checking the Application

Check the application often to keep it at the right temperature throughout the treatment. Suggested times for checking the temperatures of different kinds of applications are:

- Every 5 minutes — soaks and intermittent compresses
- Every 10 minutes — heat lamps
- Every 30 minutes — continuous compresses
- Every hour — warm water bottles and ice bags

Keeping the Patient Safe

Avoid accidents. Be sure the patient is not in a position where he might fall. Be careful not to spill any water. Be sure the bed is properly protected. Put the side rails in the upright position during the treatment.

Check the patient's skin under warm applications. Watch for too much redness. Look for a darker discoloration that might mean the patient is being burned. Listen when the patient complains. If you think a patient is being burned, remove the heat application immediately and call your head nurse or team leader.

Check the patient's skin where cold is being applied. If the area appears to be blanched, very pale, white, or bluish, tell the nurse right away. Watch for changes in the color of parts of the patient's body. For example, if the patient's lips, fingernails, and eyelids look blue or turn a dark color, this is *cyanosis*, which usually is a sign of shock. Stop the treatment immediately and call your head nurse or team leader.

Always apply the ice cap and warm water bottle with its metal or plastic stopper away from the patient's body. The stopper should never touch the patient's skin. It will be much warmer or colder than the application. It could burn the patient. Remember, ice can burn the patient's skin. You may be working with an unconscious patient. If so, you may be directed to protect him from a burn by putting a blanket between his skin and the warm water bottle or ice cap.

Keeping the Patient Comfortable

Make sure the patient is in a position that is comfortable for him and convenient for your work. Keep the patient covered and warm during the treatment. Otherwise the patient might become chilled and uncomfortable. If a

OBSERVE THE PATIENT FOR SIGNS OF CYANOSIS

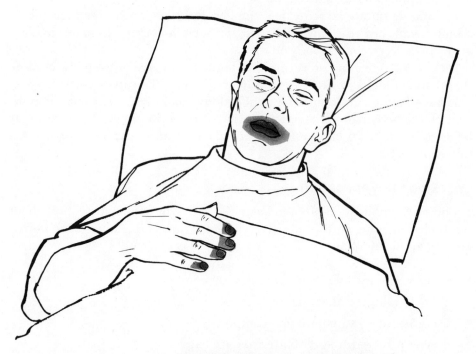

Watch for blueness or darkening of the lips, fingernails, and eyelids

patient shivers during the cold application, stop the treatment. Cover him with a blanket. Then report this at once to your head nurse or team leader. She will tell you what to do.

Never put the warm water bottle or ice bag on top of the painful area. The weight will probably increase the pain. Never fill a warm water bottle or ice bag more than half full. It gets too heavy.

Always dry the bottle or bag. Also check it for leaks by turning it upside down. Always place it in a flannel cover. Never let the patient lie on the warm water bottle or ice bag.

When you have finished with an application of moist heat or cold, dry the patient's skin thoroughly and gently, using patting motions. Don't rub the patient's skin to dry it.

Procedure: Applying the Warm Compress (Moist Heat Application)

1. Assemble your equipment:
    a. Disposable bed protector
    b. Basin
    c. Water at 115° F (46.1° C)
    d. Washcloth, towel, or gauze pads (compress)

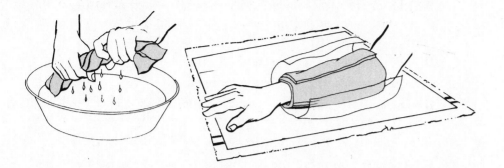

e. Bath thermometer
f. Large sheet of plastic
g. Bath towel
h. Bath blanket
i. Pitcher

2. Wash your hands.

3. Identify the patient by checking the identification bracelet.

4. Ask visitors to step out of the room.

5. Tell the patient you are going to apply a warm compress.

6. Pull the curtain around the bed for privacy.

7. Help the patient into a comfortable, safe position. Have the area exposed that is to be given a warm compress.

8. Place a disposable bed protector under the body area that is to be given the warm compress.

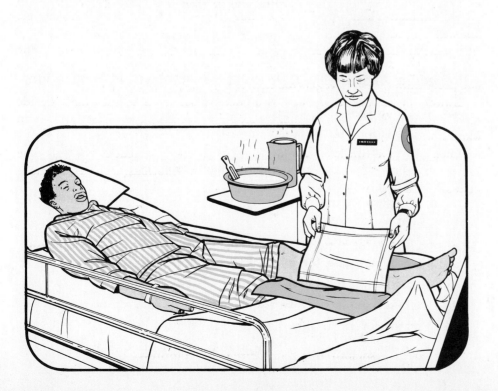

9. Fill the pitcher with warm water. Check the temperature of the water with a bath thermometer. Then pour the water into the basin.

10. Dip the compress into the water and wring it out thoroughly.

11. Apply the compress gently to the proper area.

12. Cover the entire compress with a plastic sheet. This keeps the compress warm.

13. If the patient is cold or chilly, cover him with a blanket.

14. Change the compress and remoisten it, as necessary, to keep it warm.

15. Sometimes a patient is able to apply the compress himself. If your head nurse or team leader gives permission for this, position and assist the patient as necessary.

16. Check the skin under the application every 5 minutes. If the skin appears red, remove the compress. Cover the area with a towel or blanket. Report to your head nurse or team leader.

17. A warm compress is usually applied for 15-20 minutes. However, follow the instructions of your head nurse or team leader as to how long the warm compress is to be applied.

18. After the treatment is completed, remove the compress and gently pat the area dry with a towel. Help the patient into a comfortable position in bed. Cover him with a blanket if he requests it.

19. Clean your equipment and put it in its proper place. Put disposable supplies in the proper container.

20. Wash your hands.

21. Report to your head nurse or team leader:
    - The time the warm compress was started
    - How long the compress was in place
    - The area of application
    - Your observations of anything unusual

Procedure: Applying the Cold Compress (Moist Cold Application)

1. Assemble your equipment:
    a. Disposable bed protector
    b. Basin
    c. Washcloth, towel, or gauze pads (compress)
    d. Bath towel
    e. Bath blanket
    f. Cold water

2. Wash your hands.

3. Identify the patient by checking the identification bracelet.

4. Ask visitors to step out of the room.

5. Tell the patient that you are going to apply a cold compress.

6. Pull the curtain around the bed for privacy.

7. Help the patient into a comfortable, safe position. Have the area exposed that is to receive the cold compress.

8. Place a disposable bed protector under the body area that is to be given the cold compress.

9. Put cold water in the basin.

10. Dip the compress into the water and wring it out thoroughly.

11. Apply the cold compress to the proper area of the patient's body as quickly as possible. If you are slow, the compress will absorb heat from your hands and the air.

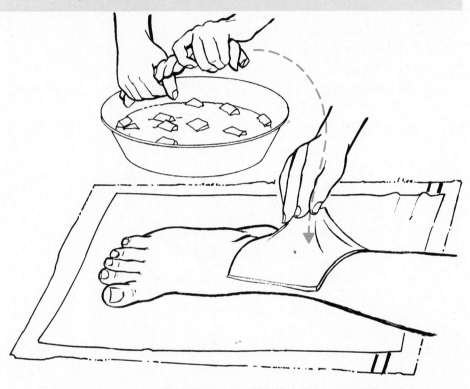

12. If the patient is cold or chilly, cover him with a blanket. Don't cover the compress or the area being treated.

13. Change the compress and remoisten it, as necessary, to keep it cold.

14. Sometimes a patient is able to apply the compress himself. If your head nurse or team leader gives permission for this, position and assist the patient as necessary.

15. Check the patient's skin under the application every 5 minutes. If the skin appears to be blanched or white, remove the compress. Cover the area with a towel or blanket. Report to your head nurse or team leader.

16. A cold compress is usually applied for 15-20 minutes. However, follow the instructions of your head nurse or team leader as to how long the cold compress is to be applied.

17. When the treatment is finished, remove the compress and gently pat the area dry with a towel. Help the patient into a comfortable position in bed. Cover him with a blanket if he requests it.

18. Clean your equipment and put it in its proper place. Put disposable supplies in the proper container.

19. Wash your hands.

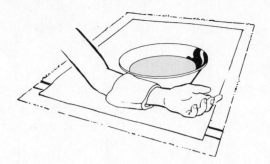

20. Report to your head nurse or team leader:
     - The time the cold compress was started
     - How long it remained in place
     - The area of application
     - Your observations of anything unusual

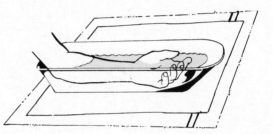

Procedure: Applying the Cold Soak (Moist Cold Application)

1. Assemble your equipment:
    a. Basin, foot tub, or arm basin
    b. Pitcher
    c. Disposable bed protectors
    d. Bath towel
    e. Bath blanket
2. Wash your hands.
3. Identify the patient by checking the identification bracelet.
4. Ask visitors to step out of the room.
5. Tell the patient that you are going to apply a cold soak.
6. Pull the curtain around the bed for privacy.
7. Help the patient into a safe, comfortable position. Have the area exposed that is to be treated.
8. Fill the pitcher with cold water. Then fill the basin half full.
9. Protect the bed with disposable bed protectors.
10. Put the basin in a position so the patient's arm, leg, foot, or hand can be dipped into the basin easily.
11. Put the patient's arm or leg into the water gradually.
12. When you need to change the water, take the patient's arm or leg

out of the basin. Wrap it with a bath towel or bath blanket to keep it warm.

13. If the patient says he feels weak or cold, stop the treatment. Cover the patient with extra blankets and report to your head nurse or team leader.

14. Check the skin every 5 minutes. If the skin is blanched or white, stop the treatment. Report to your head nurse or team leader.

15. When the treatment is finished, dry the patient's arm or leg by gently patting it with a towel.

16. Make the patient as comfortable as possible.

17. Remove the equipment from the patient's room. Clean and put it back in its proper place. Put disposable supplies in the proper container.

18. Wash your hands.

19. Report to your head nurse or team leader:
    - The time the cold soak was started
    - The length of treatment
    - The area of application
    - Your observations of anything unusual

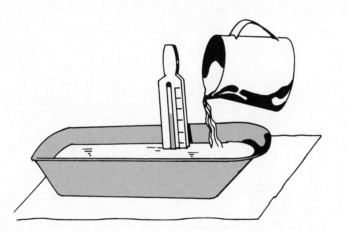

Procedure: Applying the Warm Soak (Moist Warm Application)

1. Assemble your equipment:
    a. Basin, foot tub, or arm basin
    b. Pitcher
    c. Bath thermometer
    d. Disposable bed protectors
    e. Bath towel
    f. Bath blanket

2. Wash your hands.

3. Identify the patient by checking the identification bracelet.

4. Ask visitors to step out of the room.

5. Tell the patient that you are going to apply a warm soak.

6. Pull the curtain around the bed for privacy.

7. Help the patient into a safe, comfortable position. Have the area to be treated exposed.

8. Fill the pitcher with warm water.

9. Check the temperature of the water with the bath thermometer. It should be 100° F (37.8° C).

10. Fill the basin about half full of water at 100° F (37.8° C).

11. Protect the bed with disposable bed protectors.

12. Put the basin in a position so the patient's arm, hand, leg, or foot can be placed in it easily.

13. Put the arm or leg into the water gradually.

14. Check the temperature of the water with the bath thermometer every 5 minutes to be sure it is at the right temperature. When you need to change the water, take the patient's arm or leg out of the basin. Wrap it with a bath blanket or bath towel to keep it warm.

15. If the patient says he feels weak or cold, stop the treatment. Cover the patient with extra blankets and report to your head nurse or team leader.

16. Check the skin every 5 minutes. If the skin is red, stop the treatment. Report to your head nurse or team leader.

17. When the treatment is finished, dry the patient's arm or leg by patting gently with a towel.

18. Make the patient as comfortable as possible.

19. Remove your equipment from the patient's room. Clean and put it back in its proper place. Put disposable supplies in the proper container.

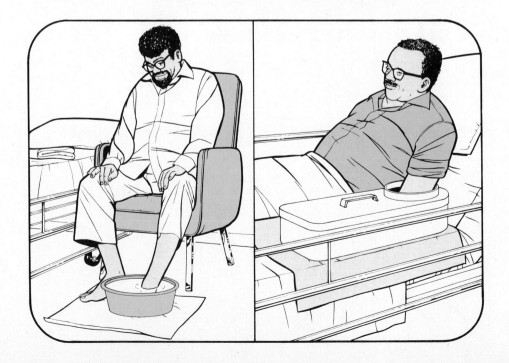

20. Wash your hands.

21. Report to your head nurse or team leader:
    - The time the warm soak was started
    - The length of treatment
    - The area of application
    - Your observations of anything unusual

Procedure: Applying the Warm Water Bottle (Dry Heat Application)

1. Assemble your equipment:
   a. Warm water bottle (may be disposable)
   b. Pitcher of water at 120° F (48.9° C)
   c. Bath thermometer
   d. Flannel cover

2. Wash your hands.

3. Identify the patient by checking the identification bracelet.

4. Ask visitors to step out of the room.

5. Tell the patient that you are going to apply a warm water bottle.

6. Pull the curtain around the bed for privacy.

7. Fill the pitcher with water. Check the temperature with a bath thermometer. The water should be 120° F (48.9° C).

8. Fill the warm water bottle one-half full.

9. To squeeze the air out of the bottle:
   a. Put the bag on the edge of a counter. Have the part of the bag containing water hanging down. Have the part of the bag without the water lying on the countertop.
   b. Put your hand on top of the bag at the edge of the table. Move your hand slowly toward the opening of the bag, pressing out the air. With your other hand, close the bag.
   c. Place the warm water bottle in a horizontal position on a flat surface. Hold the neck of the warm water bottle upright until you can see water in the neck of the bottle.

10. Fasten the top tightly.

11. Dry the warm water bottle. Check for leaks by turning it upside down.

12. Put it into a flannel cover.

13. Apply it gently to the proper body area.

14. Never put the warm water bottle on top of a painful area. The weight will increase the pain. Put it on the side.

15. Check the warm water bottle every hour to be sure the temperature is correct. Change the water in the bottle, when necessary, to continue the treatment at the same temperature.

16. Check the skin under the warm water bottle every hour. If the skin is red, remove the warm water bottle and report to your head nurse or team leader.

17. After the treatment is finished, clean and return your equipment to its proper place. Put disposable supplies in the proper container.

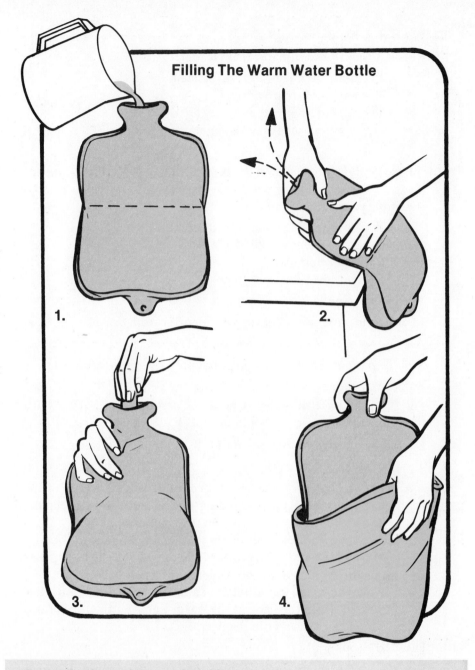

Filling The Warm Water Bottle

1.

2.

3.

4.

18. Make the patient comfortable.

19. Wash your hands.

20. Report to your head nurse or team leader:
   - The time the warm water bottle was applied
   - The length of treatment
   - The area of application
   - Your observations of anything unusual

Procedure: Applying the Ice Bag, Ice Cap, and Ice Collar (Dry Cold Application)

1. Assemble your equipment:
   a. Ice bag, ice cap, or ice collar (may be disposable), bowl of ice
   b. Flannel cover

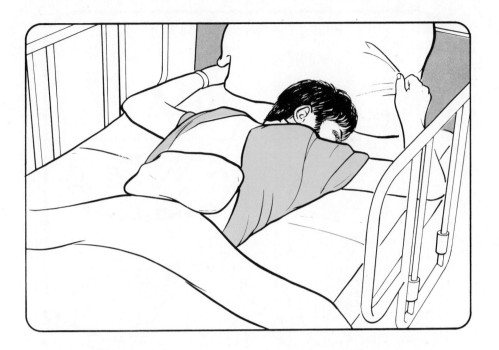

2. Wash your hands.

3. Identify the patient by checking the identification bracelet.

4. Ask visitors to step out of the room.

5. Tell the patient that you are going to apply the ice bag, ice cap, or ice collar.

6. Pull the curtain around the bed for privacy.

7. Pour cold water over the ice cubes to melt the sharp edges.

8. Fill the ice collar, ice bag, or ice cap one-half full of ice.

9. Squeeze the sides of the ice bag to force the air out of it.

10. Fasten the stopper tightly.

11. Dry the outside of the ice bag with a paper towel.

12. Invert the ice bag to test for leaking.

13. Put the ice bag into the flannel cover.

14. Apply the ice bag to the proper area of the patient's body.

15. If the patient is cold or chilly, cover him with a blanket. Don't cover the ice bag or the area being treated.

16. Don't leave the ice bag on an area of the body for more than 2 hours at a time. After 2 hours, remove the ice bag for a half hour before continuing the cold application. Replace the ice in the ice bag every hour. This will keep it cold enough for proper application.

17. Check the skin under the application every hour. If the skin appears to be blanched or white, remove the ice bag. Cover the area with a towel and report to your head nurse or team leader.

18. Clean your equipment and put it in its proper place. Put disposable supplies in the proper container.

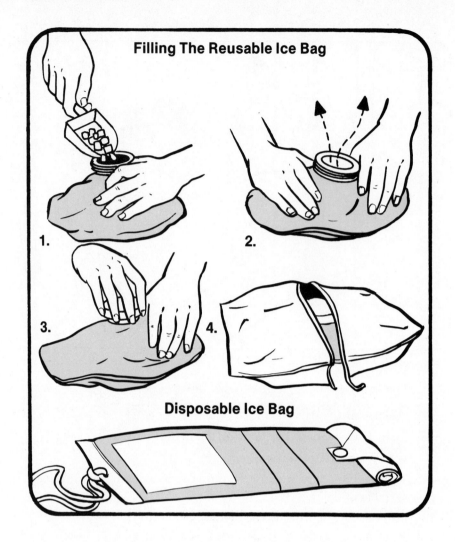

Filling The Reusable Ice Bag

1.

2.

3.

4.

Disposable Ice Bag

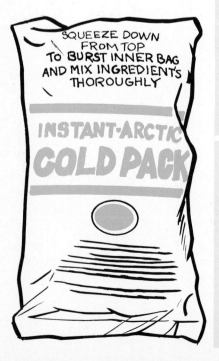

SQUEEZE DOWN FROM TOP TO BURST INNER BAG AND MIX INGREDIENTS THOROUGHLY

INSTANT-ARCTIC COLD PACK

19. Make the patient comfortable.

20. Wash your hands.

21. Report to your head nurse or team leader:
   - The time the ice bag was applied
   - The length of treatment
   - The area of application
   - Your observations of anything unusual

Procedure: Applying the Commercial Unit Cold Pack (Dry Cold Application)

1. Assemble your equipment:
   a. Commercial unit single-use cold pack
   b. Cloth cover

2. Wash your hands.

3. Identify the patient by checking the identification bracelet.

4. Ask visitors to step out of the room.

5. Tell the patient that you are going to apply a cold pack.

6. Pull the curtain around the bed for privacy.

7. Place the cloth cover on the unit. Hit the unit with your hand. A single blow to the surface activates the unit.

8. Apply the pack to the proper area of the patient's body.

9. Check the skin under the application every 10 minutes. If the skin appears blanched or white, remove the pack and report to your head nurse or team leader.

10. If the treatment is continuous, replace it as necessary with a new cold pack.

11. Put disposable supplies in the proper container.

12. Make the patient comfortable.

13. Wash your hands.

14. Report to your head nurse or team leader:
    - The time the cold pack was applied
    - The length of treatment
    - The area of application
    - Your observations of anything unusual

Procedure: Applying the Commercial Unit Heat Pack (Moist Warm Application)

1. Assemble your equipment:
   a. Commercial unit single-use warm pack (gauze pad and cover)
   b. Heating lamp unit
   c. Disposable bed protectors

2. Wash your hands.

3. Place the commercial unit single-use warm pack in the heating lamp unit for 10 minutes.

4. Identify the patient by checking the identification bracelet.

5. Ask visitors to step out of the room.

6. Tell your patient that you are going to apply a warm pack.

7. Pull the curtain around the bed for privacy.

8. Place the bed protector under the body part that is to receive the warm pack.

9. Remove the warm pack from the heating lamp unit.

10. Tear the foil covering off the warm pack.

11. Place the moist warm gauze pad on the proper body area.

12. Cover the gauze.

13. Check the skin under the application every 10 minutes. If the skin appears red, remove the pack and report to your head nurse or team leader.

14. If the treatment is continuous, replace it as necessary with a new warm pack.

15. When the treatment is finished, remove disposable supplies and put them in the proper container.

16. Make the patient comfortable.

17. Wash your hands.

18. Report to your head nurse or team leader:
- The time the warm pack was applied
- The length of treatment
- The area of application
- Your observations of anything unusual

Procedure: Applying a Heat Lamp (Dry Warm Application)

1. Assemble your equipment:
    a. Heat lamp
    b. Bath blanket
    c. Bath towel
    d. Tape measure

2. Wash your hands.

3. Identify the patient by checking the identification bracelet.

4. Ask visitors to step out of the room.

5. Tell the patient that you are going to apply a heat lamp.

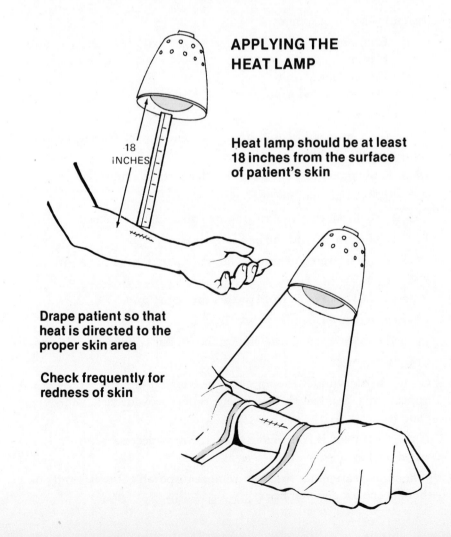

APPLYING THE HEAT LAMP

18 INCHES

Heat lamp should be at least 18 inches from the surface of patient's skin

Drape patient so that heat is directed to the proper skin area

Check frequently for redness of skin

6. Pull the curtain around the bed for privacy.

7. Expose only the body area that is to receive the heat. Drape the patient so that heat is directed to the proper area of the skin. Cover the rest of the patient's body with a bath blanket or bath towel.

8. The part of the patient's body that is being treated should be at least 18 inches away from the heat lamp. Use a tape measure to check the distance.

9. Check the skin every 5 minutes. If the patient's skin becomes red, stop the treatment and report to your head nurse or team leader.

10. There is a danger of fire when a heat lamp is being used. Therefore, keep all linen away from the lamp.

11. Leave the heat lamp on the patient for no more than 10 minutes, unless you have other instructions from your head nurse or team leader.

12. After the treatment, remove the lamp and put it back in its proper place.

13. Make the patient as comfortable as possible.

14. Wash your hands.

15. Report to your head nurse or team leader:
    - The time the heat was applied
    - The length of treatment
    - The area of application
    - Your observations of anything unusual

Note. When you are using the heat lamp as a perineal, or "peri," lamp, help the patient into the lithotomy position. Place her feet on the mattress. Bend the knees and separate them. Place the lamp 12 to 18 inches from the perineum. Remove the peripad to expose the perineal area. Remove the pillow. Instruct the patient to keep her head flat, exposing more of the perineum. Watch for excessive heat. The light should be on for only 10 minutes. When the treatment is finished, remove the lamp. Put a new peripad in place and refasten.

Procedure: Applying the Aquamatic K-Pad (Dry Heat Application)

1. Assemble your equipment:
   a. Aquamatic K-pad and control unit. The temperature is preset by CSR (central supply room). The container is filled with distilled water by CSR.
   b. Cover for pad (pillowcase or flannel case)

2. Wash your hands.

3. Identify the patient by checking the identification bracelet.

4. Ask visitors to step out of the room.

5. Explain to the patient that you are going to apply the K-pad.

6. Pull the curtain around the bed for privacy.

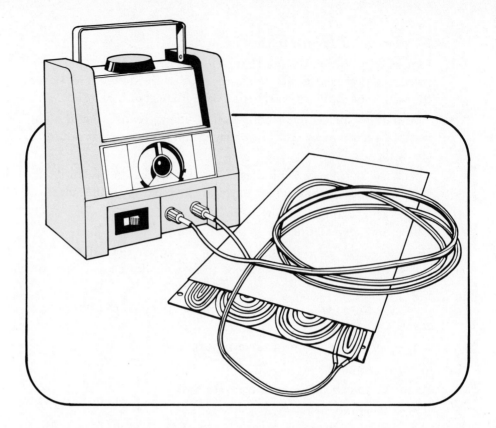

7. Inspect the K-pad for leaks and to make sure the cord and plug are in good condition.

8. Plug the cord into an electrical outlet.

9. Place the pad in the cover. Don't use pins.

10. Put the container on the bedside table. Arrange the tubing at the level of the pad. Don't allow the tubing to hang below the level of the bed.

11. Apply gently to the proper body area.

12. Check the skin under the pad every hour.

13. When the treatment is finished, return the equipment to its proper place.

14. Wash your hands.

15. Report to your head nurse or team leader:
    - The time the K-pad was applied
    - The length of treatment
    - The area of application
    - Your observations of anything unusual

Procedure: Applying the Cool Wet Pack (Moist Cold Application)

1. Assemble your equipment:
    a. Two sheets
    b. Large basin of cool water
    c. Two bath blankets
    d. Disposable bed protectors

     e.   Bath towels

     f.   Plastic laundry bag

2. Wash your hands.

3. Identify the patient by checking the identification bracelet.

4. Ask visitors to step out of the room.

5. Tell the patient that you are going to apply a cool wet pack.

6. Pull the curtain around the bed for privacy.

7. Soak both sheets in the cool water.

8. Remove the patient's gown.

9. Put one bath blanket over the bedspread. Ask the patient to hold the blanket. Without uncovering the patient, remove the top sheet and bedspread, leaving the blanket in place. Put the bedclothes on a chair nearby for replacement later.

10. Put the disposable bed protectors and bath blanket under the patient by having the patient turn from side to side.

11. Wring out one wet sheet. Place it under the patient. Put one wet sheet over the patient, removing the top blanket.

12. As the sheets get warm, remove them, covering the patient with the bath blanket. Soak the sheets again in cool water. Reapply to the patient's body every 5 minutes.

13. Don't dry the patient's skin until the entire procedure is finished.

14. Continue the procedure for the length of time specified by your head nurse or team leader.

15. When the treatment is finished, dry the patient by patting the skin gently. Put his gown back on. Remake the bottom of the bed if it is wet. Replace the top sheet and bedspread.

16. Cover the patient with extra blankets if he complains of being cold.

17. Put the soiled sheets and towels in the plastic laundry bag.

18. Clean and put the large basin in its proper place.

19. Wash your hands.

20. Report to your head nurse or team leader:

- The time the cool wet pack treatment was started
- The length of treatment
- Your observations of anything unusual

Procedure: Using the Disposable Sitz Bath
(Moist Warm Application)

1. Assemble your equipment:

     a.   Disposable sitz bath containing:

          (1)   Plastic bowl (Some models clip on. Other models have a large brim that keeps it in place. The disposable bowl is sometimes called a "Hi-hat" or "Sitz-ette.")

          (2)   Plastic bag

          (3)   Plastic tubing

          (4)   Stopcock (clamp)

          (5)   Plastic laundry bag

DISPOSABLE SITZ BATH KIT

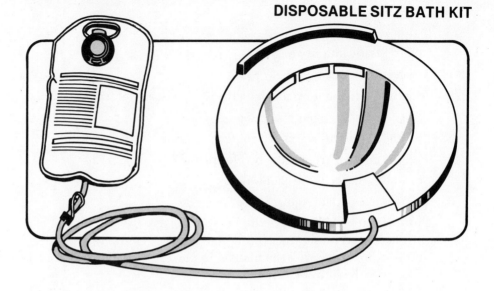

    b.   Bath thermometer
    c.   Bath towels
    d.   Pitcher

2. Wash your hands.

3. Identify the patient by checking the identification bracelet.

4. Ask visitors to step out of the room.

5. Tell the patient that you are going to give him a sitz bath.

6. Pull the curtain around the bed for privacy.

7. Help the patient into the bathroom.

8. Raise the toilet seat.

9. Fill the pitcher with water and check the temperature with the bath thermometer. It should be 105° F (40.5° C).

10. Put the plastic bowl into the toilet bowl.

11. Pour the water at 105° F (40.5° C) into the bowl, filling it one-half full.

12. Be sure that the opening for overflow is toward the front of the toilet.

13. Close the stopcock on the tubing. Fill the plastic container with water at 115° F (46.1° C) from the pitcher. Close the bag.

14. Hang the container for water 12 inches higher than the bowl.

15. Help the patient sit down in the sitz bath. Be sure the patient can reach the signal light.

16. Place the tubing inside the bowl between the patient's legs with the opening under the water level.

17. Open the stopcock and adjust the flow if necessary.

18. Have the patient sit in the sitz bath with water running in for 10 to 20 minutes.

19. If the patient says he feels weak or faint, stop the treatment. Turn on the signal light for help in getting the patient out of the bathroom.

20. When the treatment is finished, remove the tubing. Help the patient out of the sitz bath.

21. Pat the patient's body gently with a towel to dry.

22. Help the patient back into bed. Make him as comfortable as possible.

23. Clean your equipment and return it to its proper place. If it is not to be used again, put it in the proper container. Dispose of the sitz bath kit.

24. Put the used towels in the plastic laundry bag.

25. Wash your hands.

26. Report to your head nurse or team leader:
    - The time the sitz bath was started
    - The length of time the patient was in the sitz bath
    - Your observations of anything unusual

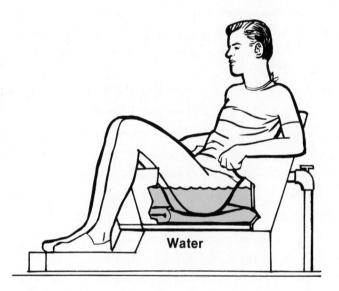

Water

Procedure: Using the Portable Chair-Type or Built-In Sitz Bath (Moist Warm Application)

1. Assemble your equipment:
    a. Portable chair or built-in sitz bath
    b. Disinfectant cleanser
    c. Bath towels
    d. Bath blankets
    e. Plastic laundry bag

2. Wash your hands.

3. Identify the patient by checking the identification bracelet.

4. Ask visitors to step out of the room.

5. Tell the patient that you are going to give him a sitz bath.

6. Pull the curtain around the bed for privacy.

7. Bring the portable chair-type sitz bath into the patient's room. Or help the patient (using a wheelchair if necessary) to the room with the built-in chair-type sitz bath.

8. Clean the sitz bath with disinfectant cleanser.

9. Rinse it well.

10. Fill it half full with water at 105° F (40.5° C).

11. Place a towel on the seat and on the front edge of the sitz bath.

12. Help the patient to undress, except for his gown.

13. Help the patient to sit down in the tub. Hold his gown up so it doesn't get wet.

14. Cover the patient's shoulders with a bath blanket if he complains of being cold.

15. Continue the treatment for 10–20 minutes, unless you have other instructions from your head nurse or team leader.

16. Check the patient every 5 minutes.

17. If the patient says he feels weak or faint, stop the treatment. Put the signal light on for help in getting the patient out of the tub. Let the water out of the tub.

18. When the treatment is finished, help the patient out of the tub.

19. Pat his body gently with a towel to dry.

20. Help the patient back to bed. Make him as comfortable as possible.

21. Clean the sitz tub with disinfectant cleanser.

22. Put the portable chair-type tub back in its proper place.

23. Put used towels in the plastic laundry bag.

24. Wash your hands.

25. Report to your head nurse or team leader:
    - The time the sitz bath was started
    - The length of time the patient was in the sitz bath
    - Your observations of anything unusual

KEY IDEAS: THE ALCOHOL SPONGE BATH

You have had the experience of perspiring on a warm summer day. You often feel cooler as the moisture evaporates from your skin. As perspiration evaporates into the air, it carries some heat with it. This cools the body. An alcohol sponge bath cools a patient's body in the same way. Alcohol is applied to the patient's body because it will evaporate from the skin much faster than water. The purpose of the alcohol sponge bath is to lower the patient's body temperature.

When you are giving the alcohol sponge bath:

- You will put ice caps on certain areas of the patient's body. Often the areas are the armpits or the groin (the area where the thighs meet the trunk of the body). These are places where many blood vessels are close to the surface of the body.

- You will put warm water bottles around the patient's feet. This prevents the patient from becoming chilled. The feet are the area of the body farthest from the heart. Therefore they have the poorest circulation.

- Never apply alcohol to the patient's face.

- You may add ice cubes to the cooling solution. This is done only if you are given this instruction by your head nurse or team leader.

- If the patient becomes chilled and starts to shiver, stop the treatment. Call the nurse. If the patient's shivering can't be controlled, the alcohol sponge bath will do no good. This is because the shivering causes increased cell and muscle activity. This produces more heat and causes the body temperature to rise.

- Alcohol sponge baths are never given without the doctor's orders.

- Alcohol sponge baths are not given to children. This treatment is too severe for a child.

Two other methods are sometimes used for generalized cold applications. These are thermal blankets and oxygen tents. Such applications also lower the patient's body temperature. A cool-mist air tent is sometimes used if an infant or child has a fever. The coolness and increased humidity from the fine mist help to reduce the fever.

Procedure: Giving the Alcohol Sponge Bath (Moist Cold Application)

1. Assemble your equipment:
   a. Alcohol 70% (one cup of alcohol mixed with one cup of cool water)
   b. Basin
   c. Two bath blankets
   d. Two warm water bottles with covers
   e. Six ice caps with covers
   f. Ice cubes, if ordered
   g. Bath towels
   h. Two washcloths
   i. Thermometer
   j. Two small towels
   k. Disposable bed protectors
   l. Plastic laundry bag
2. Wash your hands.
3. Identify the patient by checking the identification bracelet.
4. Ask visitors to step out of the room.
5. Tell the patient that you are going to give him an alcohol sponge bath.
6. Pull the curtain around the bed for privacy.
7. Take the patient's temperature, pulse, and respiration.
8. Record the information in the proper place.
9. Put the bath blanket on top of the bedspread and top sheet.
10. Ask the patient to hold the blanket. Without uncovering the

patient, remove the top sheet and bedspread from under the blanket the patient is holding.

11. Remove the patient's gown without uncovering him.

12. Fold and place the top sheet, the bedspread, and the gown on a chair nearby. These will be replaced after the treatment.

13. Place the disposable bed protectors and bath blanket under the patient by turning him from side to side.

14. Help the patient to move close to the side of the bed where you will be working.

15. Place a small dry towel between the patient's legs to cover the genital area.

16. Fill the ice caps with ice cubes. Cover them with flannel covers. Place one on each side of the patient's neck, one in each armpit, one on the groin, and one on top of the patient's head.

17. Wet one small towel with cold water and place it under both knees.

18. Fill both warm water bottles. Place one at the bottom of each of the patient's feet.

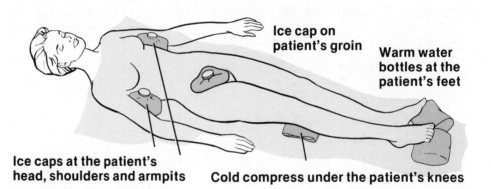

Ice cap on patient's groin

Warm water bottles at the patient's feet

Ice caps at the patient's head, shoulders and armpits

Cold compress under the patient's knees

19. Mix the solution as instructed, or put one cup of alcohol with one cup of water into the basin.

20. Put both washcloths in the water-alcohol solution.

21. Alternate the washcloths throughout this procedure.

22. Place a bath towel under the arm farther away from you.

23. Make a mitt with a washcloth. Dip it into the solution. The washcloths should not be wrung out. They should be dripping wet.

24. Sponge the entire arm and underarm with long, even strokes. Do not dry the area. Place the arm under the blanket wet. Then remove the towel.

25. Repeat the step on the arm closer to you.

26. Fold the bath blanket down to the patient's waist. Place a towel across the blanket to keep it dry.

27. Sponge the front of the patient's neck and chest to the waistline. Do not dry, but cover with a towel.

28. Fold the bath blanket to the groin. Place a second towel across the groin area.

29. Sponge the entire abdomen with the alcohol solution. Then cover the abdomen and chest with a blanket. Remove both towels as you cover him with the blanket.

30. Expose the leg farther from you. Place a towel under the leg. Sponge the entire leg with the alcohol solution. Do not dry, but cover the leg with the blanket and remove the towel.

31. Repeat the process on the leg closer to you.

32. Turn the patient on his side. Spread a towel over the mattress near his back. Sponge the back of his neck, his back, and his buttocks with long, even strokes.

33. Do not dry. Turn the patient on his back. Cover him with the blanket. Remove the towels.

34. Repeat this entire process for 20 minutes.

35. Add more alcohol and water as needed.

36. Stop the treatment if the patient complains of being cold or if he shivers. Stop if he becomes cyanotic or if you observe anything unusual. Report to your head nurse or team leader.

37. When the treatment is finished, remove the bath blankets. Change the sheets if they have become damp. Remove all ice bags and warm water bottles. Replace the gown, the top sheet, and the bedspread. Cover the patient with extra blankets if you are instructed to do so by your head nurse or team leader.

TAKING VITAL SIGNS

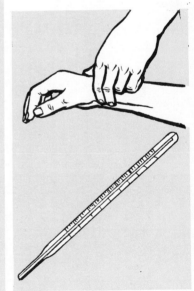

38. Put all soiled linen in the plastic laundry bag.

39. Clean your equipment and put it in its proper place. Put any disposable supplies in the proper container.

40. Take the patient's vital signs twice: 10 minutes after the treatment has been completed and one-half hour after the treatment is completed.

41. Wash your hands.

42. Report to your head nurse or team leader:
   - The time the alcohol sponge bath was started
   - How long it was given
   - The patient's vital signs
   - The time they were taken
   - Your observations of anything unusual

WHAT YOU HAVE LEARNED

You have studied the principles and purposes of warm and cold and dry and moist applications. You have been given the procedures for applying warm and cold compresses; warm and cold soaks; warm water bottles; ice bags, caps, and collars; heat lamps; the aquamatic K-pad; the commercial unit cold pack; the portable chair-type and built-in sitz bath; cool wet packs; and alcohol sponge baths. Keep alert and observe the patient carefully during applications of warmth and cold.

Preoperative and Postoperative Nursing Care

15

Section 1: Preoperative Nursing Care

OBJECTIVES: WHAT YOU WILL LEARN

When you have completed this section, you should be able:

- To complete a preoperative checklist accurately
- To shave a patient in preparation for surgery
- To help the preoperative patient feel calm and relaxed
- To get the patient's unit ready for his return from the operating room or recovery room

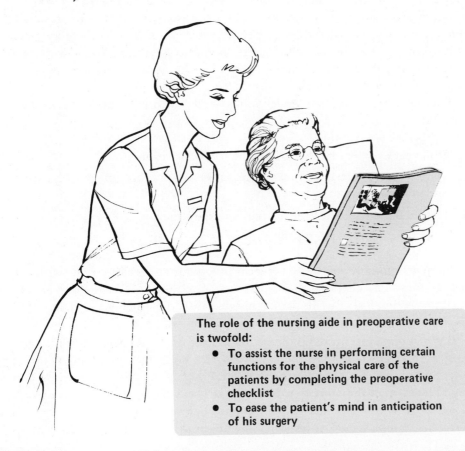

The role of the nursing aide in preoperative care is twofold:
- To assist the nurse in performing certain functions for the physical care of the patients by completing the preoperative checklist
- To ease the patient's mind in anticipation of his surgery

KEY IDEAS

Two very important words are used often in this chapter. They are: *preoperative* and *postoperative*.

- The word *operative* means an operation or surgery
- *Pre* means before
- *Post* means after
- Therefore, *preoperative* means before surgery
- *Postoperative* means after surgery

Almost every patient who enters a hospital for an operation will be a little nervous and upset. Part of your job as a nursing aide is to make the patient feel as calm and relaxed as possible.

Some things that might upset the preoperative patient are:

- Concern for his family
- Being away from work
- How soon he may return to his job
- A possible disability because of the operation
- The possibility of death or serious complications
- Fear of the unknown

Good physical and emotional preoperative care can help to reduce anxiety and fears. Give the patient all your attention. Make him feel that you care about him and how the operation comes out. Listen and show interest in what the patient says. Many frightened people relieve their tension by talking a lot and by asking lots of questions. Others do not say anything. You can give support to your patient just by being there when he needs assistance, by staying calm if he seems upset, and by being tactful.

Your head nurse or team leader will give you the preoperative checklist and tell you:

- What each patient has been told about his operation
- What you are to tell and teach the patient to prepare him for his surgery and postoperative care
- How to handle and answer the patient's questions
- What nursing care to give the patient

In most hospitals, you will be given a preoperative checklist along with your instructions. The checklist shown here is a sample. It is like the one actually used in the hospital. By filling out this checklist, the nursing staff can be sure the patient has been properly prepared for surgery.

Before an operation, the patient's skin in the operative area must be free of hair and as clean as possible. Hair on the body is a breeding place for microorganisms. Because hair can't be sterilized, it must be removed by shaving. The area on the body that is shaved is where the operation is going to be done. When you are shaving a patient before an operation, watch for scratches, pimples, cuts, sores, or rashes on the skin. If you see anything on the

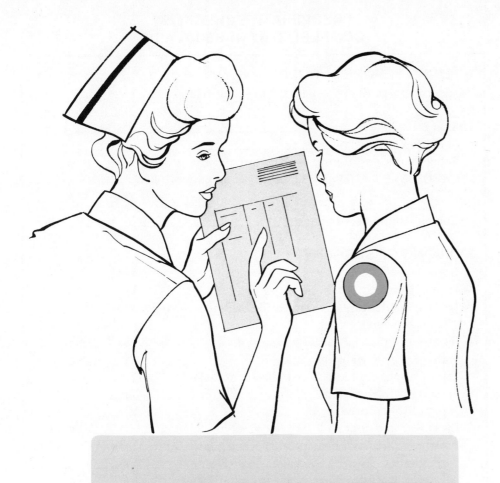

YOUR HEAD NURSE OR TEAM LEADER WILL GIVE YOU THE PREOPERATIVE CHECKLIST

skin that looks abnormal, be sure to report this to the head nurse or team leader.

In some hospitals, the patient is sent to the operating room suite one hour before he is scheduled for surgery. At that time the nurses in the operating room will *prep* the patient (shave him or her in preparation for surgery). This is done in those hospitals that have anterooms to the operating rooms. In the anteroom, each patient has his own cubicle, which is merely a curtained-off area. In other hospitals, the staff does the prep the evening before surgery. The operating room staff does another complete prep after the patient is on the operating room table.

The prep is done with a special prep kit. This is obtained from the central supply room for each patient. After it is used, it is discarded in the dirty utility room. There is a sponge in each kit or pack with soap and a safety razor. Most hospitals have a special place to dispose of razors in the dirty utility room, usually a covered metal container. If your hospital does not supply a disposable prep kit, get the individual items from CSR.

PREOPERATIVE CHECKLIST
COMPLETED BY NURSING AIDE

EVENING BEFORE SURGERY

Identify the patient by checking his identification bracelet . . . .
Yes_____ No_____

Skin prep done by _____ at_____ p.m.
Skin prep checked by _____ at_____ p.m.
Food restrictions, if any, explained to patient . . . . . Yes_____ No_____
"NPO AFTER MIDNIGHT" sign put on patient's bed . . . .
Yes_____ No_____

Enema administered by _____ at_____ p.m.

MORNING OF SURGERY

Bath . . . . Yes_____ No_____
Oral hygiene . . . . Yes_____ No_____
False teeth (dentures) & removable bridges removed . Yes_____ No_____

Jewelry and pierced earrings removed . . . . Yes_____ No_____
Hairpiece, wig, hairpins removed . . . . Yes_____ No_____
Lipstick, makeup, and false eyelashes removed . . . . Yes_____ No_____
Sanitary belts removed . . . . Yes_____ No_____
Nail polish removed . . . . Yes_____ No_____
Eyeglasses and contact lenses removed . . . . Yes_____ No_____
Prosthesis (artificial hearing aid, eye, leg, arm, and so forth)
removed . . . . Yes_____ No_____
All clothing removed except clean hospital gown . . . Yes_____ No_____
Patient allergic or sensitive to drugs . . . . Yes_____ No_____
Pre-op urine specimen obtained and sent to lab . . . . Yes_____ No_____
Urinary drainage bag emptied . . . . Yes_____ No_____
Side rails in up position . . . . Yes_____ No_____

Temperature _____ Pulse _____ Respiration _____
Blood Pressure _____ Weight _____ lbs. Height _____ ft. _____ in.
Time patient leaves for the operating room _____
Observations_____

Signature and title _____

Procedure: Shaving a Patient in Preparation for Surgery

1. Assemble your equipment:
   a. Disposable prep kit containing:
      (1) Razor and razor blades
      (2) Sponge filled with soap
      (3) Tissues
   b. Basin of water at 115° F (46.1° C)
   c. Bath blanket
   d. Towels

DISPOSABLE PREP KIT

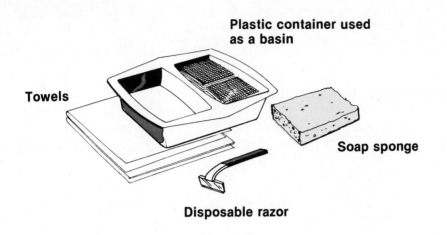

Plastic container used as a basin

Towels

Soap sponge

Disposable razor

2. Wash your hands.

3. Identify the patient by checking his identification bracelet.

4. Ask visitors to step out of the room.

5. Explain to the patient that you are going to shave him.

6. Pull the curtain around the bed for privacy.

7. Place the bath blanket over the bedspread and top sheet. Ask the patient to hold the blanket in place. Fanfold the top sheets to the foot of the bed. Do this from underneath the blanket without exposing the patient's body.

8. Adjust the bedside lamp so that the area is well lighted. Make sure there are no shadows where you will be working.

9. Open the disposable prep kit.

10. Wet the soap sponge in the basin of water. Then soap the area to be shaved. Work up a good lather with the sponge.

11. Check to be sure the razor blade is in the correct position in the razor.

12. Hold the skin taut with a dry tissue. Shave in the direction the hair grows. Rinse the razor often. Keep the razor and the patient's skin wet and soapy throughout the shaving procedure.

13. Clean the patient's umbilicus (navel), if it is in the area to be shaved.

14. Wash the soap off the patient's skin. Dry thoroughly with the towel.

15. Clean your equipment and put it in its proper place. Discard disposable supplies in the proper container.

16. Cover the patient with the top sheet and bedspread. Ask him to hold them while you take the bath blanket from underneath, without exposing the patient.

17. Make the patient comfortable.

18. Wash your hands.
19. Report to your head nurse or team leader the time at which you shaved the patient. Also report your observations of anything unusual.

PREP FOR BREAST SURGERY

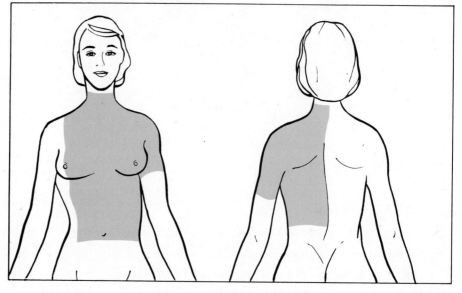

The area not being operated on is called the *unaffected* side. The area where the operation will be done is called the *affected side*. Shave from the nipple line of the unaffected side to the middle of the patient's back on the affected side. On the affected side, shave from the chin down to the umbilicus (navel), the axilla (armpit), and part of the upper arm.

CHEST PREP FOR THORACIC SURGERY

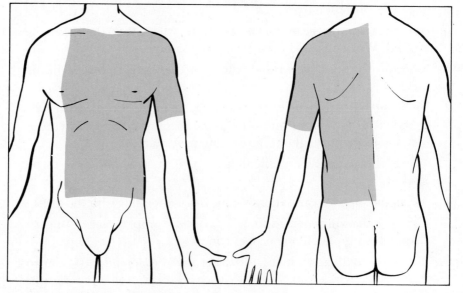

Shave the area extending from the nipple on the unaffected side, across the chest area of the affected side, and across the back, from the top of the shoulders down to the pubic hair.

ABDOMINAL PREP

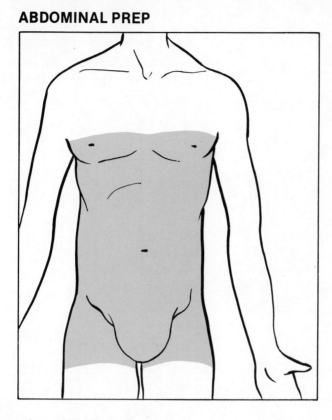

Shave from the nipple line on male patients, and from below the breasts on female patients, down to and including the pubic area. Shave the width of this area to each side of the body.

PREP FOR SURGERY OF EXTREMITY (ARM OR LEG)

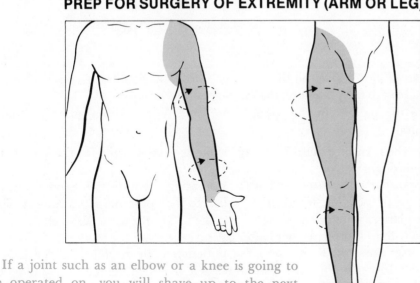

If a joint such as an elbow or a knee is going to be operated on, you will shave up to the next joint above and down to the next joint below. For example, if the patient's elbow is going to be operated on, you will shave his entire arm from the shoulder down to the wrist. If an area between joints is going to be operated on, you will shave the entire area, including the joints above and below. Shave all around an arm or a leg.

The words *vaginal prep* mean the preparation of the genital area of female patients.

VAGINAL PREP

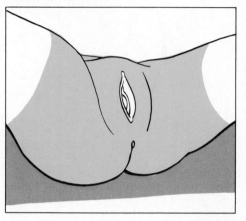

SCROTAL PREP

Preparation of the genital area of male patients is called the *scrotal prep*.

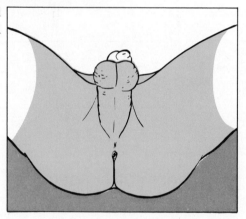

An enema also is given to the patient, if ordered. Food restrictions, if any, are explained to the patient on the evening before surgery.

• Dress the patient in the special operating room clothing used in your hospital.

• Move the furniture out of the way. Make the room ready for the stretcher to be brought in.

The transportation attendant or the operating room aide will come to the floor at the proper time to take the patient to the operating room suite. Help this attendant in moving the patient from the bed to the stretcher. Tell the patient you will see him in his room after the surgery.

The attendant will then wheel the patient on the stretcher to the head nurse's desk. At this time, the head nurse will give the attendant the patient's chart. She will check the name on the identification bracelet against the name on the chart.

The attendant then takes the patient to the operating room. Your next task is to strip the linen from the bed, make the operating room bed, and prepare the unit to receive the patient postoperatively.

BACK PREP

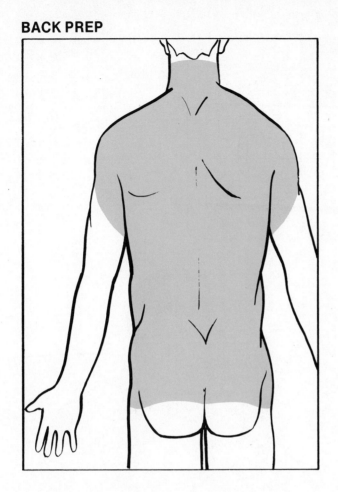

Shave the patient's entire back from the hairline on the neck down to the middle of the buttocks, including the axillary area.

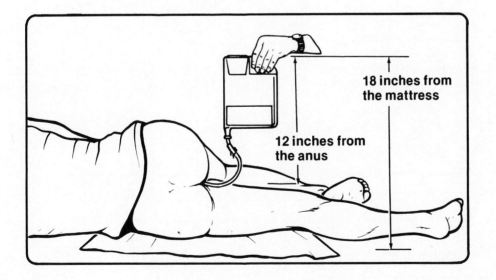

If ordered by a physician, an enema is given on the evening before surgery. Your head nurse or team leader will tell you if the enema is to be given.

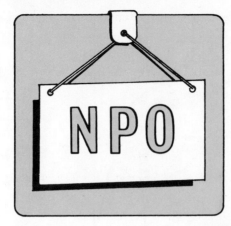

You may be asked to take away the patient's water pitcher and glass at midnight and to post a sign saying *NPO*. NPO is taken from the Latin, *nils per os,* which means "nothing by mouth." The sign is usually put at the head or foot of the bed; your instructor will tell you where.

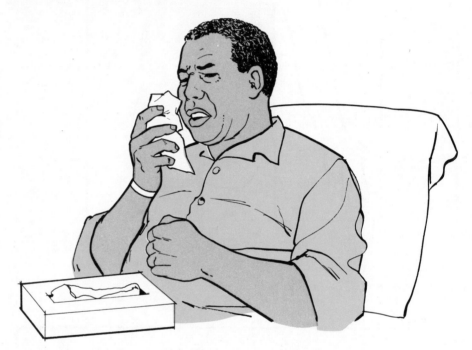

To prevent chest complications following surgery, watch for these symptoms in preoperative patients:

- Signs of respiratory infection
- Sneezing, sniffling, or coughing
- Complaints or signs of chest pains
- Elevated temperature

Report any of these immediately to your head nurse or team leader.

After the patient has been given his preoperative medications by the medication nurse:

- Keep the side rails in the up position.
- Remind the patient that he is not to smoke.

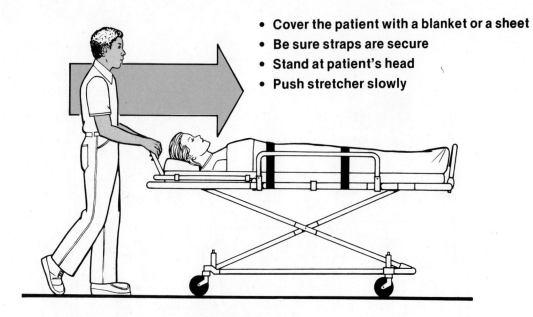

- Cover the patient with a blanket or a sheet
- Be sure straps are secure
- Stand at patient's head
- Push stretcher slowly

Section 2: Postoperative Nursing Care

OBJECTIVES: WHAT YOU WILL LEARN

When you have completed this section, you should be able:

- To observe the patient for signs of postoperative trouble
- To provide a safe environment for the postoperative patient

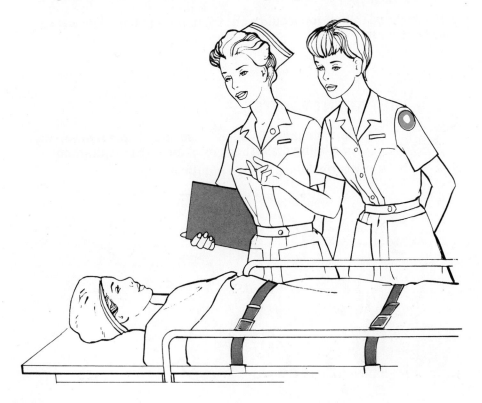

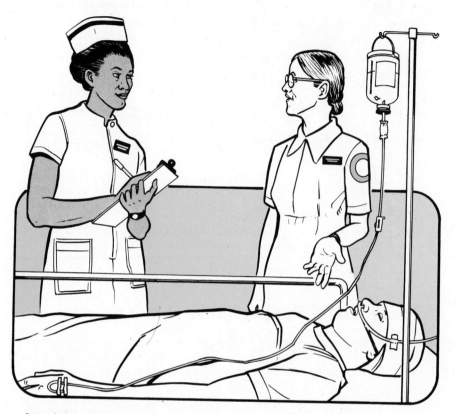

- A patient may *appear* to be unconscious, but not really be . . . He may be able to hear you!
- Say only those things you would want the patient to hear if he were fully conscious.

IF THE PATIENT VOMITS

- Turn the patient's head to one side to prevent vomitus from being drawn back into the lungs (aspiration)
- Wipe off the patient's mouth and chin

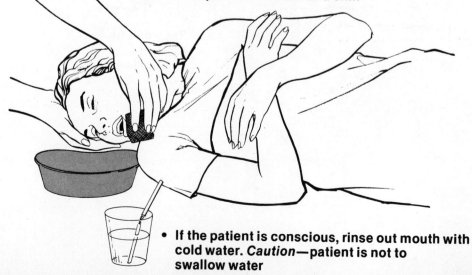

- If the patient is conscious, rinse out mouth with cold water. *Caution*—patient is not to swallow water

SIGNAL FOR YOUR HEAD NURSE OR TEAM LEADER IMMEDIATELY IF YOU NOTICE ANY OF THESE SYMPTOMS

Observe the patient for

- Choking
- Pulse: Fast (above 100), slow (below 60) or an irregular pulse beat
- Respirations: Rapid (above 30), labored
- Skin, lips, fingernails: Very pale or turning blue (CYANOSIS)
- Thirst: Patient asks for water often
- Unusual or extreme restlessness
- Moaning or complaining of pain
- Sudden bright red bleeding

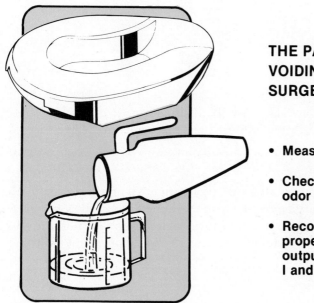

THE PATIENT'S FIRST VOIDING AFTER SURGERY SHOULD BE

- Measured for amount

- Checked for odor and color

- Recorded in proper place on output side of I and O sheet

You are expected to measure the amount of urine the patient produces the first time he voids after surgery. The amount should be entered on the output side of the Intake and Output (I and O) sheet. Most hospitals collect a routine urine specimen from this first voiding following surgery. Report to the head nurse or team leader if the urine has an unusual odor or color or if the patient voids only a few drops of urine. If a urinary catheter is present, be sure it is unclamped and draining. Observe the amount and color of urine in the drainage bag.

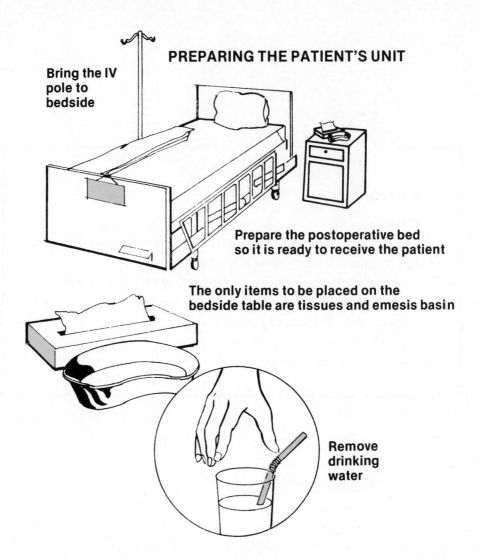

PREPARING THE PATIENT'S UNIT

Bring the IV pole to bedside

Prepare the postoperative bed so it is ready to receive the patient

The only items to be placed on the bedside table are tissues and emesis basin

Remove drinking water

The patient will be coming back to his unit on a stretcher. Get the furniture out of the way, and make sure the bedside area is clear. The stretcher then can be brought easily and quickly to its place next to the bed.

KEY IDEAS

Postoperative care means taking care of a patient right after surgery. Most patients are taken to a surgical recovery room immediately following surgery. They remain in the recovery room until they begin to recover from the effects of anesthesia. When the patient returns to his room, you will begin postoperative nursing care.

Anesthesia

Before they have surgery, patients are given special medications that cause a loss of feeling in all or part of the body. This loss of feeling means the patient feels no pain. When the patient is under the influence of these special medications called *anesthetics,* he is in a state of anesthesia. Some anesthetics cause the patient to become unconscious. Others, however, do not. Some anesthetics cause the loss of sensation in the whole body. These are called *general anesthetics.* Some anesthetics cause a numbness or loss of feeling in only a part of the body. These medications are called *local* anesthetics. A spinal anesthetic causes loss of feeling in a large area of the body, usually from the umbilicus down to and including the legs and feet.

The doctor who administers the anesthetic to the patient in the operating room is known as an *anesthesiologist.* The registered nurse who administers the anesthetic to the patient in the operating room is known as an *anesthetist.*

Chest complications following anesthesia may happen for several reasons:

- The anesthetic may irritate the patient's respiratory passages (mouth, nose, trachea, lungs) and cause the secretions in these passages to increase. This might raise the chance of an infection in the lungs or other parts of the respiratory system.
- Smoking tends to irritate the whole respiratory system. Smoking may increase the secretion of mucus, which also could raise the chance of an infection.
- After surgery, many patients are so sore they can't breathe deeply. They can't cough up the increased amount of mucous material being secreted in the lungs. This could cause a respiratory infection, such as pneumonia.
- A patient might vomit while he is still unconscious after surgery. The vomitus (vomited material) might be aspirated, that is, drawn back into the lungs. This could very quickly cause an infection or even the patient's death. Saliva might also be drawn into the throat and block the air passages, which could cause an infection.
- Unconsciousness and inactivity during anesthesia allow mucus to accumulate in the patient's respiratory passages.

At the doctor's order, your head nurse or team leader will call the inhalation therapy department. Staff persons from that department will treat the patient with chest complications.

When the Patient Comes Back

When your patient is brought back to his unit, you will do the following things:

- Help to move the patient from the stretcher to the bed.
- Be sure the patient is covered with blankets to keep him warm.
- Be sure the bedside rails are raised after the patient is in his bed.

KEY IDEAS: DEEP-BREATHING EXERCISES

Deep-breathing exercises expand the lungs by increasing lung movement and assist in bringing up lung secretions. These exercises will help in preventing postoperative pneumonia or pneumonitis.

Procedure: Helping with Deep-Breathing Exercises

1. Assemble your equipment:
   a. Pillow
   b. Specimen container, if a specimen is ordered
   c. Tissues

WHEN A PATIENT IS RECEIVING IV FLUIDS:

- Check the IV solution or blood transfusion for proper flow of fluid
- Check the skin for swelling, bleeding,
  or pain around the needle
- Do not adjust the clamps or flow
  rate
- Send for the nurse if adjustments
  are required
- Signal for your head nurse or team
  leader immediately if the patient's skin
  around the needle is swollen or
  bleeding, or if the fluid is not running
  properly

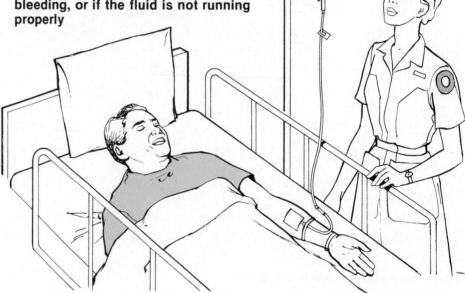

2. Report to the medication nurse that you are ready to start deep-breathing exercises. If she wishes to give the patient medication to relieve him of any discomfort or pain, she will do so at this time.

3. Wash your hands.

4. Identify the patient by checking the identification bracelet.

5. Ask visitors to step out of the room.

6. Tell the patient that you are going to help him with deep-breathing exercises.

7. Pull the curtain around the bed for privacy.

8. Offer the patient a bedpan or urinal.

9. Dangle the patient, if allowed. If not, place the patient in as much of a sitting position as possible.

10. Place the pillow on the patient's abdomen for support.

11. Ask him to breathe deeply 10 times.

12. Count the respirations out loud to the patient as he inhales and exhales. If the patient can't breathe deeply, ask him to cough. Coughing is just another way of breathing deeply.

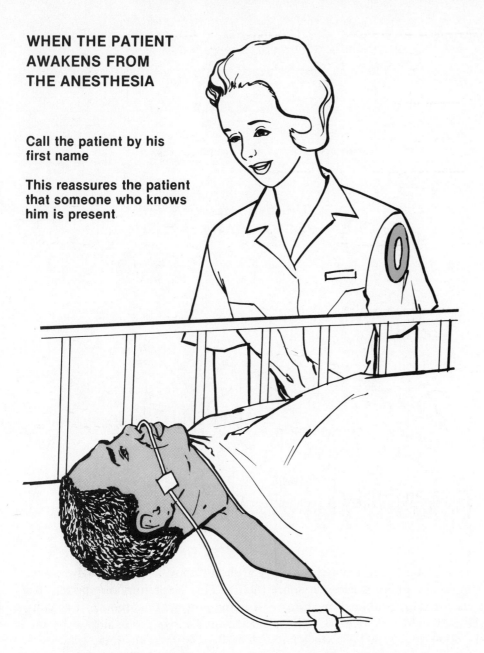

WHEN THE PATIENT AWAKENS FROM THE ANESTHESIA

Call the patient by his first name

This reassures the patient that someone who knows him is present

13. Ask the patient to feel his chest as he breathes to encourage deeper breathing.

14. Tell the patient to cough up all loose secretions into the tissues, if a specimen is not necessary, or into a specimen container, if a specimen is needed.

15. Return the patient to a comfortable and safe position in bed.

16. If a specimen has been collected, label it and attach a laboratory requisition slip.

17. Dispose of the tissues.

18. Replace the pillow under the patient's head.

19. Wash your hands.

20. Report to your head nurse or team leader:
   - That you have helped the patient with his deep-breathing exercises
   - The time during which you helped him
   - The number of exercises
   - Your observations of anything unusual

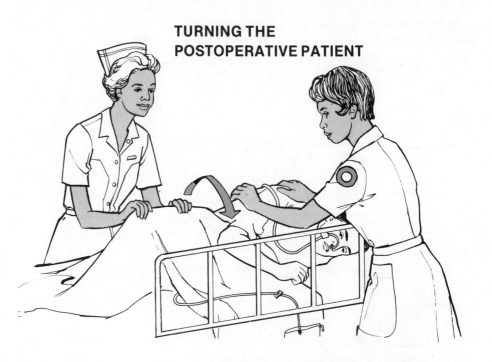

TURNING THE POSTOPERATIVE PATIENT

Unless you are instructed not to, you should move a postoperative patient into a new position every 2 hours (Q2h). This helps him rest better, protects his skin, promotes healing, and helps prevent pneumonia. Each time the patient is moved he should be turned onto his opposite side so he faces the other side of the bed. Move the patient's legs at the same time.

If the patient's gown becomes wet, change it immediately. Change the bed linens whenever they become damp and soiled. Take the blankets off the bed if the patient complains of being too warm. Keep the side rails up at all times.

Section 3: Binders and Elastic Bandages

OBJECTIVES: WHAT YOU WILL LEARN

When you have completed this section, you should be able:

- To apply the five types of binders
- To apply elastic bandages and anti-embolism elastic stockings

KEY IDEAS

Binders are wide cloth bandages, usually made of cotton. They are used on different parts of a patient's body for several reasons. Binders can be used postoperatively, or after childbirth, or whenever it is desirable to:

- Give support to a weakened body part
- Hold dressings and bandages in place
- Put pressure on parts of the body to make the patient more comfortable

The nurse will tell you if a particular patient is to have a binder applied and what kind of binder is to be used. Remember that, unless the binder is put on properly, it can be more uncomfortable for the patient than if it had not been used at all. Binders are obtained from the central supply room (CSR) in most hospitals.

Rules To Follow

- Keep the binder smooth and clean. Otherwise it will be uncomfortable in the same way that crumbs or wrinkles in the patient's bed are uncomfortable. Bedsores (decubitus ulcers) can be caused by wrinkles or wetness in a binder.
- Watch for reddened areas on the patient's skin. Report these to your head nurse or team leader right away.
- Use the correct type of binder. Be sure it is the correct size.

There are five different types of binders:

- The scultetus (many-tailed) binder
- The straight abdominal binder
- The T binder
- The double T binder
- The breast binder

Using Elastic Stockings and Ace Bandages

Binders are applied mainly to the torso of the patient. Anti-embolism elastic stockings and elastic bandages are applied to the body extremities (arms, hands, legs, feet). In postoperative care, they are most often used on the lower extremities, or legs. They are used either as treatment for thrombophlebitis (blood clots of the leg) or as a prevention against that condition. The purpose of anti-embolism elastic stockings and elastic bandages is to compress veins and therefore improve the return of venous blood to the heart. They are also used to improve circulation and therefore prevent thrombophlebitis. In cases of sprain or strain at the joint, they are used to provide support and comfort.

Applying Anti-embolism Elastic Stockings.   Anti-embolism elastic stockings can be either knee-length or full-length. Be careful to smooth out all the

**SCULTETUS
BINDER**

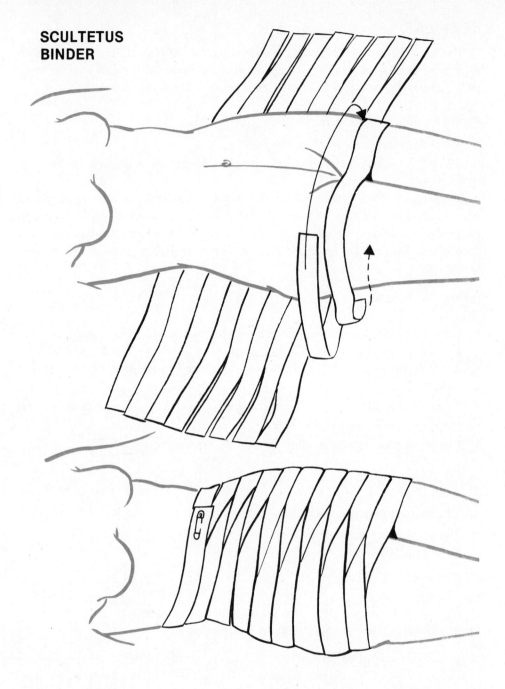

The scultetus binder is called the many-tailed binder because of its shape. It is used to hold dressings in place and to provide pressure and support. It is applied from the bottom up (or toward the heart) and is fastened with one safety pin at the top tail.

wrinkles. Be sure the stocking is pulled up firmly. Elastic stockings must be removed and reapplied at least once every day and more often if the doctor has so ordered.

The T binder is used to keep dressings in place on the perineal (genital) area and rectal area. This binder often is used after a hemorrhoidectomy (an operation to remove hemorrhoids), or after the delivery of a baby. The binder is first wrapped around the patient's waist. Part of the binder then goes between the patient's legs and is brought back up to be fastened at the waist.

T BINDER

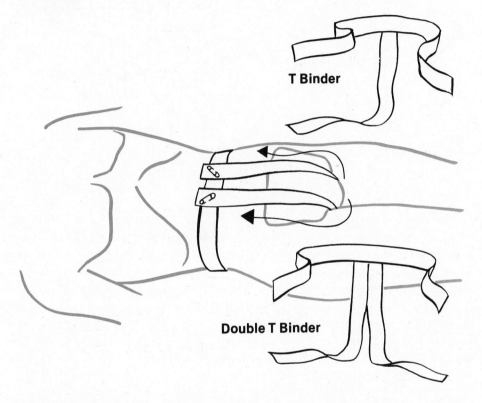

T Binder

Double T Binder

The double T binder is also used for holding perineal dressings in place. Double T binders are always used for holding these dressings on male patients. They sometimes are used on female patients if rectal surgery is extensive and calls for a very large dressing.

Applying Elastic Bandages.   Elastic bandages are long strips of elasticized cotton. They have been neatly wound into rolls.

They provide support, hold dressings in place, apply pressure to a body part, and improve return circulation. Bandages may be ordered "toes to knees" or "toes to mid-thighs," or "toes to groin," or "heel free, toes to groin." Use as many bandages as necessary to cover the area.

If the bandage has been wrapped too tightly, the patient's circulation may be impaired. He may develop such symptoms as paleness, coldness, blueness, pain, swelling, or tingling or numbness in the extremities.

BREAST BINDER

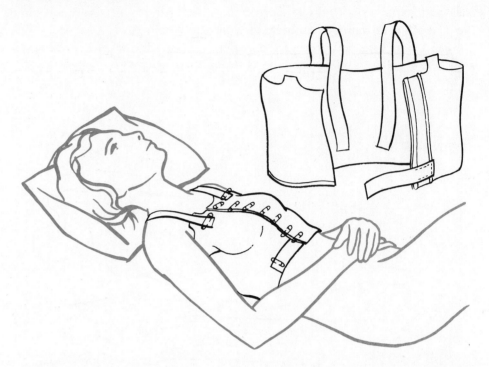

The breast binder sometimes is used with female patients after childbirth or after breast surgery. The binder gives support to the breasts and holds dressings in place. Sometimes the binder is used to compress the breasts when it is necessary to dry up the patient's milk, as with a patient who will not be breast feeding her baby. The binder is first fastened at the shoulders. It then is fastened along the front, working from the middle to the top and bottom. Darts are pinned at the waist to provide room and support for the breasts and also to help make the binder fit better. Ask the patient to support her breasts inward and upward with her hands, outside the binder, as you pin it together.

STRAIGHT ABDOMINAL BINDER

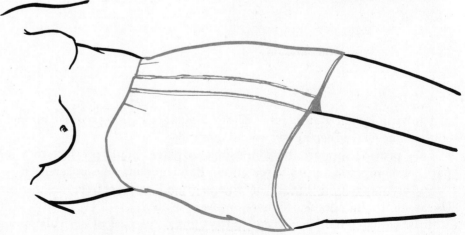

The straight abdominal binder is used for the same purposes as the scultetus binder. It usually is applied from the bottom up (toward the heart), and darts are pinned to the top of the binder to make sure it will fit snugly. The straight abdominal binder may be fastened with velcro.

ELASTIC STOCKINGS AND BANDAGES

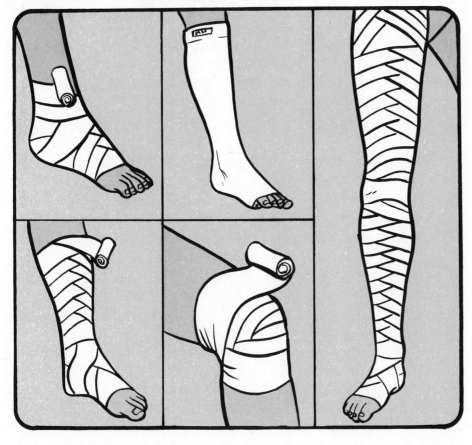

Procedure: Applying Elastic Bandages

1. Assemble your equipment:
    a. Elastic bandages
    b. Clips
2. Wash your hands.
3. Identify the patient by checking the identification bracelet.
4. Ask visitors to step out of the room.
5. Tell the patient that you are going to wrap his leg or arm (or whatever area is to be wrapped) with an elastic bandage.
6. Pull the curtain around the bed for privacy.
7. Place the patient in a comfortable position that is convenient for you to work. Expose the area to be wrapped.
8. Extend the part of the body to be bandaged. Support the patient's heel.
9. Stand directly in front of the patient or facing the part to be bandaged.

10. Roll the bandage smoothly.

11. Hold the bandage with the loose end coming off the bottom of the roll.

12. Anchor the bandage by two circular turns around the body part at its smallest point. This usually is the ankle or the wrist. Wrap firmly but not too tightly.

13. Apply the bandage in the same direction as venous circulation, that is toward the heart.

14. Exert even pressure. Keep the bandage smooth. Be sure no skin areas show between the turns.

15. If possible, leave the toes or fingers exposed for observation of circulatory changes.

16. Continue wrapping upward with a spiral turn. Each turn should overlap the one before about one-half width of the bandage.

17. After applying the bandage, secure the terminal end by pinning it with safety pins or by applying bandage clips.

18. If more than one bandage is used, overlap them to prevent the bandages from slipping.

19. To remove the bandage, unwind it gently. Gather it into a loose mass, passing the mass from hand to hand as the bandage is unwound. Then roll the bandage smoothly so it is ready for the next application.

20. Wash your hands.

21. Report to your head nurse or team leader:
   - That you have applied (or removed) the elastic bandages
   - The area of application
   - Your observations of anything unusual

WHAT YOU HAVE LEARNED

As a nursing aide, you will be part of both preoperative and postoperative care. Giving good care before, during, and after surgery is very important for the well-being of the patient.

Shaving the operative area in preparation for surgery, filling in all blanks on the preoperative checklist, and following the instructions of your head nurse or team leader are your main duties in working with surgical patients.

Care of the Dying Patient 16

Section 1: Care of the Dying Patient

OBJECTIVES: WHAT YOU WILL LEARN

When you have completed this section, you should be able:

- To make the dying patient as comfortable as possible
- To help meet the emotional needs of the patient
- To help meet the special needs of the patient's family
- To identify signs of approaching death

KEY IDEAS

Some of the patients who enter the hospital are terminally ill, that is, dying. Sometimes death is sudden or unexpected. More often it is not. Your first responsibility is to help make the patient comfortable for as long as possible. Your second responsibility is to assist in meeting the emotional needs of the patient and his family.

The most important single fact to remember when you are caring for a dying patient is that he is just as important as the patient who is going to recover. You will not have the satisfaction of contributing to his recovery. But you will know that you have helped a human being to end his life in peace, comfort, and dignity. Everyone must die. Surely we would all prefer to die in reassuring and comfortable surroundings.

Try to be very understanding. The patient may want to believe he will get well. He may want people around him to reassure him that he won't die. When a dying patient talks to you, listen. But don't give him false hopes. Don't tell him that he is getting better. If you did that, the patient sooner or later would know that you had lied to him. He might resent you for this.

People have different ideas about death and the hereafter. These ideas depend on the patient's beliefs and background. You must show respect for the patient's beliefs. Be careful not to impose your own beliefs on him or his family.

When it is known that death is approaching, the dying patient's family may want to spend a lot of time with him. This is usually permitted by the hospital as much as possible.

347

THE PATIENT'S EMOTIONAL NEEDS

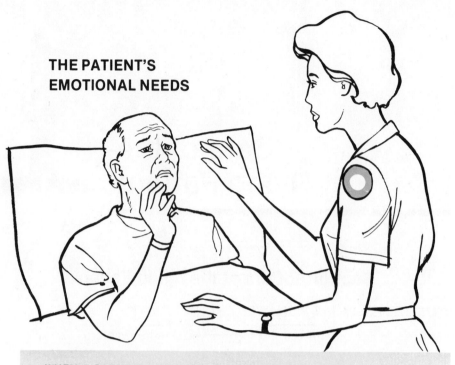

WHEN A PATIENT SUSPECTS HE IS GOING TO DIE, HE MAY REACT IN VARIOUS WAYS:

- HE MAY ASK EVERYONE ABOUT HIS CHANCES FOR RECOVERY
- HE MAY BE AFRAID TO BE ALONE, AND WANT A LOT OF ATTENTION FROM YOU
- HE MAY ASK A LOT OF QUESTIONS
- HE MAY SEEM TO COMPLAIN CONSTANTLY
- HE MAY OFTEN SIGNAL MEMBERS OF THE STAFF
- HE MAY MAKE MANY APPARENTLY UNREASONABLE REQUESTS

Everyone on the staff should respect the family's need for privacy during their visits. If a private room is not available, the patient should be screened so he and his family will have the privacy they need.

Don't stop doing your work just because the patient's family is present. Carry out your job quickly, quietly, and efficiently. Don't wait until the family has gone before taking care of the patient. They might think that, because he is dying, he is being neglected by the hospital staff.

The patient's family may ask you many questions. Don't ignore their questions. Answer any you can. Also, do whatever is asked of you, if it is allowed.

There will be some questions that you can't answer. For example, you may be asked, "What did the doctor say today about his condition?" Refer the family to your head nurse or team leader.

Even if the patient becomes unconscious, the family may want to stay with him. Family members may continue to hope for his recovery. They will watch you perform your patient care procedures. They will want you to make the patient comfortable, even if you cannot help him recover.

Unconscious patients require as thorough care as those who are conscious. Their needs must still be met. Sometimes you must ask the family to leave the bedside while you are giving care to the patient. Explain this to the family. Tell them that you will let them know when you have finished.

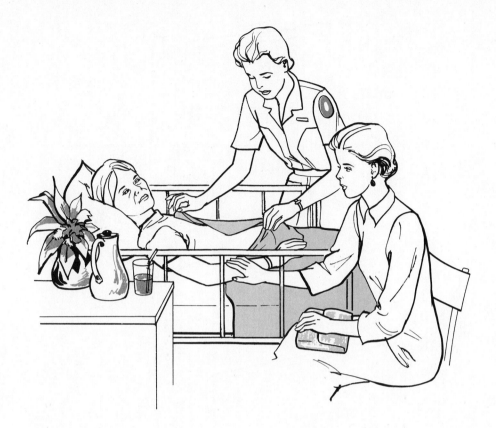

Make an effort to respect the family's wishes for privacy. Screen the unit well to ensure privacy for the patient and family whenever this is desired. When the patient is visited by his pastor (priest, rabbi, or minister), assure them they will not be disturbed.

Some visitors stay with the patient for many hours at a time. Be as helpful to them as you can. You might suggest that they have a cup of coffee. Tell them where the coffee shop is. Also, learn the policy in your hospital on serving meals to visitors. You may be able to arrange for trays to be delivered to the patient's family at mealtimes. If this is not allowed, tell the visitors where they can find the hospital cafeteria or a nearby restaurant. Make sure the visitors know the location of the washrooms, lounge, and telephones.

Remember at all times to be quietly courteous, understanding, sympathetic, and willing to help. These are the marks of a competent nursing aide. Don't feel helpless or guilty because you can't improve the patient's condition. You can help the patient and his family most by maintaining a concerned and efficient approach to your work.

A patient approaching death continues to be given routine personal care, such as baths and mouth care. That is, he is given the same care he would receive if he were expected to recover. Members of the nursing staff should stay calm and sympathetic. This may help to relieve some of the patient's fears and make this time easier for him. As the patient becomes weaker and finally helpless, his condition may require more of your time. You will probably be doing many things for him that he had earlier taken care of himself.

Rules To Follow

1. Keep the room well ventilated and lighted as usual. Because the dying patient's eyesight is usually failing, a dark room may frighten him.

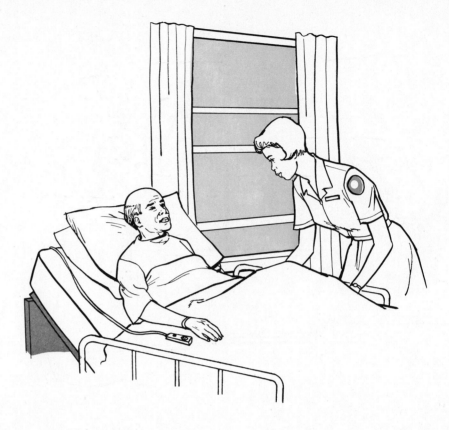

2. Change the patient's position often to keep him comfortable and prevent irritation of his skin.

3. As long as the patient is conscious, speak to him in your normal voice. Even if he seems to be unconscious, use your normal voice when you are talking to someone else in the room.

4. Don't say things you wouldn't want the patient to hear. The dying patient's hearing usually is one of the last senses to fail.

5. Respect the patient's need for spiritual support. Learn the policy in your hospital concerning religious observances and requirements at the time of death. For example, if a Roman Catholic patient wishes to see a priest or appears to be in danger of dying, a priest should be called. Because the body of an Orthodox Jewish patient should not be touched after death until the rabbi or proper religious authority arrives, it is important to straighten the patient's limbs before death occurs.

6. The patient may be most comfortable lying on his back. He may have his head slightly raised and have a pillow under his knees for support. Every 2 hours, change the patient's position. Pillows should be placed at his back for support.

7. Change the bedding whenever necessary. This will keep the patient's skin from becoming irritated and will help to keep the patient comfortable. You may also be giving the patient more back rubs than usual.

8. The dying patient may be incontinent, that is, unable to control the elimination of urine or feces. He may soil the bed often. Your job is to keep the patient's body clean at all times.

9. The patient may be given softer food and in smaller amounts than usual. The amount and consistency of food will depend on what the patient's

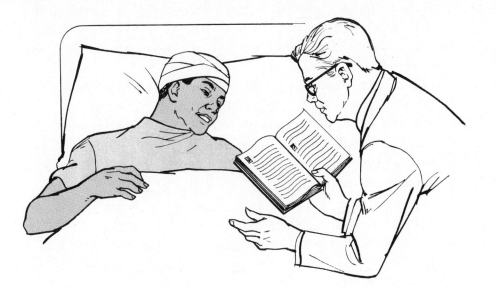

digestive system can tolerate. He may be given liquids as long as he can swallow. This helps to keep his mouth moist.

10. Report any observations that will tell your head nurse or team leader that a change has taken place in the patient's condition.

11. The patient approaching death needs special mouth care. His mouth may be dry because he is breathing through it. His mouth also may be dry because a nasogastric tube is being used. In this case, you might use an applicator with glycerine (or other lubricant) to swab the patient's mouth and lips. If the patient's mouth has a lot of secretions in it, tell the head nurse. She may use suction to remove the secreted material. If the patient has dentures, ask your head nurse or team leader if you should leave them in the patient's mouth or take them out. If you remove dentures, place them in a denture cup with the patient's name on the cover.

A patient may be receiving oxygen through a nasal catheter or mask. If so,
12. check his nostrils from time to time. Tell your head nurse or team leader if the nostrils are dry and encrusted.

A patient's nostrils also may become dry and encrusted because he has
13. difficulty in breathing. If you notice dryness, clean the nostrils with cotton swabs moistened slightly with glycerine (or other lubricant), with your head nurse's or team leader's permission.

Signs of Approaching Death

Death comes to patients in different ways. It may come quite suddenly after a patient has seemed to be recovering. Or it may come after a long period during which there has been a steady decline of body functions. Death also may result from complications during convalescence. Here are some signs showing that death may be near:

1. Blood circulation slows down. The patient's hands and feet are cold to the touch.

2. If the patient is conscious, he may complain that he is cold. Keep him well covered.

3. The patient's face may become pale because of decreased circulation.

4. His eyes may be staring blankly into space. There may be no eye reaction when you move your hand across his line of vision.

5. The patient may perspire heavily, even though his body is cold.

6. The patient loses muscle tone, and his body becomes limp. His jaw may drop, and his mouth may stay partly open.

7. Respirations may become slower and more difficult.

8. Mucus collecting in the patient's throat and bronchial tubes may cause a sound that is sometimes called the "death rattle."

9. The pulse often is rapid, but it becomes weak and irregular.

10. Just before death, respiration stops and the pulse gets very faint. You may not be able to feel the patient's pulse at all.

11. Contrary to popular belief, a dying person is rarely in great pain. As the patient's condition gets worse, less blood may be flowing to the brain. Therefore the patient may feel little or no pain.

12. If you notice any of these signs or any change in the patient's condition, report to your head nurse or team leader immediately.

13. Try to be with the patient as much as possible, even if you cannot do a lot. Your presence often is comforting.

Section 2: Postmortem Care (PMC)

OBJECTIVES: WHAT YOU WILL LEARN

When you have completed this section, you should be able:

- To give postmortem care gently and respectfully
- To protect the patient's valuables
- To remove the patient's body from the unit discreetly

KEY IDEAS

If you observe any signs of approaching death, tell your head nurse or team leader immediately. The nurse will examine the patient and confirm what you have found. Until you have received direct instructions from your head nurse or team leader, no postmortem care can be given to a patient. The word *postmortem* means after death.

In some hospitals, when the head nurse or team leader confirms that a patient has no pulse or has stopped breathing, she calls a *Blue Code*. A Blue Code (or whatever code is used in your hospital) is an emergency announcement to the staff of the hospital. A team that has been assigned to Blue Code will come to the patient within one minute. Then every means available to keep the patient alive is used by the Blue Code team. Only when the team fails to keep the patient alive is the patient declared by a physican to be dead.

After a patient has died, his body still must be treated with respect and must be given gentle care. If family members are present, they usually wait outside the room until the doctor has finished his examination. The patient's family will probably be allowed to view the body if they wish to do so.

Sometimes the family is not present when the patient dies. In this case, the nurse calls the doctor and tells him the family is not there. Either the doctor or the nurse then notifies the family and finds out whether they wish to view the body before it is sent to the morgue. If so, the body stays in the room until the family arrives.

When the family is present, they are given the patient's personal belongings. These items are checked against the clothing list to be sure that everything is accounted for. You will learn the procedure in your hospital for taking care of the deceased patient's clothes. If the members of the family do not wish to view the body, you will then proceed with postmortem care.

Postmortem care should be done before *rigor mortis* sets in. Rigor mortis means that the body and limbs become stiff.

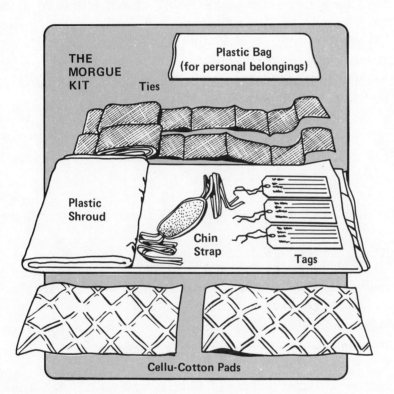

Procedure: Giving Postmortem Care

1. Assemble your equipment:

   a. Postmortem care kit from CSR (central supply room)
      - Plastic shroud or sheet
      - Chin strap (if used in your hospital)
      - Cellulose pads
      - Three identification tags, to be filled out by your head nurse or team leader

- Roll of 1-inch bandage or ties
- Large bag for personal belongings
- Plastic laundry bag
- Disposable bed protector

   b. Stretcher

2. Wash your hands.

3. Identify the patient by checking the identification bracelet.

4. Ask visitors to step out of the room.

5. Pull the curtain around the bed for privacy.

6. Lower the backrest on the bed.

7. Remove all pillows except one.

8. Place the patient's body in the supine or dorsal recumbent position, straightening the arms and legs. Move the body gently to avoid bruising.

9. Place a pillow under the patient's head.

10. In some institutions the arms are crossed and laid over the body at the waist.

11. Close the person's eyes if they are open:
       a. Take the lashes and pull the eyelids down over the eyes.
       b. Avoid touching the eyelids. Pressure may give them an unnatural appearance.

12. Replace dentures in the patient's mouth. Or leave the dentures in a denture cup labeled with the patient's name for the mortician to take.

13. The patient's mouth should be closed. You can do this by cupping your hand under his chin and applying slight pressure. If the patient's mouth will not stay closed, roll up a towel and place it under the chin as a support.

14. Bathe the patient's body, if necessary, to remove any discharges or secretions.

15. Comb the patient's hair, if necessary.

16. Remove all soiled dressings, bandages, and tubes if so instructed. Be sure that wounds or open incisions are covered with fresh dressings and are held in place with adhesive tapes. Old marks from adhesive tape should be removed with adhesive remover.

17. Remove all jewelry and give it to the head nurse. She will have the family sign a release form before giving the jewelry to them. If the rings cannot be removed because of swelling, they should be tied in place with a 1-inch bandage. This should be reported to your head nurse or team leader.

18. Fasten the chin strap in place, protecting the face with a cellulose pad.

19. Fold the patient's arms over the abdomen. Tie the wrists and ankles, loosely, with bandages or ties. Place cellulose pads under the bandages to prevent bruising.

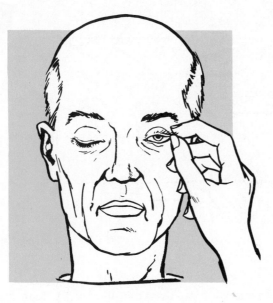

20. Attach identification tags to the bandage on the patient's wrist and to the right big toe. The tags are filled out by your head nurse or team leader with the patient's name, sex, hospital number, room number, and age.

21. Place the deceased patient's body on the shroud or sheet with a disposable bed protector under the buttocks. Cover the body with the shroud.

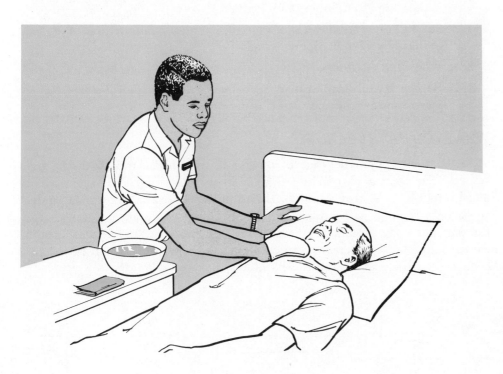

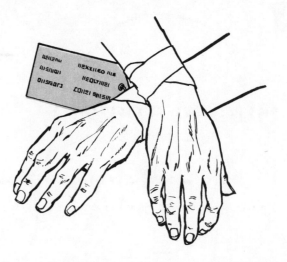

22. Fold the shroud or sheet over the deceased person and tie it with bandages at the waist, above the elbows, and below the knees.

23. Attach the third identification tag to the shroud at the waist bandage.

24. Move the body onto a stretcher and cover it with a sheet.

25. Move the stretcher to the morgue. Try to give the appearance of simply moving a patient to another place. It is important that other patients not be disturbed, so far as is possible, by seeing a patient who has died.

26. Every item belonging to the deceased patient is placed in a large bag. The bag is labeled with all needed information—patient's name, hospital number, and so forth.

27. Strip all linen from the bed. Place it in a plastic laundry bag. Put it in the dirty linen hamper.

28. Wash your hands.

29. Report to your head nurse or team leader that postmortem care was given and that the body was transferred to the morgue.

WHAT YOU HAVE LEARNED

As a patient approaches death, you should treat him sympathetically and respectfully. Personal care should be given in the usual way. The dying patient and his family have strong emotional and physical needs. As a nursing aide, you should respond with understanding and quiet confidence. After death, the patient's body should be treated with gentleness and reverence. Special care should be taken to avoid bruises. Remember that throughout these procedures the patient's body must be handled gently and carefully.

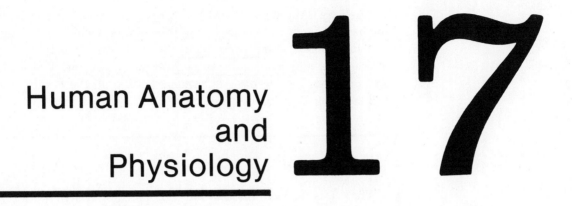

Human Anatomy and Physiology

17

OBJECTIVES: *WHAT YOU WILL LEARN*

When you have completed this chapter, you should be able:

- To demonstrate a basic understanding of human anatomy and physiology by applying their principles to each clinical procedure
- To use the medical terminology necessary to carry out the instructions of your head nurse or team leader
- To demonstrate your ability to answer questions about the human body because each member of the health team is also a teacher
- To describe the body systems
- To explain how the body systems are interrelated

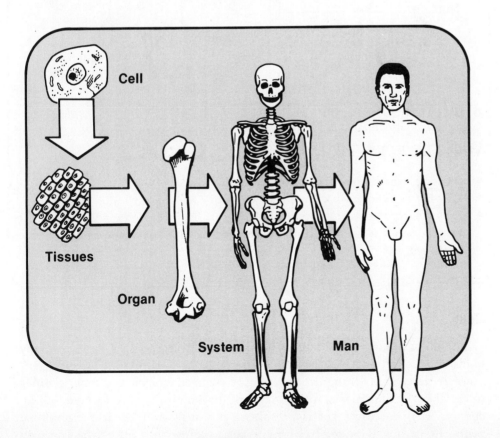

Cell

Tissues

Organ

System   Man

KEY IDEAS

Anatomy is the study of the structure of the body. *Physiology* is the study of the bodily functions. Knowledge of these subjects will help give better care to your patients. The *vocabulary* of these subjects will help you understand the instructions your head nurse or team leader gives you. The study of anatomy and physiology is the basis for understanding all the clinical procedures you will be doing as a nursing aide.

THE CELL

The cell is the fundamental building block of all living matter. You should understand its structure and function. First, cells are all microscopic in size. Second, all living body cells need food and oxygen and must be able to rid themselves of wastes to remain alive. All living cells perform several basic functions:

- They produce energy and perform work.
- They grow and repair themselves.
- They reproduce themselves.
- They die of old age or disease.

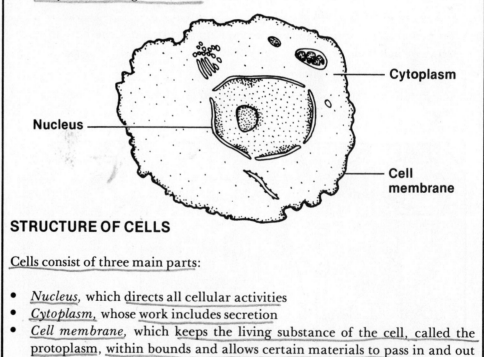

STRUCTURE OF CELLS

Cells consist of three main parts:

- *Nucleus,* which directs all cellular activities
- *Cytoplasm,* whose work includes secretion
- *Cell membrane,* which keeps the living substance of the cell, called the protoplasm, within bounds and allows certain materials to pass in and out of the cell

---

Cells

The human body is made up of millions of living cells. There are many kinds of cells, all of which perform different jobs in the body. All of them, however, have many things in common. They need oxygen and food in order to metabolize. This means to do the work for which they are formed—using energy. They all must get rid of waste products from their metabolism, primarily carbon dioxide. It is important to know that all of the complex systems of the entire body function so that each cell is provided with what it needs in an environment or area suitable for its work, growth, repair, and reproduction.

Each cell is surrounded by tissue fluid. It is this watery environment that acts as a place where gases, food, and waste products are exchanged, This environment stays pretty much the same. But it always changes a little, within limits. This state of normal conditions is known as *homeostasis*. All physiology is directed toward keeping the cells of the body in a homeostatic environment in which they can function best.

Except for the red blood cells, each cell has a nucleus. It is here that the work of the cell is determined by a substance known as *DNA*. This substance

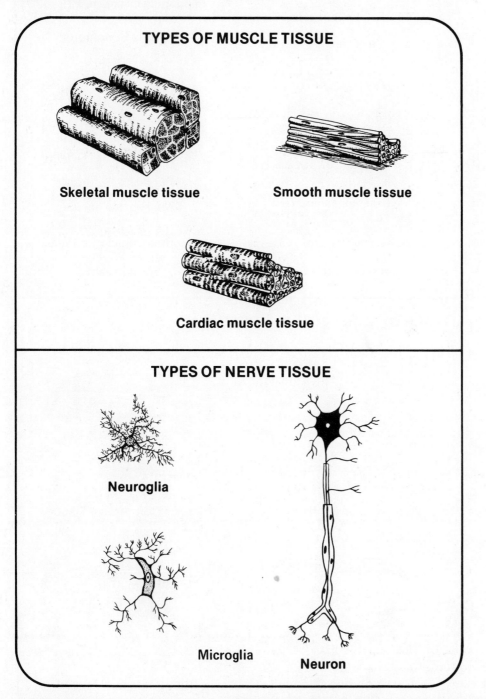

A Programmed Approach to Anatomy and Physiology. The Cell. 2d ed. Robert J. Brady Co., Bowie Md, 1972

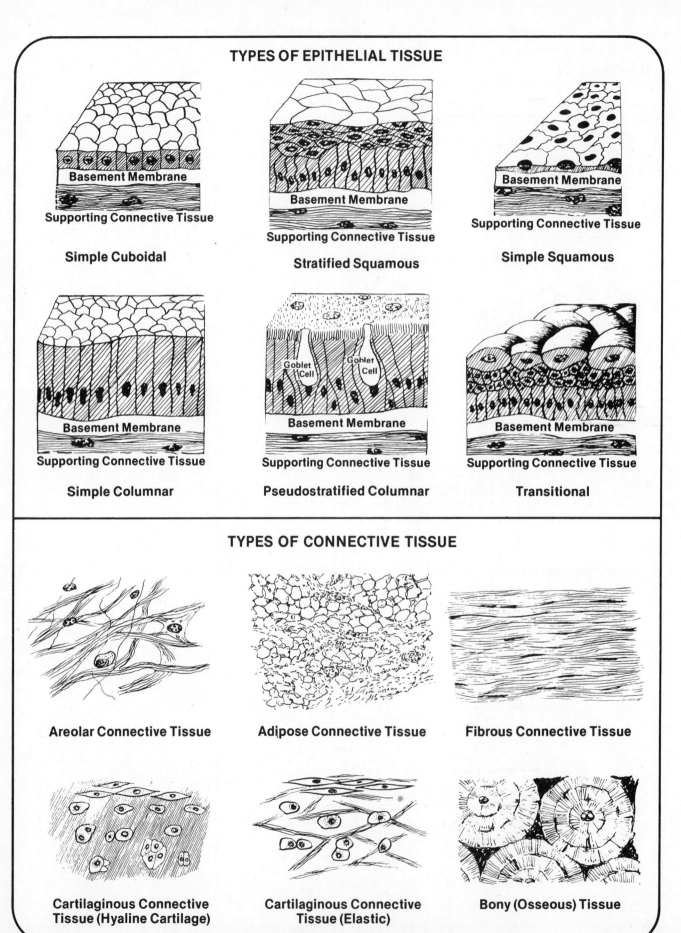

TYPES OF EPITHELIAL TISSUE

Simple Cuboidal

Basement Membrane

Supporting Connective Tissue

Stratified Squamous

Basement Membrane

Supporting Connective Tissue

Simple Squamous

Basement Membrane

Supporting Connective Tissue

Simple Columnar

Basement Membrane

Supporting Connective Tissue

Pseudostratified Columnar

Goblet Cell

Goblet Cell

Basement Membrane

Supporting Connective Tissue

Transitional

Basement Membrane

Supporting Connective Tissue

TYPES OF CONNECTIVE TISSUE

Areolar Connective Tissue

Adipose Connective Tissue

Fibrous Connective Tissue

Cartilaginous Connective Tissue (Hyaline Cartilage)

Cartilaginous Connective Tissue (Elastic)

Bony (Osseous) Tissue

A Programmed Approach to Anatomy and Physiology. The Cell. 2d ed. Robert J. Brady Co., Bowie Md, 1972.

EPITHELIAL TISSUE

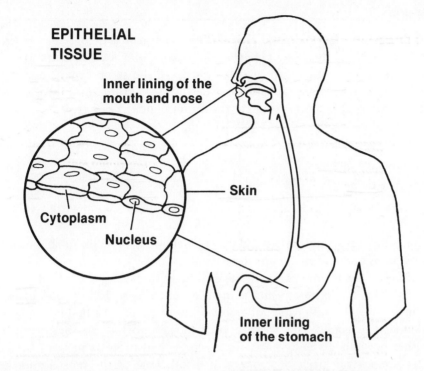

Inner lining of the mouth and nose

Skin

Cytoplasm

Nucleus

Inner lining of the stomach

sends messages to the organelles (little organs) in the cells, telling them what to do, how often, and how much. It is surprising that such important activity takes place in a structure that is usually so small you need a microscope to see it. Most current research to discover what is causing diseases involves studying the cell and its immediate environment, the tissue fluid. We are living in a time when there is an explosion of scientific knowledge about the cell. It is from this kind of study that the scientist will someday find out what causes cancer or the common cold.

CONNECTIVE TISSUE

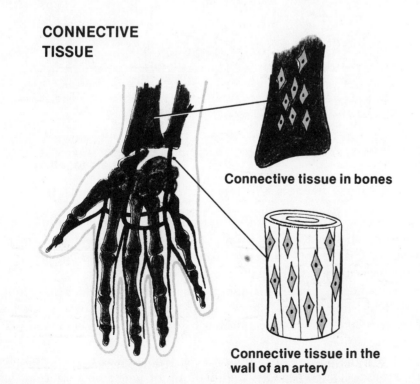

Connective tissue in bones

Connective tissue in the wall of an artery

Tissues

Cells usually do not work alone. They are grouped together in tissues. Groups of cells of the same type that do a particular kind of work are called *tissues*. A tissue is made up of cells that have the same origin during their development in the fetus. A tissue may be a mass, a group, or a sheet of cells.

There are four primary tissues in the human body. They are:

- Epithelial tissue
- Connective tissue
- Muscle tissue
- Nerve tissue

Epithelial cells may be irregular, cube-shaped, or column-shaped. They always are found on top of connective tissue.

Epithelial tissue makes up the skin and is the lining for all of the body cavities. This tissue has special properties, such as secreting substances, absorbing material, and protecting many of the organs of the body.

Connective tissue forms the supporting framework of the body and binds together or connects body parts. It also pads and protects parts of the body. There are several kinds of connective tissue. One of the most important is loose, or areolar, connective tissue. This is found underneath the skin and throughout the whole body. Because it is continuous, it can act as a place in which infection spreads.

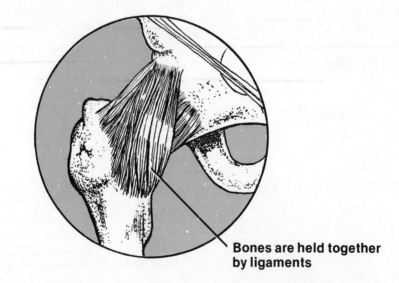

Bones are held together by ligaments

Elastic and white fibrous tissues are strong but flexible. These hold parts of the body together in a compact way. Ligaments, which hold bones together, are made of this type of connective tissue. Adipose tissue, or fat, helps to support and protect organs, especially the kidneys.

Other connective tissues include blood and lymph, which are liquid in nature. They, like all tissue, have cells in them. The septum of the nose is made of cartilage, which is a connective tissue. Bone, or osseous tissue, is also a connective tissue.

There are three kinds of muscle tissue. The first is called *voluntary* or *striated* muscle. These muscles are made up of long fibers, or cells, joined together in bundles. They are connected to one another and surrounded by

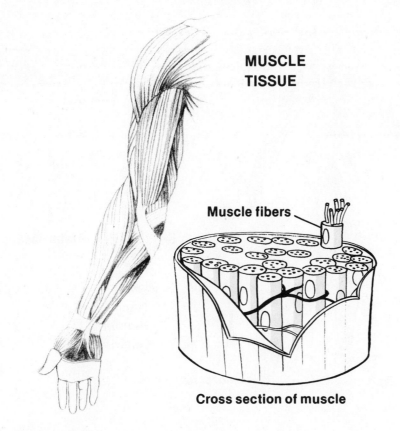

MUSCLE TISSUE

Muscle fibers

Cross section of muscle

connective tissue. This type of muscle tissue makes up the large skeletal muscles, the ones you can move consciously.

A second type of muscle tissue is called smooth, or involuntary, muscle. This is made of long, spindle-shaped cells that are found primarily in the

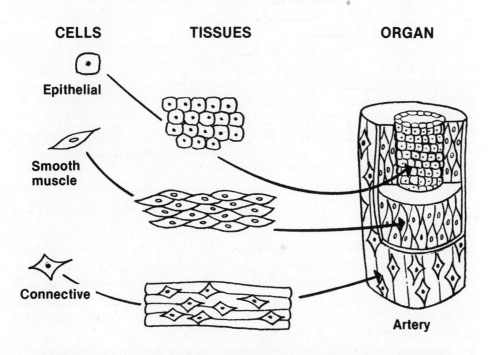

CELLS   TISSUES   ORGAN

Epithelial

Smooth muscle

Connective

Artery

Cells combine to form tissues, and tissues combine to form organs

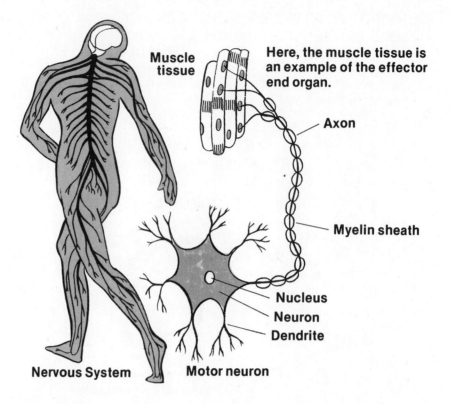

Muscle tissue

Here, the muscle tissue is an example of the effector end organ.

Axon

Myelin sheath

Nucleus
Neuron
Dendrite

Nervous System   Motor neuron

organs of the abdominal cavity. They are very helpful in pushing food and water through the gastrointestinal tract, the long tube that runs from your mouth to your anus.

The third type of muscle tissue is cardiac muscle tissue, which is found in the heart wall. In this tissue the cells are joined together much like branches of a tree. This is because it is necessary for them to contract together in order for your heart to beat regularly.

Nervous tissue is made up of cells called *neurons* and other supporting cells called *neuroglia*. Although this tissue is made up of cells that look very different from one another, they all do the same job. They carry nervous impulses from a portion of the brain or spinal cord to all parts of the body.

Tissues are grouped together to form *organs,* such as the heart, lungs, and liver. Each organ has specific jobs. Organs that work together to perform similar tasks make up *systems.* It is easier to study anatomy and physiology by systems. Always remember that a system cannot work by itself. Systems are dependent, one upon the other.

THE WHOLE BODY

Before we begin the study of each system, it would be wise to take an overall look at the body and to become familiar with the names given to body areas and cavities. In any demonstration or diagram, the body or body part shown is in the anatomical position. The person is standing up straight, facing you, palms out and feet together. When you look at a person in the anatomical position, remember that the left side is always on your right, as in a mirror. This is especially important in studying diagrams. The front of a person is referred to as the *anterior* side. The back, containing the backbone, is called the *posterior* side. The areas of the body closer to the head are called *superior.*

WORDS THAT SHOW WHERE BODY PARTS ARE LOCATED

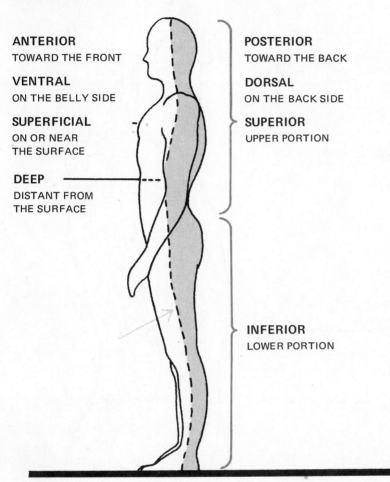

ANTERIOR
TOWARD THE FRONT

VENTRAL
ON THE BELLY SIDE

SUPERFICIAL
ON OR NEAR
THE SURFACE

DEEP
DISTANT FROM
THE SURFACE

POSTERIOR
TOWARD THE BACK

DORSAL
ON THE BACK SIDE

SUPERIOR
UPPER PORTION

INFERIOR
LOWER PORTION

Those closer to the feet are called *inferior*. These terms may also be used to describe the position of an organ in the body. For example, the liver is inferior to the diaphragm. The shoulder is superior to the elbow.

The body has two major cavities—the *dorsal* cavity and the *ventral* cavity. The dorsal cavity is divided into the *cranial* and *spinal* cavities. The cranial cavity is in the head. It contains the brain, its protecting membranes, large blood vessels, and nerves. The spinal cavity contains the spinal cord.

The ventral cavity is divided by a large, dome-shaped muscle—called the *diaphragm*—into the *thoracic* and *abdominal* cavities. The thoracic cavity is in your chest. It contains the lungs, the heart, the major blood vessels, and a portion of the esophagus. The esophagus is the food tube. It penetrates the diaphragm and enters the stomach, which is in the abdominal cavity.

Other organs in the abdominal cavity include the liver, spleen, pancreas, small and large intestines, and, in the female, the ovaries and uterus.

The kidneys are located in the dorsal portion of the abdominal cavity. The kidneys are outside the large membrane that envelops all of the other organs. This membrane is known as the *peritoneum*. When this membrane becomes infected, the disease is known as *peritonitis*. The peritoneum, like all membranes in the body, is made up of both epithelial and connective tissue. It protects organs and prevents friction when they move.

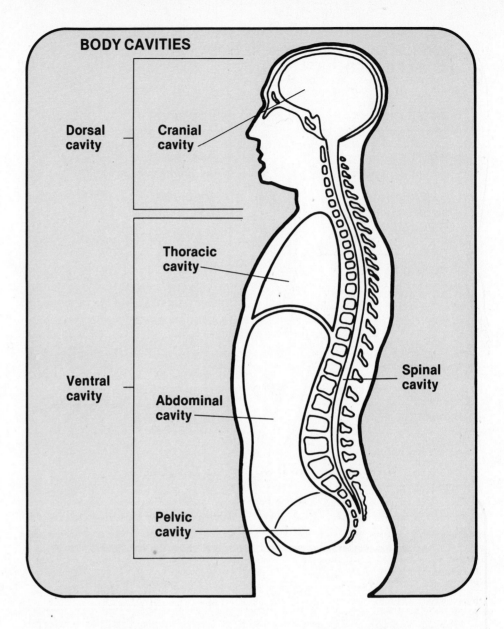

BODY CAVITIES

Dorsal cavity

Cranial cavity

Thoracic cavity

Ventral cavity

Spinal cavity

Abdominal cavity

Pelvic cavity

The Skeletal System

The skeletal system is made up of 206 bones. The bones act as a framework for the body, giving it structure and support. They are also the passive organs of motion. They do not move by themselves. They must be moved by muscles, which shorten or contract. A muscle is stimulated to contract by a nerve impulse. This is an example of how systems interact. It is necessary to learn the names of the bones because they are like landmarks. Many parts that cover them take their names from the bones.

There are four types of bones:

1. Long bones, such as the big bone in your thigh, the femur
2. Short bones, like the bones in your fingers, the phalanges
3. Irregular bones, such as the vertebrae that make up the spinal column
4. Flat bones, like the bones of the rib cage

Long bones give shape to the body and support body parts

TYPES
OF
BONES

Flat bones protect soft tissues and vital organs within the skeleton

Short and small bones give flexibility to the body

Irregular bones

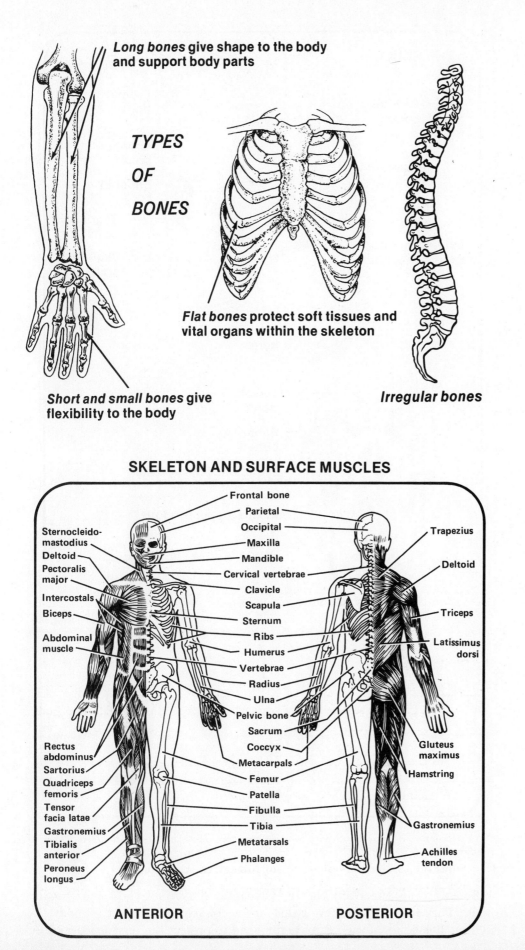

SKELETON AND SURFACE MUSCLES

Sternocleido-mastodius
Deltoid
Pectoralis major
Intercostals
Biceps
Abdominal muscle

Rectus abdominus
Sartorius
Quadriceps femoris
Tensor facia latae
Gastronemius
Tibialis anterior
Peroneus longus

Frontal bone
Parietal
Occipital
Maxilla
Mandible
Cervical vertebrae
Clavicle
Scapula
Sternum
Ribs
Humerus
Vertebrae
Radius
Ulna
Pelvic bone
Sacrum
Coccyx
Metacarpals
Femur
Patella
Fibulla
Tibia
Metatarsals
Phalanges

Trapezius
Deltoid
Triceps
Latissimus dorsi
Gluteus maximus
Hamstring
Gastronemius
Achilles tendon

ANTERIOR

POSTERIOR

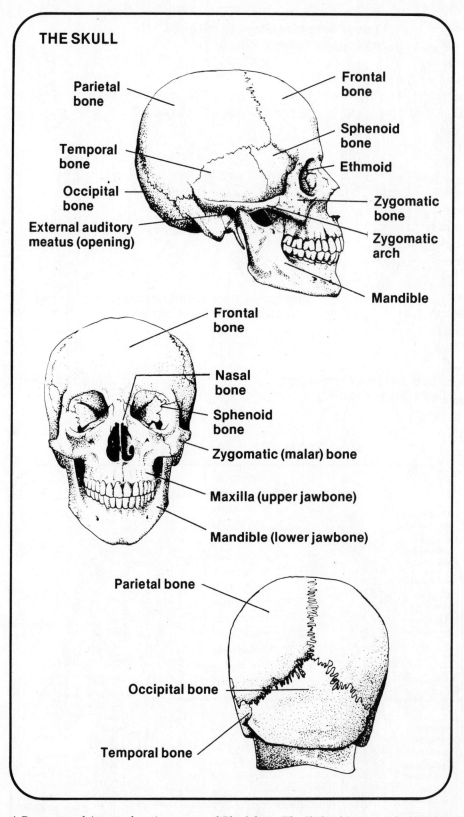

THE SKULL

Parietal bone

Frontal bone

Temporal bone

Sphenoid bone

Occipital bone

Ethmoid

External auditory meatus (opening)

Zygomatic bone

Zygomatic arch

Mandible

Frontal bone

Nasal bone

Sphenoid bone

Zygomatic (malar) bone

Maxilla (upper jawbone)

Mandible (lower jawbone)

Parietal bone

Occipital bone

Temporal bone

A Programmed Approach to Anatomy and Physiology. The Skeletal System. 2d ed. Robert J. Brady Co., Bowie Md, 1972

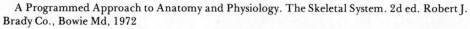

Bones are not inactive. They are dynamic and usually busy parts of the body. They store vital minerals that are necessary for many other body activities. The bones of the head are designed to protect the very delicate tissue of the brain. They are joined by sutures, similar to a zigzag embroidery pattern, and totally surround the brain and cranial nerves.

When the fetus is developing in the uterus, the entire skeleton is formed in cartilage by about two and one-half months after conception. From this cartilage, bone is formed, much as if you replaced a wooden bridge, piece by piece, with steel. The bones of the head are formed from strong membranes. They do not completely undergo *ossification* (which means development of bone) until after the child is born. This is a great aid during childbirth, when the baby's bones can overlap a little.

Joints (Motion). The systems of the body must all work together. No one system can stand alone. All the systems operate simultaneously in a healthy human body. The skeletal system, muscular system, nervous system, and circulatory system are all interacting during each body movement. Movement of the body occurs at the joints. This is a perfect example of how several systems must work together.

Joints are areas in which one bone connects with one or more bones. They are necessary levers in all motion. Joints are made up of many structures. The tough white fibrous cord, the *ligament,* connects bone to bone. The *tendons* connect muscle to bone. The meeting place of two bones—the *joint*—especially those in the shoulder, hip, and knee, is enclosed in a strong capsule. This capsule is lined by a membrane that secretes a fluid called *synovial fluid.* This fluid acts as a buffer, very much like a water bed, so the ends of the bones do not get worn out with a lot of motion. Other structures that protect the bone include the pad of cartilage at the end of the bone, a sac of synovial fluid (which is known as a *bursa*), and a disc of cartilage called the *meniscus.* Many such safeguards are built into the body. Injury to joints may

SYNOVIAL (MOVABLE) JOINTS

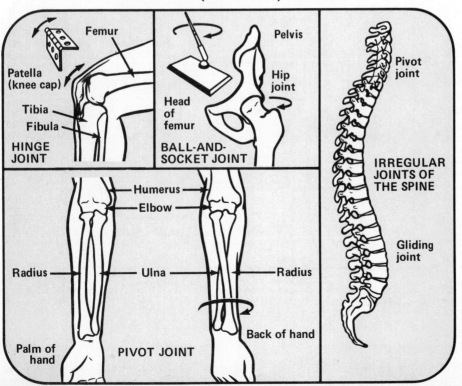

ADDUCTION   **ABDUCTION**

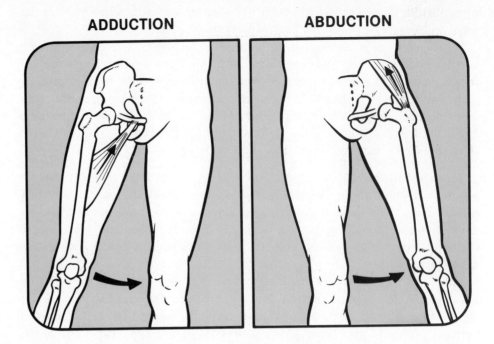

cause a ligament or tendon to be strained in what we call a *sprain*. Inflammation of the bursa causes *bursitis*.

There are several kinds of joints in the human body. The hinge joint, such as in the knee, is freely movable. There are also less-movable joints, such as those between the vertebrae. Some joints do not move at all. An example is joints between the bones of the head, which protect the brain.

COORDINATION OF MUSCLES

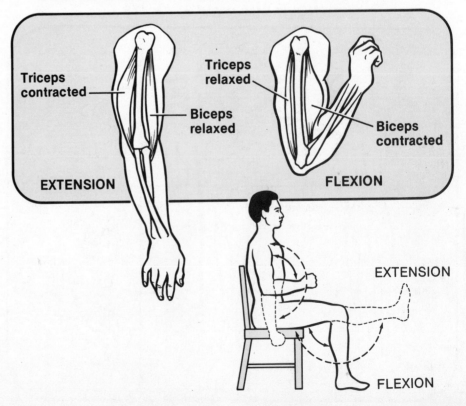

Triceps contracted
Biceps relaxed
Triceps relaxed
Biceps contracted
EXTENSION
FLEXION
EXTENSION
FLEXION

The Muscular System

The muscular system makes all motion possible, either that of the whole body, or that which occurs inside the body. Learning about the large skeletal muscles is important to you as a nursing aide.

Groups of muscles work together to perform a body motion. Other groups perform just the opposite motion. These two groups are called antagonistic groups. For example, flex your forearm, which means bringing it toward your shoulder. Your biceps brachii contract, and the triceps brachii relax. Extend your forearm. The biceps muscle relaxes while the triceps contracts. *Flexion* and *extension* are the two terms you should know. Two others are *abduction*, which means moving a part away from the body midline, and *adduction*, which means moving it toward the body.

When you are helping to lift a patient or when you are making a bed, remember to use the strong muscles of your legs rather than those of your back. This will prevent you from seriously hurting yourself. Use the large thigh muscles, the quadriceps femoris, on the ventral portion of the thigh, and the hamstrings on the dorsal portion. This will also save you from straining your muscles.

The Nervous System

The nervous system controls and organizes all body activity, both voluntary and involuntary. The nervous system is made up of the brain, the spinal cord, and the nerves. The nerves are spread throughout all areas of the body in an orderly way.

Nervous tissue is made up of cells called *neurons* and other supporting cells called *neuroglia*. A typical neuron is made up of a cell body with one long column called the *axon* and many small outbranchings called *dendrites*. Nerve impulses move from the dendrites through the cell body along the axon. Inside and outside our bodies, we have structures called receptor-end organs. Any change in our external or internal environment that is strong enough will set up a nervous impulse in these receptor-end organs. This impulse is carried by a sensory neuron to some part of the brain or spinal cord where it connects with an *interneuron*. The connection is called a *synapse*. This interneuron often makes hundreds of synapses (particularly in the cerebrum, the part of the brain in which we think) before a decision is made. Once that happens, the proper impulses are sent down a motor neuron to the effector-end organs, those organs that are going to respond to the nerve impulse.

Most nerve cells outside the brain and spinal cord have a protective covering known as the *myelin sheath*. This sheath helps prevent damage to the cells and often helps the nerve return to healthy function, or regenerate, if it has been injured. Nerve cells with a myelin sheath also carry an impulse faster than those without myelin. The neurons in the brain do not have this kind of protection. When they are injured, as they are by a stroke, or cerebral vascular accident (CVA), it is necessary for another part of the brain to take over the function of the part that has been damaged. The rehabilitation department in your hospital helps patients learn to do things again after such damage has been done.

The brain is perhaps the last frontier of man's scientific exploration. It is interesting to think that we are using our brains to study our brains. There is still so much to be learned about the tissue that makes up this organ, which organizes all of our activity.

THE NERVOUS SYSTEM

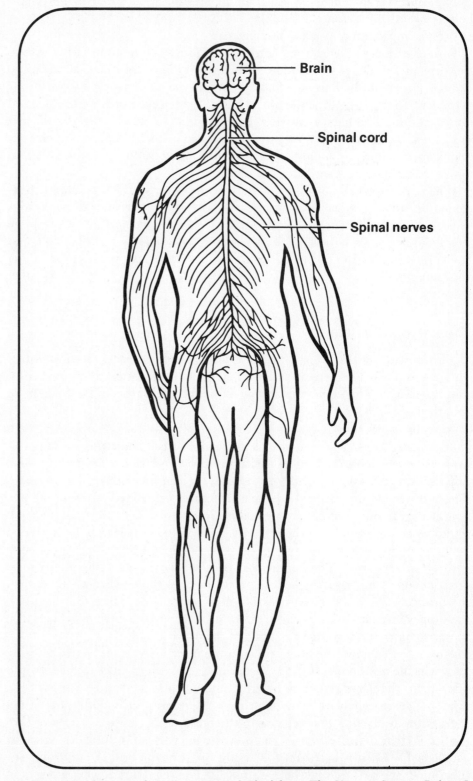

Brain

Spinal cord

Spinal nerves

A Programmed Approach to Anatomy and Physiology. The Nervous System. Robert J. Brady Co., Bowie Md, 1974

The brain is well protected by bones, membranes, the meninges, and a cushion of fluid called cerebral spinal fluid. This fluid circulates outside of and within the brain as well as around the spinal cord.

THE NEURON

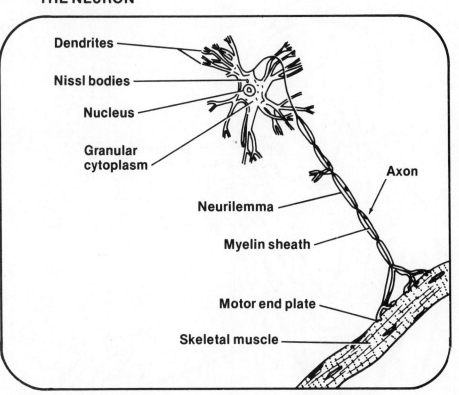

Dendrites

Nissl bodies

Nucleus

Granular
cytoplasm

Axon

Neurilemma

Myelin sheath

Motor end plate

Skeletal muscle

This is an example of a typical neuron. Note the motor end plate, which is the point of contact between the axon and the skeletal muscle.

The brain is a very complicated organ. It is made up of five portions. The *cerebrum* is divided into two halves, called *hemispheres*. They are connected to one another by white material known as *corpus callosum*. The right hemisphere controls most of the activity on the left side of the body. And the left hemisphere of the cerebrum controls the activity on the right side of the body. The cerebrum has many indentations, which are known as *convolutions*. It is here that all learning, memory, and associations are stored so that thought is possible. Also, it is here that decisions are made for voluntary action. Certain areas of the cerebrum seem to perform special organizing activities. For example, the *occipital* lobe is the place where what you see is interpreted. The *frontal* lobe is the primary area of thought and reason. The *cerebellum* is the part of the brain that controls voluntary motion. It works with part of the inner ear, the semicircular canals, to enable us to walk and move smoothly through our world. The *midbrain, pons,* and *medulla* are primarily pathways through which nervous impulses reach the brain from the spinal cord.

Nerves throughout the body send messages into the tracts of white matter in the spinal cord, from which they rise to higher centers in the brain. There are 12 pairs of cranial nerves and 32 pairs of spinal nerves. These have many branches, which go to all parts of the body.

SENSORY AND MOTOR PROCESSES IN OPERATION

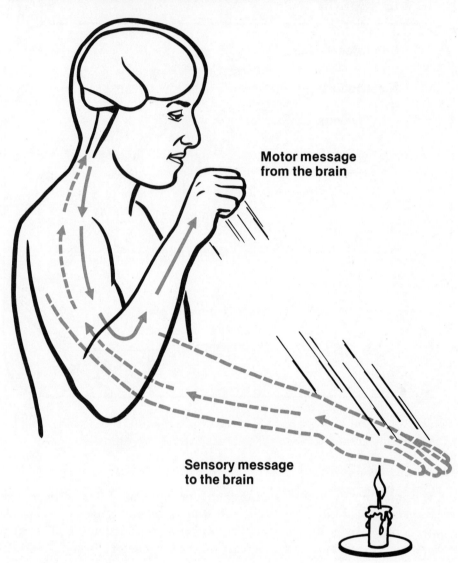

Motor message from the brain

Sensory message to the brain

One of the most important areas of the brain is an area called the *diencephelon.* It is here that small structures surround one of the ventricles of the brain. These structures help circulate cerebral spinal fluid and exercise an almost dictatorial control over the body's activities. They screen all nervous impulses going to the brain, either getting them there faster or slowing them down. One of these tiny structures is the *hypothalamus.* In times of stress or emergency, excitement, or danger, this structure actually takes over control of the body. This is because it keeps its control over the body's master gland, the *pituitary* gland. Although it can be mapped, like the subways of a great city, we still know very little about its actual activity. We do know that it has tremendous control over most body activities. It seems to be the link between the mind and the body. It receives messages from the cerebrum, from the cerebellum, and from impulses coming up the spinal cord, and it has direct control over all the *endocrine* glands.

Much of the activity of the organs of the body is *involuntary.* In other words, we do not think about it. Or, for the most part, we have no conscious control over this activity. The part of the nervous system that controls such things as digestion and the functions of other visceral (abdominal) organs is the *autonomic nervous system*. This is really not separate from the brain and the spinal cord. The neurons that make up the autonomic nervous system use the same pathways as those neurons that control our voluntary actions. However, the two divisions of this part of the nervous system direct and control the activity of our internal organs. Each organ is supplied with neurons from each division of the autonomic nervous system.

One division is called the *sympathetic* division. The neurons that make up this division become active during stress, danger, excitement, or illness. These neurons cause the pupils of our eyes to become larger, so we can see more clearly and can see better at a distance. These neurons also cause the heart to beat more strongly and to send more oxygen to the large muscles of the body in case it is necessary to fight or run. In today's fast-paced world, we are all subject to stress, and sometimes we cannot run away from it or fight it. The action of the neurons from the sympathetic system then causes changes in the shape or activity of some of our organs. This action may also cause illness.

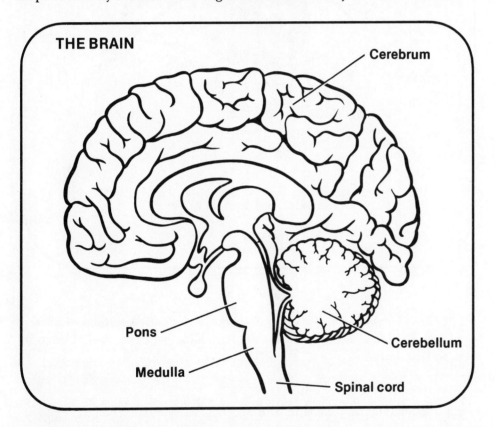

THE BRAIN

The *parasympathetic* division of the autonomic nervous system is in control when we are relaxed. It is known to conserve our energy.

Fortunately, there is a checks-and-balances system between the two divisions. When one has been in action too long, the other automatically switches on. We have all had the experience of eating a large meal after being emotionally upset and feeling as if we had lead in our stomach. This is because of the sympathetic division of the autonomic nervous system. *Peristalsis* (which is movement of the gut) lessens, and digestion does not go on. The sympathetic nervous system can also cause contractions of the uterus to decrease. Sometimes during labor a woman can be so frightened that the sympathetic division causes the contractions that will help her baby to be born to slow down. This is one of the reasons it is so important for pregnant women to attend prenatal classes. When they know all about labor and delivery, they will lose much of their fear, and the contractions will remain steady and even.

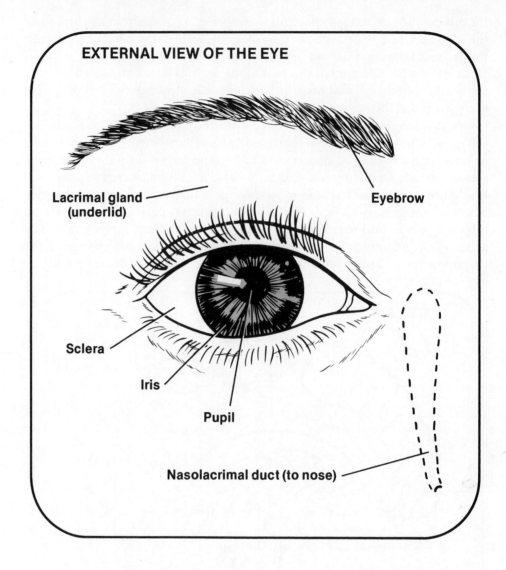

EXTERNAL VIEW OF THE EYE

Lacrimal gland
(underlid)

Eyebrow

Sclera

Iris

Pupil

Nasolacrimal duct (to nose)

The Sense Organs. The sense organs contain specialized endings of the sensory neurons. These are excited by sudden changes in the outside environment, called *stimuli*.

- *Eyes* respond to visual stimuli.
- *Ears* respond mainly to sound stimuli.
- *Membranes of the nose* respond to smells.
- *Taste buds,* located chiefly on the tongue, respond to sweet and sour and other sensations.
- *Skin* responds to touch, pressure, heat, cold, and pain.

Hormones and the Endocrine System

The *endocrine glands* secrete liquid substances called *hormones.* These help the nervous system organize and direct the activities of the body. The hormones are secreted (flow) directly into the bloodstream. *Exocrine glands,* such as the salivary glands, deliver their products through ducts into a body cavity.

The hormones from the pituitary gland, both the anterior and posterior portions, regulate all *metabolism* of our billions of cells. The anterior portion manufactures and releases seven hormones.

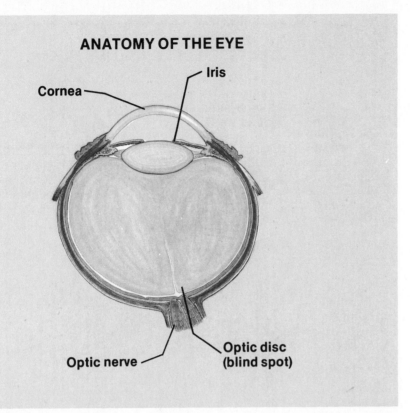

ANATOMY OF THE EYE

Iris

Cornea

Optic nerve

Optic disc
(blind spot)

A Programmed Approach to Anatomy and Physiology. The Special Senses. Robert J. Brady
Co., Bowie Md, 1972

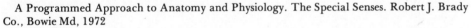

The *pituitary* gland is the master gland. Its hormones directly affect the
other endocrine glands, stimulating them to produce their hormones. Its hormones are especially important in reproduction and in all functions leading to
puberty. This is the time at which a child takes on the physical characteristics
of an adult man or woman. Hormones from the pituitary gland regulate the
menstrual cycle in the female and sperm production in the male. Without
these hormones, it would not be possible for us to reproduce our own kind.

The pituitary gland and all of these important hormones are under the
direct control of the *hypothalamus*, a tiny fragment of tissue lying near the
base of the brain. This structure seems to be the real link between our thinking, our emotions, and our body functions.

The *thyroid* gland produces a hormone that regulates growth and general
metabolism. The *thymus* gets smaller after puberty, but it plays an important
part in the body's immunity system. It is this immunity system that prevents us
from getting many diseases.

The *parathyroids* are located within the capsule of the thyroid. They produce a hormone that regulates, along with one of the hormones in the thyroid
gland, the level of calcium and potassium in the blood. Calcium is important
for many functions of the body, such as muscle contraction and conduction of
nerve impulses.

The *pancreas* is both an endocrine gland and an exocrine gland, or a gland
that has a duct. Its endocrine portion produces the hormone *insulin.* Insulin
regulates the sugar content of the blood. If the body does not have enough insulin, the person becomes diabetic. He must be treated by reducing the carbohydrate or sugar intake and by regulating the balance between insulin and
blood sugar.

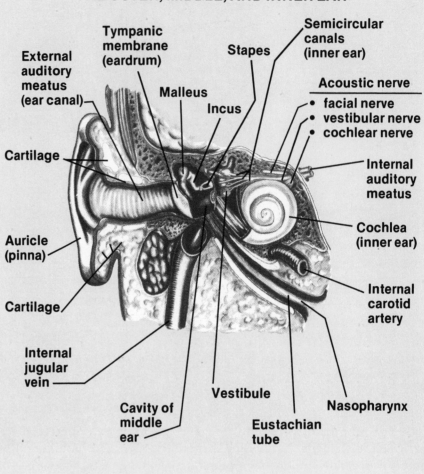

THE OUTER, MIDDLE, AND INNER EAR

A Programmed Approach to Anatomy and Physiology. The Special Senses. Robert J. Brady Co., Bowie Md, 1972

Diabetes Mellitus. When the body cannot change starches and sugar into energy and cannot store them because of an imbalance of hormones (insulin), the result is the chronic disease known as *diabetes mellitus,* which is a disturbance of carbohydrate metabolism.

Signs and symptoms of diabetes mellitus:

- Fatigue, tiredness
- Loss of weight
- Vaginitis—inflammation of the vagina
- Skin erosions—sores heal poorly and slowly
- Poor vision—eyesight affected
- Hyperglycemia—high blood sugar
- Glycosuria—sugar in the urine
- Polyuria—frequency and large amounts of urine
- Polyphagia—excessive appetite
- Polydipsia—excessive thirst

ENDOCRINE GLANDS

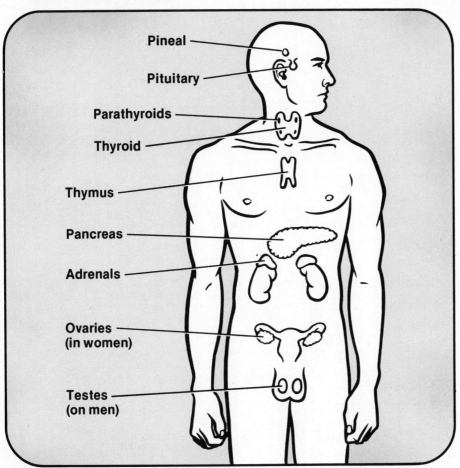

Pineal
Pituitary
Parathyroids
Thyroid
Thymus
Pancreas
Adrenals
Ovaries
(in women)
Testes
(on men)

Terms often used with diabetes mellitus:

- FBS—fasting blood sugar
- GTT—glucose tolerance test
- Ketone bodies
- Gangrene—necrosis
- S&A test—sugar and acetone test
- Pancreas—Islands of Langerhans—endocrine and exocrine glands
- PPBS—Postprandial blood sugar

Signs and symptoms of insulin shock:

- Low blood sugar
- No sugar in urine
- Coma—unconsciousness
- Stupor
- Numbness of tongue and lips
- Tremors
- Nervousness
- Weakness

- Blurred vision
- Headache
- Perspiration
- Dizziness
- Hunger

Signs and symptoms of diabetic coma:

- Abdominal pain or discomfort
- Vomiting or nausea
- Sweet or fruity odor of the breath
- Flushed skin
- Air hunger
- Increased respirations
- Dry skin
- Parched tongue
- Soft eyeballs
- Dulled senses

THE HEART

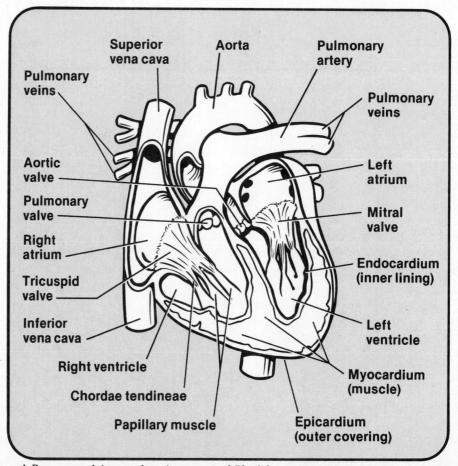

A Programmed Approach to Anatomy and Physiology. Robert J. Brady Co. Bowie Md, 1972

The *adrenal* glands lie on top of the kidneys. They are very important in helping the body adapt to stress conditions, giving a lot of help to the autonomic nervous system.

The *ovaries* in the female are responsible for secreting the hormones *estrogen* and *progesterone*. The rise and fall of the levels of these hormones in the blood determines the menstrual cycle. The hormones are also important in causing an ovum, or egg, to develop and in maintaining a pregnancy.

The *testes* in the male produce *testosterone,* the primary sex hormone of the male, which also causes the production of sperm.

The Circulatory System

The circulatory system is made up of the blood, the heart, and the blood vessels—arteries, veins, and capillaries. The heart actually acts as a pump for the blood, which carries the nutrients, oxygen, and other elements needed by the cells. Important facts to know about blood include:

- The blood carries oxygen from the lungs to the cells.
- Carbon dioxide is carried by the blood from the cells to the lungs.
- Nutrients (food) are picked up (absorbed) by the blood from the duodenum (small intestine) and brought to the cells.
- Waste products from the cells are carried by the blood to the kidneys to be eliminated in urine.
- The hormones from the endocrine glands are transported by the blood.
- Dilation (enlargement) and contraction (narrowing) of the blood vessels help regulate body temperature.
- The blood helps maintain the fluid balance of the body.
- The white cells of the blood defend the body against disease.

The heart is made up of four chambers—two *auricles* (the *atria*) and two *ventricles*. The atria are the two smaller chambers. They have thinner walls because their contractions send the blood only as far as the lungs. Here, in the pulmonary circulation, the blood picks up oxygen and gets rid of carbon dioxide. This blood then returns to the heart, carrying its load of oxygen, which is pushed into systemic circulation by the ventricles.

The ventricles have thick walls of muscle. When they contract, the left ventricle pushes the blood through the largest blood vessel, the aorta, to all parts of the body. The blood vessels that carry blood having a lot of oxygen are called *arteries.* The only exception is the pulmonary artery, which carries the blood to the lungs. Arteries branch into a vast network throughout the body. As they branch, the blood vessels become smaller and smaller until finally they are so thin they become *capillaries.* The walls of the capillaries are only one cell-layer thick. Through these walls, gases, nutrients, waste products, and other substances are exchanged among the blood in the capillaries, the tissue fluid, and the individual cell. After the blood has given up its oxygen, which is carried on the surface of the red blood cells, it is returned to the heart through the *veins.*

Other important points are:

- All arteries carry blood away from the heart.
- All veins carry blood back to the heart.
- All arteries carry oxygenated blood (red) except the pulmonary artery.

- All veins carry deoxygenated blood (blue) except the four pulmonary veins.

It is necessary that the heart muscle be supplied with blood carrying oxygen. The first branches of the aorta, which comes from the heart's left ventricle, are the coronary arteries, which surround the heart. These carry needed oxygen to cardiac (heart) muscle tissue. If one of these branches of the coronary arteries is blocked by a blood clot (embolism), the patient has had a heart attack (coronary thrombosis). This can result in the death of some heart tissue. The event is called a *myocardial infarction* (MI).

Blood is a kind of connective tissue. The liquid portion of it is called *plasma*. The cells are red blood cells, which carry oxygen, and white blood cells, which fight infection. If a patient has an inflammation in some area of the body, a physician often prescribes warm, moist compresses. These are applied to dilate (widen) the blood vessels in the area and to bring more of those important white blood cells to the place of infection, to help fight it. People who have too few red blood cells have some type of anemia. People with two few white blood cells have a lowered resistance to disease. An increase in white blood cells in the blood means that an infection is present somewhere in the body.

A patient's circulation of blood tends to slow down when he is in bed. Sometimes this can cause clotting of the blood. A blood clot is dangerous.

If you have orders to help a patient out of bed for the first time after an illness or after surgery, remember that his circulation is slower. Therefore make sure he moves carefully and slowly. Allow the patient to sit at the edge of the bed until his circulation stabilizes, that is, comes back to normal. Then assist him carefully to a standing position. Sometimes this procedure will cause the blood to leave the brain suddenly. Then the patient may be dizzy or feel faint.

The circulatory system is responsible for getting all of the necessary ingredients to a cell for its metabolism and for carrying away its products and waste material. The circulatory system works in close harmony with the respiratory system.

The Respiratory System

The respiratory system provides a route or pathway for oxygen to get from the air into the lungs, where it can be picked up by the blood. The organs that make up this system include the nose and mouth, the *pharynx* (throat), the *trachea* (windpipe), *larynx* (voicebox), *bronchi,* and *lungs.* Because we must have oxygen to live, it is necessary to keep this pathway open. The structures themselves help to do this. The trachea and bronchi are kept open by incomplete cartilage rings.

On top of the trachea, opening from the pharynx (the throat), is a structure known as the *larynx.* It is not only the opening to the trachea, it also contains the vocal cords, which make it possible for us to talk. An important piece of cartilage, the *epiglottis,* covers the opening to the trachea when food is swallowed, preventing the food from going into the lungs. A very weak patient, or one who is having trouble breathing, must be watched carefully when you are feeding him so that food does not get into the trachea. This is known as *aspiration* of food. An unconscious patient who vomits may also be in danger of aspirating that material. Turn the patient's head to one side at once. You must watch the patient with great care, because if the pathway for oxygen is blocked, the patient will not live without immediate treatment.

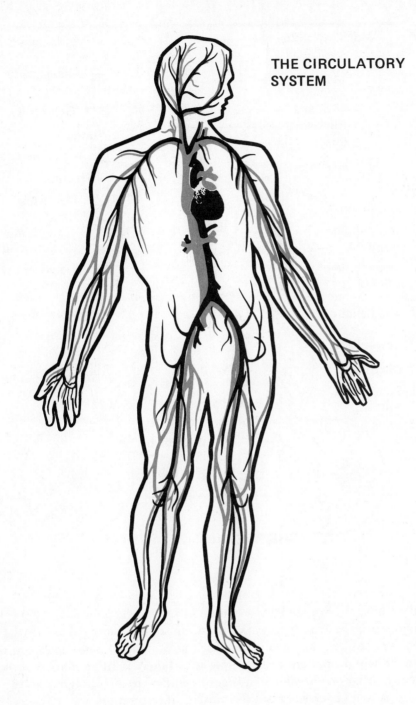

THE CIRCULATORY SYSTEM

As in our other systems, the important work of the respiratory system is done at the level of the cell. The exchange of oxygen and carbon dioxide occurs in an area of the lungs that is so small you must use a microscope to see it. The last branch of the bronchus is called the *alveolar duct*. At its end is a small sac, the *alveolus*. Many oxygen molecules fill this sac after you breathe in. The blood has less oxygen and therefore is able to pick up a lot of oxygen from the alveolar sac. The blood is then returned to the heart to be sent around the body beginning in the largest artery, the aorta.

The respiratory system, then, is responsible for getting oxygen to the blood. Internal respiration occurs when those cells that need the oxygen receive it in exchange for carbon dioxide, which is the cells' gas waste product. Both functions are equally important.

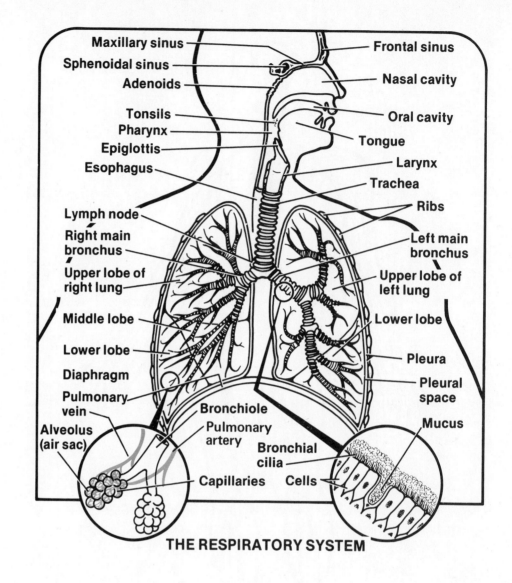

THE RESPIRATORY SYSTEM

Breathing is regulated by a center in the *medulla,* a part of the brain. Often, especially after surgery, a patient must be encouraged to breathe deeply in order to keep all the air sacs open and inflated. Sometimes you will be asked to help the patient cough, especially if there is inflammation of the lung tissue. Placing one of your hands gently under the diaphragm and the other on the patient's back will assist the muscles of respiration.

The Digestive System (Gastrointestinal System)

The digestive system is responsible for breaking down the food that is eaten into a form that can be used by the body cells. This action is both chemical and mechanical. The digestive tract is about 30 feet long. All of it is important in reducing food to simple compounds.

Digestion begins in the mouth, where food is chewed and mixed with the substance called *saliva.* During swallowing, the food moves in a moistened ball down the esophagus to the stomach. The stomach churns and mixes the food at the same time it is being broken down chemically. The most important area of digestion is the *duodenum.* This is the first loop of the small intestine. It is here that the digestive juices, not only from the duodenum itself but also from the *pancreas,* finish the job of breaking down food into usable parts. In addi-

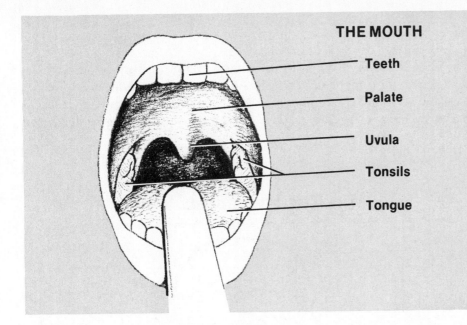

THE MOUTH

- Teeth
- Palate
- Uvula
- Tonsils
- Tongue

tion, *bile,* which has been stored in the gallbladder after being manufactured in the liver, also enters the duodenum and helps the reduction process.

A lot of water is necessary for the chemical reduction of food into its end products. It is moved by the rhythmic contraction, called *peristalsis,* of the muscle walls of the several organs of digestion.

Some of the final products of digestion are also absorbed in the area of the duodenum. These end products are:

- Amino acids, the building blocks for all growth and repair of body tissue, which come from dietary proteins
- Fatty acids and glycerols, from fat
- Simple sugars, such as glucose, from carbohydrates
- Water and vitamins

The lining of the duodenum is composed of thousands of tiny fingerlike projections called *villi.* Each villus is capable of absorbing these end products of digestion. The products are then moved into the bloodstream, where they are carried to individual cells.

Some digestion continues to take place in other parts of the small intestine. What is left of the food moves through the large intestine, where water is reabsorbed into the body. The material that cannot be used by the body is excreted from the rectum through the anus as feces.

The *liver* has important responsibilities aside from manufacturing bile. The liver is a storage area for glucose. This form of sugar is released in large amounts when the cells need it for energy to carry on their activities. The liver also is the place where toxins, or poisons, are removed from the blood. Damage to the liver can be caused by eating certain substances or taking drugs that are harmful to its tissues, such as alcoholic beverages. The liver is also responsible for production and storage of some proteins, which are necessary for proper circulation of the blood and for blood clotting. Blood clots aren't all bad. When a blood vessel has been injured, a clot may form that holds the blood within a closed tube (the blood vessel) until healing occurs.

On the right side of the *colon,* at the junction between the small intestine and the large intestine, there is a pouch with a projection of tissue called the *appendix*. Because there is very little peristalsis in this area, the appendix has a tendency to become infected, in a disease known as *appendicitis*. Surgery is usually performed to correct this condition.

The lowest portion of the large intestine curves in an S-shape into the rectum. The rectum is made of very delicate tissue. It has an internal sphincter muscle and an external sphincter muscle. Sometimes blood vessels that supply this area become enlarged and filled with blood clots, causing *hemorrhoids*.

THE DIGESTIVE SYSTEM

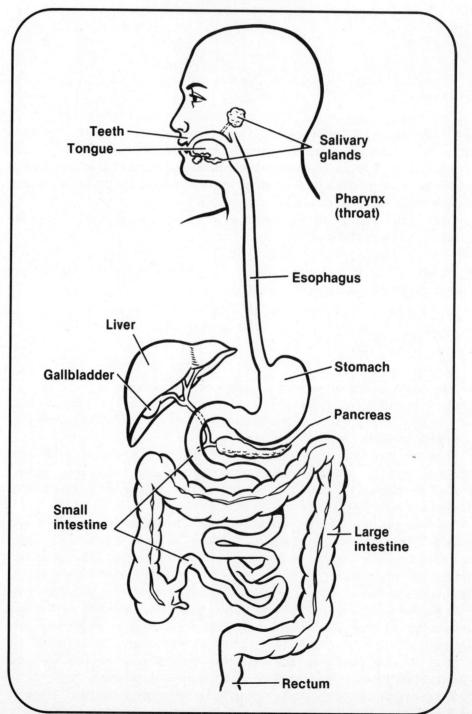

INTERNAL VIEW OF
STRUCTURE OF SMALL INTESTINE

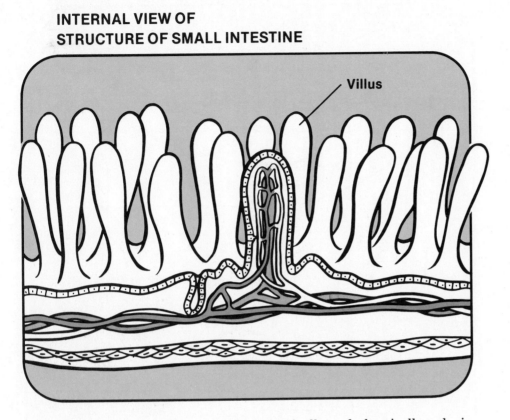

Villus

The digestive system takes care of mechanically and chemically reducing the food we eat into simple substances that can be used by the cells for their metabolism.

The Excretory System

A vital body system in maintaining homeostasis is the excretory system (which gets rid of waste products). The organs that make up this system include:

- The kidneys
- The ureters (tubes leading from the kidneys)
- The urinary bladder
- The urethra (which leads from the bladder to the outside of the body)

The other organs that help rid the body of waste material include the lungs, which get rid of carbon dioxide by exhalation (breathing out); the skin, which not only is protective but contains glands that secrete moisture and so help maintain body temperature; and, of course, the large intestine.

The functional unit of the kidneys is called a *nephron*. An exchange of substances takes place between the blood capillaries and a part of the nephron. A network of capillaries, called the *glomerulus,* lies withing a cupping of a tube, known as Bowman's capsule. Materials from the blood that are not needed by the body are filtered into Bowman's capsule. They are then carried through a series of tubules, which help make up the nephron. As the filtered material flows through these tubules, the blood vessels surrounding them reabsorb those materials still needed by the body, particularly the water. Near the end of the winding tubules, substances from the blood, such as toxins and some drugs, pass into the urine. The filtrate that is left is collected in a

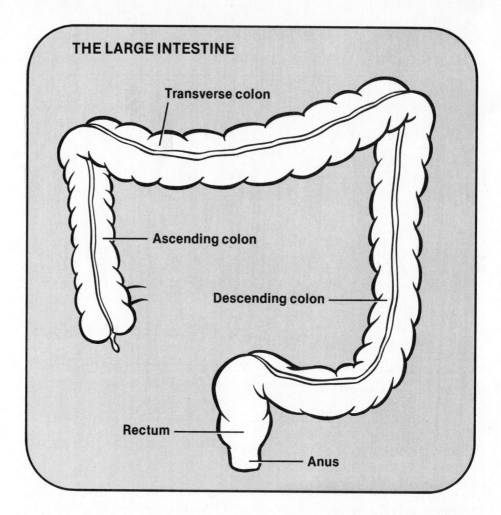

larger tube. This tube joins those of all the other nephrons in a basin-like portion of the kidney. From here it drips steadily through the ureter, helped by a peristaltic motion very similar to that of the gastrointestinal tract, to the urinary bladder. There are stretch receptor-end organs in the muscular wall of the bladder. The bladder is capable of expanding greatly. When these receptors are stimulated by a full bladder, messages are sent to the brain that cause the person to urinate.

Because the urethra is open to the outside of the body, it may also provide a passageway for disease-causing organisms. These organisms may go up to the bladder, infecting it and causing a disease known as *cystitis*. The infection may also spread through the ureters to the kidney, causing kidney damage.

The urinary system is perhaps the most important system for maintaining homeostasis. This is because the system determines the content of the blood. The blood content, in turn, determines the content of the tissue fluid, which is the immediate environment of the cells. Many changes in kidney function, some normal, can be found in urine samples. Such changes are also revealed in accurate measurement of intake and output. Sometimes in illness, especially after surgery, the patient is unable to void or urinate.

The Reproductive System

In the female the primary reproductive organ is the ovary. There are two of them. Once each month—usually 14 days before the onset of the next menstrual period—an ovum (egg) is released from the surface of one or the other ovary. During this time a woman is fertile, that is, she is able to get preg-

THE URINARY SYSTEM

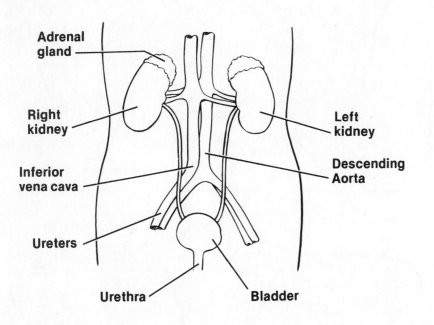

nant. During the time the egg is developing, it lies in a lake of *estrogen*. Estrogen is a hormone manufactured by a body structure called the *graffian follicle*. It is being poured into the blood stream during ovulation. This hormone causes a buildup of the lining of the uterus, the *endometrium*, preparing it for a possible pregnancy. When the ovum is released during ovulation, it is picked up by the fringes (or *fimbriae*) of the *oviduct* (fallopian tube). Then it is carried very slowly through the oviduct to the *uterus*. Another name for the uterus is *womb*.

During sexual intercourse, millions of sperm are released during each ejaculation. The sperm move through the vagina and uterus and up the oviduct (fallopian tube). If the timing is right and contraception has not been used, one sperm will unite with the ovum, causing conception. Rapid division of the fused cells (ovum plus sperm) takes place and an embryo is formed, the beginning of a baby.

Menstruation is simply the periodic (monthly) loss of some blood and a small part of the lining of the uterus, an organ that is full of blood vessels. The discharge flows out of the vagina for a period of 2 to 5 days. The process of ovulation is controlled by hormones from the pituitary gland, under the control of the hypothalamus. The hormones from the pituitary gland are involved in the development of the ovum and in maintaining pregnancy.

In the human female there are three openings in the perineal area. One is the external urinary *meatus*, the end of the urethra. One is the *vagina*, which is not only the organ for intercourse but also the main part of the birth canal. The last one is the *anus*. Many women who find it necessary to have a hysterectomy, or surgical removal of the uterus, are afraid of what will happen to their bodies after surgery. Although such women will not be able to become pregnant, they usually are not affected in any other way.

THE MENSTRUAL CYCLE

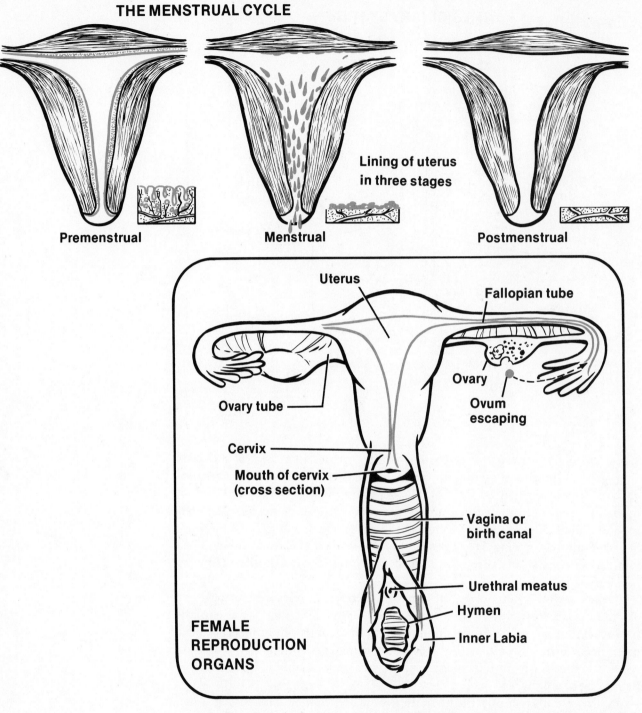

Lining of uterus in three stages

Premenstrual
Menstrual
Postmenstrual

Uterus
Fallopian tube
Ovary tube
Ovary
Ovum escaping
Cervix
Mouth of cervix (cross section)
Vagina or birth canal
Urethral meatus
Hymen
Inner Labia

FEMALE REPRODUCTION ORGANS

The most important area of sexual sensation for the female is the *clitoris*. This small organ is located where the *labia minora* come together. It has a shaft and roots, which run deeply into the labia minora and labia majora. The vagina has receptor-end organs for sexual pleasure only at its edges and about an inch down.

In the male the primary reproductive organs are the *testes*. Testicles, or testes, are paired glands that lie in a sac called the *scrotum* outside the body, posterior to the *penis,* which is the primary male sex organ. Each testicle is divided into lobes, in which there are tightly coiled tubes called *seminiferous tubules.* It is here that the *sperm* come to full development. They are stored in a structure on top of each testis, the *epididymis.* During intercourse, the sperm travel up the *vas deferens,* or sperm duct, to a point where they enter

FEMALE PELVIC ORGANS

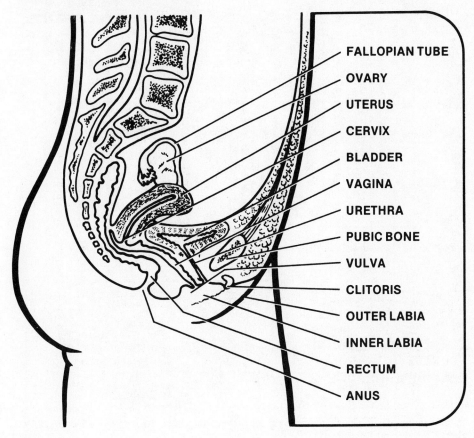

FALLOPIAN TUBE
OVARY
UTERUS
CERVIX
BLADDER
VAGINA
URETHRA
PUBIC BONE
VULVA
CLITORIS
OUTER LABIA
INNER LABIA
RECTUM
ANUS

FERTILIZATION AND CELL DIVISION

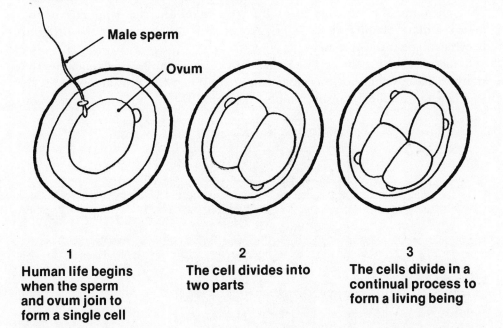

Male sperm
Ovum

1
Human life begins
when the sperm
and ovum join to
form a single cell

2
The cell divides into
two parts

3
The cells divide in a
continual process to
form a living being

the urethra. The entrance is made along with secretions from other glands in
the male reproductive system. These glands—the seminal vesicles, the prostate
gland, and Cowper's glands—contribute water, nutrients, and vitamins,
which, added to the sperm, make up the semen, a fluid that is ejaculated (ex-

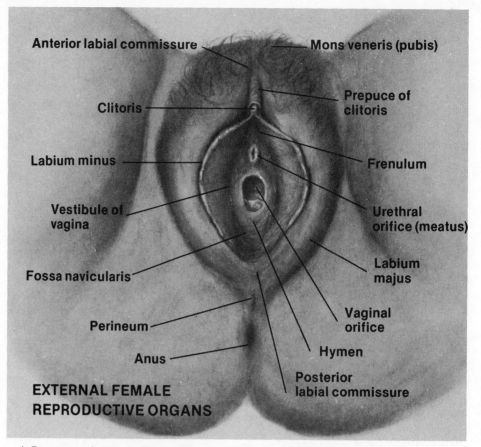

Anterior labial commissure

Mons veneris (pubis)

Clitoris

Prepuce of clitoris

Labium minus

Frenulum

Vestibule of vagina

Urethral orifice (meatus)

Fossa navicularis

Labium majus

Perineum

Vaginal orifice

Anus

Hymen

Posterior labial commissure

EXTERNAL FEMALE REPRODUCTIVE ORGANS

A Programmed Approach to Anatomy and Physiology. The Reproductive System. 2d ed. Robert J. Brady Co., Bowie Md, 1970

pelled) at the time the male has an orgasm. There is only one duct in the penis. It is used for the flow of urine and for the ejaculation of sperm in its carrying medium, the semen. During intercourse the internal sphincter of the male's urinary bladder closes tightly, so there is no chance for the urine to become mixed with the semen.

Sometimes during the aging process the prostate gland, which encircles the urethra like a doughnut, becomes enlarged. When the prostate expands, it squeezes the urethra, causing painful urination. Many men fear surgery on

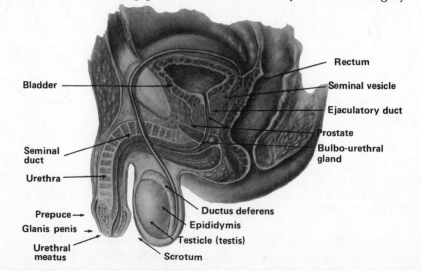

Bladder

Rectum

Seminal vesicle

Ejaculatory duct

Prostate

Bulbo-urethral gland

Seminal duct

Urethra

Prepuce →

Ductus deferens

Glanis penis →

Epididymis

Urethral meatus

Testicle (testis)

Scrotum

A Programmed Approach to Anatomy and Physiology. The Reproductive System. 2d ed. Robert J. Brady Co., Bowie Md, 1970

their prostate glands, because they believe it will end their sex life. The amount of semen ejaculated will be less, but otherwise men who have had a prostatectomy are almost always capable of having normal sexual relations.

The penis has three columns of spongy or cavernous tissue. During sexual excitement, blood rushes in through the penile artery and the veins constrict, trapping the blood so it fills these spaces. Then the penis becomes erect and turgid. All of this activity occurs under the influence of *testosterone*, the primary male sex hormone, which is also manufactured in the testes. It is secreted into the blood through the influence of the hormones from the anterior pituitary, which is under the control of the hypothalamus.

MAGNIFIED CROSS SECTION OF THE SKIN

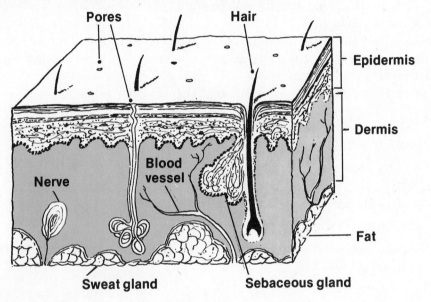

The Integumentary System (The Skin)

The skin covers and protects underlying structures from injury or bacterial invasion. Skin also contains nerve endings from the nervous system, which aid the body in awareness of its environment.

The skin helps regulate the body temperature by controlling the loss of heat from the body. To increase heat loss, the blood vessels near the skin dilate, and the increased blood flow brings more heat to the skin. Then the skin temperature rises and more heat is lost from the hot skin to the cooler environment. Even more important in heat loss is the evaporation of sweat (perspiration). It carries heat away from the skin. When the body is conserving heat, sweating stops and blood vessels contract. This prevents the blood from carrying heat to the skin. The skin temperature falls, decreasing heat loss. In this way, the body temperature is kept almost constant. The body also rids itself of certain waste products through perspiration.

Perspiration is released from the body through sweat glands, which are distributed over the entire skin surface. The glands open by ducts, or pores. Skin also secretes a thick, oily substance through ducts that lead to oil glands. In this way, the skin is lubricated and kept soft and pliable. The oil also provides a protective film for the skin, which limits the absorption and evaporation of water from the surface. In elderly persons these oil glands sometimes fail to function properly, and the skin becomes quite dry, scaly, and delicate.

Appendages of the skin, in addition to the sweat and oil glands, include the hair and the nails. Each hair has a root embedded in the skin, into which the oil glands of the skin open. Fingernails and toenails grow from the nail bed at the base underneath. If the nail bed is destroyed, the nail stops growing.

The skin covers the entire body. At certain places it joins the mucous membranes. These mucous membranes form the lining of the nose, mouth, and other body openings. The outer layer of the skin—the layer you can see—is called the *epidermis*. Tiny particles called cells are constantly flaking off or being rubbed off this outer layer of skin. Beneath the epidermis is the *dermis*. In this layer of skin are the new cells that will replace the cells that are lost from the epidermis.

Moisture on the skin can pick up dust and dirt from the air. Moisture can also mix with the skin particles being flaked off the epidermis. This process causes a condition that promotes the growth and spread of bacteria. This is the main reason for keeping the skin clean. As you know, the skin is where the battle for asepsis begins.

Watch for changes in the color of the patient's skin. Watch for blueness or darkening (cyanosis) of the lips, fingernails, or eyelids. Cyanosis is a sign of shock, or one of the effects of shock.

The primary functions of the skin are:

- To cover and protect underlying body structures from injury and bacterial invasion
- To help regulate body temperature by controlling loss of heat from the body
- Storage of energy in the form of fat and vitamins
- Elimination of wastes by perspiration
- Sensory perception—the sense of touch (The skin can sense heat, cold, pain, and pressure.)

The Body Systems

System	Function	Organs
Skeletal	Supports and protects the body	Bones; joints
Muscular	Gives movement to the body	Muscles; tendons; ligaments
Gastrointestinal (digestive, GI)	Takes and absorbs food and eliminates wastes	Mouth; teeth; tongue; esophagus; salivary glands; stomach; duodenum; intestines; liver; gallbladder; ascending, transverse, and descending colon; rectum; anus; appendix
Nervous	Controls activities of the body	Brain; spinal cord; nerves
Urinary	Removes wastes from the blood, produces urine, and eliminates urine	Kidneys; ureters; bladder; urethra
Reproductive	Allows a new human being to be born (reproduced)	Male: testes, scrotum, penis Female: ovaries, uterus, breasts, fallopian tubes, vagina
Respiratory	Eliminates carbon dioxide and gives the body air to supply oxygen to the cells through the blood	Nose; pharynx; larynx; trachea; bronchi; lungs

The Body Systems (continued)

Circulatory	Carries food, oxygen, and water to the body cells and removes wastes	Heart; blood; arteries; veins; capillaries; spleen; lymph; lymph nodes; lymph vessels
Endocrine	Secretes hormones directly into the blood	Thyroid and parathyroid glands; pineal gland; adrenal glands; testes; ovaries; thymus; pancreatic islands of Langerhans; pituitary gland
Integumentary	Provides first line of defense against infection, maintains body temperature, and provides fluids	Skin; hair; nails; sweat and oil glands

WHAT YOU HAVE LEARNED

The cell is the basic unit of all living matter. The human body is made up of millions of cells. Cells reproduce by a process called cell division, which eventually produces groups of similar cells. When the cells that are similar in form and function become specialized, they are called *tissues*. When two or more tissues work together to perform a certain function, they form an organ, such as the heart. A system, such as the circulatory system, is formed when a group of organs act together to perform complex body functions. All cells, tissues, organs, and systems operate together to form a human being.

Good reasons for studying human anatomy are: to deliver more effective health care to the patient, to understand better the instructions your head nurse or team leader gives you, and to have the knowledge necessary to act as a teacher to your patients. Perhaps the best reason of all is that an appreciation of the design of the healthy human body and how it works will help you treat each patient with tender, loving care.

Medical Terminology: Continuing to Learn

18

Section 1: Medical Terminology—Abbreviations

OBJECTIVES: WHAT YOU WILL LEARN

When you have completed this section, you should be able:

- To recognize many abbreviations commonly used in hospitals
- To correctly spell and pronounce various medical terms
- To divide words into their elements
- To define the terms *prefix, suffix,* and *root*
- To distinguish between similar word elements and define them
- To recognize word elements and their meanings (prefixes, roots, and suffixes)
- To define terms and elements relating to anatomy and physiology, diseases and diagnoses, and surgical procedures

KEY IDEAS: ABBREVIATIONS AND THEIR MEANINGS

Abbreviations are the shorthand of the medical and nursing professions. They are clear and efficient tools for the head nurse or team leader to use when writing.

The abbreviations make it easy for the head nurse or team leader to tell you quickly what they want you to do. As a nursing aide, you will use these abbreviations in your daily work. They will help you to understand instructions from your head nurse or team leader.

Abbreviations help you when you are receiving reports on your patients and in keeping your own notes on your daily assignments.

List of Abbreviations Used in Keeping Notes

Abbreviation	Meaning
aa	Of each, equal parts
ABR	Absolute bed rest
ac	Before meals
AD	Admitting diagnosis
A&D	Admission and discharge
ad lib	As desired, if the patient so desires

List of Abbreviations Used in Keeping Notes (cont.)

Abbreviation	Meaning
Adm	Admission
Adm Spec	Admission urine specimen
a.m.	Morning
amb	Ambulation (walking); ambulatory (able to walk)
Amt	Amount
AP	Appendectomy
aqua	Water
bid	Twice a day
BM	Bowel movement
BP	Blood pressure
BR	Bed rest
BRP	Bathroom privileges
°C	Centigrade (celsius)
c̄ or [c	With
Ca	Cancer
Cath	Catheter
CBC	Complete blood count
cc	Cubic centimeter, cubic centimeters
CCU	Cardiac care unit
CO	Carbon monoxide
C/O	Complains of
CO_2	Carbon dioxide
CS	Central supply
CSD	Central service department
CSR	Central supply room
CVA	Cardiovascular accident; cerebrovascular accident (stroke)
dc	Discontinue
Del Rm	Delivery room
Dis	Discharge
DOA	Dead on arrival
Dr	Doctor
DX	Diagnosis
ECG or EKG	Electrocardiogram
ED	Emergency department
EEG	Electroencephalogram
EENT	Eyes, ears, nose, and throat
ER	Emergency room
°F	Fahrenheit
F	Female
FBS	Fasting blood sugar

List of Abbreviations Used in Keeping Notes (cont.)

Abbreviation	Meaning
FF	Forced feeding; forced fluids
ft	Foot, feet
gal	gallon, gallons
GI	Gastrointestinal
gt	One drop
gtt	Two or more drops
GTT	Glucose tolerance test
GU	Genitourinary
Gyn	Gynecology
H_2O	Water
hr	Hour, hours
HS	Bedtime; hour of sleep
ht	Height
hyper	Above (high)
hypo	Below (low)
ICU	Intensive care unit
in.	Inch, inches
I&O	Intake and output
irr	Irregular
Isol	Isolation
IV	Intravenous
L	Liter, liters
Lab	Laboratory
lb	pound, pounds
Liq	Liquid; liquor
LPN	Licensed practical nurse
M	Male
Mat	Maternity
MD	Medical doctor
meas	Measure
mec	Meconium
med	Medicine
min	Minute, minutes
ml	Milliliter, milliliters
noct	At night
NP	Neuropsychiatric; nursing procedure
NPO	Nothing by mouth
Nsy	Nursery
O	By mouth (orally); oxygen
Ob	Obstetrics
Obt	Obtained
OJ	Orange juice

List of Abbreviations Used in Keeping Notes (cont.)

Abbreviation	Meaning
OOB	Out of bed
OPD	Outpatient department
OR	Operating room
Ortho	Orthopedics
OT	Occupational therapy; oral temperature
oz	Ounce, ounces
PAR	Postanesthesia room
pc	After meals
Ped or Peds	Pediatrics
per	By, through
p.m.	Afternoon
PMC	Postmortem care
PN	Pneumonia
po	By mouth
post	After
postop	After surgery
postop spec	Postoperative urine specimen
PP	Postpartum (after delivery)
PPBS	Postprandial blood sugar
pre	Before
prn	Whenever necessary, when required
preop	Before surgery
preop spec	Preoperative urine specimen
prep	Prepare the patient for surgery by shaving the skin
Pt	Patient, pint
PT	Physical therapy
q	Every
qd	Every day
qh	Every hour
q2h	Every 2 hours
q3h	Every 3 hours
q4h	Every 4 hours
QHS	Every night at bedtime
qid	Four times a day
qam	Every morning
qod	Every other day
qs	Quantity sufficient; as much as required
qt	Quart, quarts
r	Rectal temperature
Rm or R	Room
RN	Registered nurse

List of Abbreviations Used in Keeping Notes (cont.)

Abbreviation	Meaning
RR	Recovery room
R_x	Prescription or treatment ordered by a physician
s	Without
SOB	Shortness of breath
sos	Only if necessary; whenever emergency arises
SPD	Special purchasing department
Spec	Specimen
ss	One-half
SSE	Soapsuds enema
stat	At once, immediately
Surg	Surgery
tid	Three times a day
TLC	Tender loving care
TPR	Temperature, pulse, respiration
Ung	Ointment; unguentum
WBC	White blood count
w/c	Wheelchair
WC	Ward clerk
wt	Weight

KEY IDEAS: GUIDE TO PRONUNCIATION

New medical terms in this section are followed by simple guides to their pronunciation. Only long vowels are marked in the pronunciation guides. Pronunciation of other vowel sounds is shown only on words that are very difficult to pronounce correctly. As an exercise, and using the rules given in the figure, pronounce each new word aloud.

Accents. The principal accent is written in capital letters. Example: DOC tor.

Syllables. Division between syllables is indicated by a slash (/). Example: gas/TRI/tis.

Vowels.

Many medical terms are composed of several smaller, simpler words or word elements. This discussion describes and shows how to use three primary word elements that are frequently combined to form medical terms. These three word elements are the prefix, the root, and the suffix.

- The *root* is the body or main part of the word. It denotes the primary meaning of the word as a whole.
- The *prefix* is a word element combined with the root. It changes or adds to meaning of the words. A prefix is always added to the beginning of a root.
- The *suffix* is also a word element used to change or add to the meaning of a root. It is always added to the end of the root.

Symbol	Name	Example
> ā	long a	> āle
> ă	short a	> ădd
> ē	long e	> ēve
> ĕ	short e	> ĕnd
> ī	long i	> īce
> ĭ	short i	> ĭll
> ō	long o	> ōld
> ŏ	short o	> ŏdd
> ū	long u	> c̄ube
> ŭ	short u	> ūp

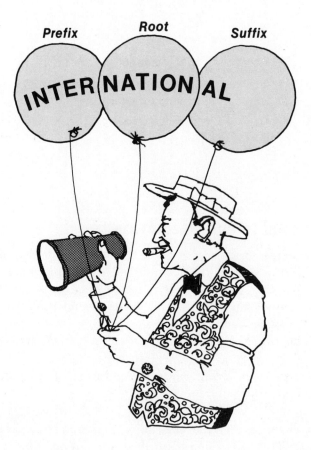

The word elements of medical terms work very much like these examples. The main difference is that most medical word elements are derived from foreign languages, mostly Latin and Greek. So before you will be able to easily recognize the meanings of medical terms, you must learn the English meanings of the word elements in those terms. A list of common word elements in medical terms, with their meanings and guides to pronunciation, is given here. (The many anatomical terms and diseases that are named for their discoverer are not listed here.)

You may encounter a few special problems as you begin your study of medical terminology. First, a word that has been created from several word elements may leave out, change, or add certain letters so that it conforms to rules of spelling and pronunciation.

This chart shows some familiar English words that are composed of common word elements. These should give you an idea of what is meant by the term *word elements*.

Examples of Combining Word Elements

Prefix	Root	Suffix	Word
dis	agree	able	disagreeable
	war	like	warlike
un	pardon	able	unpardonable
inter	nation	al	international
speed (o)	meter		speedometer
	beauty	full	beautiful

Combining Word Elements.   Medical terms (like many English words) do not necessarily contain all three elements. The medical term may be a combination of a prefix and a root.

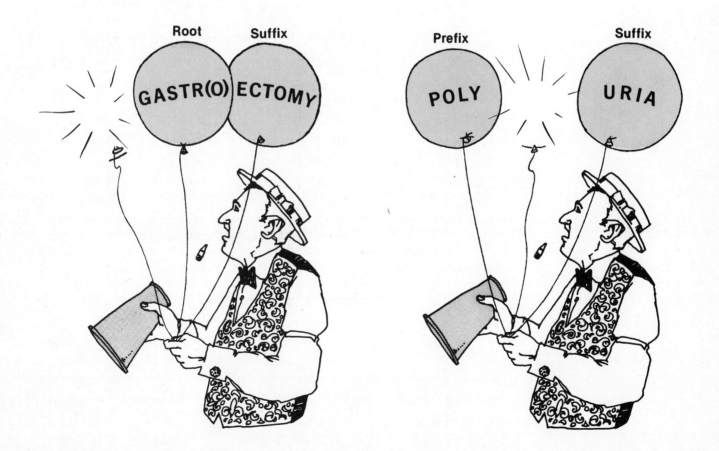

Examples of Prefixes and Roots

Prefix	+	Root	Prefix	Root
ectoderm		EC/to/derm	ecto	derm
retropubic		RE/tro/pu/bic	retro	pubic
endoskeleton		EN/do/skel/e/ton	endo	skeleton
hemiplegic		hem/i/PLE/gic	hemi	plegic
hypertension		hy/per/TEN/sion	hyper	tension

In other medical terms, the root may be combined with only a suffix.

Examples of Roots and Suffixes

Root	+	Suffix	Root	Suffix
colostomy		co/LOS/to/my	col (o)	ostomy
gastrectomy		gas/TREC/to/my	gastr (o)	ectomy
myasthenia		my/as/THE/ni/a	my (o)	asthenia
osteoma		os/te/O/ma	oste (o)	oma

Some medical terms may be formed by using prefixes and suffixes alone.

Examples of Terms Formed by Combining Prefixes and Suffixes

Prefix	+	Suffix	Prefix	Suffix
diarrhea		di/ar/RHE/a	dia	rrhea
endoscopy		en/DOS/co/py	end (o)	oscopy
excise		ex/CISE	ex	cise
epilepsy		EP/i/lep/sy	epi	lepsy
polyuria		pol/y/U/ri/a	poly	uria

Some medical terms are formed by combining two roots. The resulting word describes the disease or treatment more accurately.

Examples of Terms with Two Roots

Root	+	Root	First Root	Second Root
Bronchopneumonia		bron/cho/pneu/MO/ni/a	broncho	pneumo
gastroenteritis		gas/tro/en/ter/I/tis	gastro	enter (o)
osteoarthritis		os/te/o/ar/THRI/tis	osteo	arthr (o)
pyelonephritis		py/e/lo/neph/RI/tis	pyelo	nephr (o)

Examples of Spelling Variations

Prefix	Root	Suffix		Word	
em	pyo	ema	empyema	em/py/E/ma
endo	arterio	itis	endarteritis	end/ar/ter/I/tis
	neuro	ology	neurology	neu/ROL/o/gy
supre	renal		suprarenal	su/pra/RE/nal
	stomato	itis	stomatitis	sto/mat/I/tis

Second, many of the word elements you should be familiar with are similar in spelling but quite different in meaning. Here is a list of word elements that often present difficulties. Examine this list carefully.

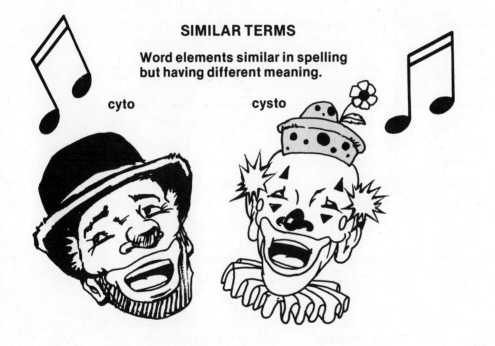

SIMILAR TERMS

Word elements similar in spelling but having different meaning.

cyto   cysto

Examples of Similarity Between Terms

Word Element	Example	Meaning
ante	*ante*febrile	*before* onset of fever
anti	*anti*febrile	used *against* fever
a	*a*dipsia	*absence* of thirst
ad	*ad*renal	*near* the kidney
a, an	*an*uria	*absence* of urine
ano	*ano*rectal	pertaining to *anus* and rectum
ad	*ad*oral	*near* the mouth
adeno	*aden*itis	*gland*ular inflammation

Examples of Similarity Between Terms (cont.)

Word Element	Example	Meaning
cyto	*cyto*genesis	production (origin) of the *cell*
cysto	*cysto*gram	x-ray record of the *bladder*
di	*di*atomic	containing *two* atoms
dia	*dia*gnosis	to know *through* (recognize) a disease
dis	*dis*sect	to cut *apart*
dys	*dys*menorrhea	*difficult* or painful menstruation
en	*en*cephalitis	inflammation *of* the brain
entero	*entero*plasty	operative revision of *intestines*
hema	*hema*ngioma	angioma consisting of *blood* vessels
hemi	*hemi*analgesia	pain relief in *half* of body
hemo	*hemo*toxin	a *blood* cell poison
hyper	*hyper*tension	*high* blood pressure
hypo	*hypo*tension	*low* blood pressure
ileo	*ileo*cecum	section of *small intestine*
ilio	*ilio*sacrum	part of hip *bone*
inter	*inter*stitial	lying *between* spaces
intra	*intra*cranial	*within* the skull
macro	*macro*scopy	seen *large*, as with the naked eye
micro	*micro*scopy	seen *small*, as by microscope
myo	*myo*logy	study of *muscle*
myelo	*myelo*ma	tumor of the *bone marrow*
necro	*necro*sis	state of tissue *death*
nephro	*nephro*sis	condition of the *kidneys*
neuro	*neuro*sis	*nervous* condition
osteo	*osteo*logy	study of *bone*
oto	*oto*logy	study of the *ear*
per	*per*cussion	a striking *through* the body
peri	*peri*cardial	*around* the heart
pre	*pre*clinical	*before* the onset of disease
pyo	*pyo*genic	*pus* producing
pyro	*pyro*genic	*fever* producing

Two groups of suffixes often contain quite similar word elements, each of which has a specific meaning.

-gram	electrocardiogram	*record* of heart action
-graph	electrocardiograph	*machine* that makes record
-graphy	electrocardiography	*process* of making record

Example: Electrocardio*graphy* is performed by a technician who connects parts of the patient's body to an electrocardio*graph*, which produces a record of the patient's heart action called an electrocardio*gram*.

-ectomy	gastrectomy	surgical *removal* of the stomach
-ostomy	gastrostomy	surgical *opening* into the stomach
-ostomy	gastrotomy	surgical *incision* into the stomach

Example: An infant who swallowed a pin requires a gastr*otomy* to remove the pin from his stomach.

A patient unable to take food by mouth has a gastr*ostomy* performed and is fed by tube directly into the stomach.

The doctor performs a gastr*ectomy* on a patient with bleeding ulcers.

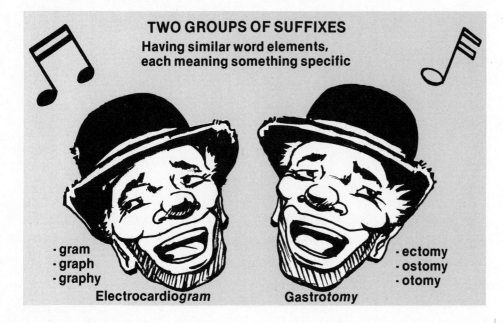

TWO GROUPS OF SUFFIXES
Having similar word elements,
each meaning something specific

· gram
· graph
· graphy
Electrocardio*gram*

· ectomy
· ostomy
· otomy
Gastr*otomy*

Word Elements

The following list of word elements is arranged in alphabetical order. Word elements most often used as prefixes are followed by a hyphen (ambi-). Suffixes are preceded by a hyphen (-algia). Remember that sometimes a term changes its function (a prefix is used as a root, for example) when it is used in a different word.

1.   Say out loud each word element and its meaning.

2.   Pronounce the words given as examples.

3.   Try to figure out the meaning of the sample word from the information given in the list. For example, the third word on the list is *adrenal*. *Ad* means *near* or *toward*. Now look up *renal*. You will find that it means *kidney*. Therefore adrenal means *near the kidney*.

4.   Make flashcards for yourself. Write the new word on little cards with the meaning on the back. Look at the cards as often as you can.

Glossary of Word Elements

Word Element	Refers to or Means	Example	
A-, AN-	without, lack of, absent, deficient	asepsis a/SEP/sis	anorexia an/or/EX/i/a
AB-, ABS-	from, away	abnormal ab/NORM/al	abscess ABS/cess
AD-	near, toward	adrenal	ad/REN/al
ADENO	gland	adenopathy	ad/en/OP/a/thy
AERO	air	anaerobe	an/A/er/obe
ALB	white	albumin	al/BU/min
-ALGIA, -ALGESIA	pain	analgesia	an/al/GE/si/a
AMBI-	both	ambidextrous	am/bi/DEX/trous
ANGIO	vessel (blood or lymph)	angioma	an/gi/O/ma
ANO	anus	anoscope	A/no/scope
ANTE-	before	antenatal	an/te/NAT/al
ANTI-	against	antiseptic	an/ti/SEP/tic
ARTERIO	artery	arteriosclerosis	ar/ter/i/o/scler/O/sis
ARTHRO	joint	arthroplasty	AR/thro/plas/ty
-ASTHENIA	weakness	myasthenia	my/as/THE/ni/a
AUTO-	self	autonomic	au/to/NOM/ic
BI-	two, twice	biweekly	bi/WEEK/ly
BRADY-	slow	bradycardia	brad/y/CAR/di/a
BRONCHO	bronchus	bronchitis	bron/CHI/tis
CARDIO	heart	myocardium	my/o/CAR/di/um
-CELE	tumor, swelling, hernia, sac	enterocele	EN/ter/o/cele
-CENTESIS	puncture	thoracentesis	tho/ra/cen/TE/sis
CEPHALO	head	hydrocephaly	hy/dro/CEPH/a/ly
CHOLE	gall	cholelithiasis	cho/e/lith/I/a/sis
CHOLECYSTO	gallbladder	cholecystectomy	cho/le/cys/TECT/o/my
CHOLEDOCHO	common bile duct	choledochostomy	cho/ed/o/CHOS/to/my
CHONDRO	cartilage	chondroma	cho/DRO/ma
-CIDE	kill	germicide	GERM/i/cide
CIRCUM-	around	circumcision	cir/cum/CI/sion
-CISE	cut	excise	ex/CISE
COLO	colon	colitis	co/LI/tis
COLPO	vagina	colporrhaphy	col/POR/rha/phy
CONTRA-	against	contraception	con/tra/CEP/tion
COSTO	rib	intercostal	in/ter/COS/tal

Glossary of Word Elements (cont.)

Word Element	Refers to or Means		Example
CRANIO	skull	craniotomy	cra/ni/OT/o/my
CYANO	blue	cyanotic	cy/an/OT/ic
CYSTO	urinary bladder	cystogram	CYS/to/gram
CYTO	cell	monocyte	MON/o/cyte
DE-	down, from	decubitus	de/CU/bi/tus
DENTI	tooth	dentistry	DEN/tis/try
DERMO, DERMATO	skin	dermatology	derm/a/TOL/o/gy
DI-	two	diataxia	di/a/TAX/i/a
DIA-	through, between, across, apart	diarrhea	di/ar/RHE/a
DIS-	apart	dissect	dis/SECT
DYS-	painful, difficult, disordered	dysmenorrhea	dys/men/or/RHE/a
ECTO-	outer, on the outside	ectoparasite	ect/o/PAR/a/site
-ECTOMY	surgical removal	prostatectomy	pros/ta/TEC/to/my
-EMESIS	vomiting	hematemesis	hem/at/EM/e/sis
-EMIA	blood	leukemia	leu/KE/mi/a
EN-	in, inside	encapsulated	en/CAP/su/la/ted
ENCEPHALO	brain	encephalitis	en/ceph/a/LI/tis
ENDO-	within, inner, on the inside	endometrium	en/do/ME/tri/um
ENTERO	intestine	enteritis	en/ter/I/tis
EPI-	above, over	epigastric	ep/i/GAS/tric
ERYTHRO	red	erythroblast	e/RYTH/ro/blast
-ESTHESIA	sensation	paresthesia	par/es/THE/si/a
EX-	out	excretion	ex/CRE/tion
FEBR	fever	afebrile	a/FEB/rile
FIBRO	connective tissue	fibroid	FI/broid
GASTRO	stomach	gastrointestinal	gas/tro-in/TEST/in/al
-GENE, -GENIC	production, origin	neurogenic	neu/ro/GEN/ic
GLOSSO	tongue	glossalgia	glos/SAL/gi/a
GLUCO, GLYCO	sugar, sweet	glycogen	GLY/co/gen
-GRAM	record	myelogram	MY/e/lo/gram
-GRAPH	machine	electroencephalograph	e/lec/tro/en/CEPH/al/o/graph
-GRAPHY	practice, process	ventriculography	ven/tri/cu/LOG/ra/phy
GYNE	woman	gynecology	gy/ne/COL/o/gy

Glossary of Word Elements (cont.)

Word Element	Refers to or Means	Example	
HEMA, HER-MATO, HEMO	blood	hematology	hem/at/OL/o/gy
HEMI-	half	hemiplegia	hem/i/PLE/gi/a
HEPA, HEPATO	liver	hepatitis	hep/a/TI/tis
HERNI	rupture	herniation	her/ni/A/tion
HISTO	tissue	histology	his/TOL/o/gy
HYDRO-	water	hydronephrosis	hy/dro/neph/RO/sis
HYPER-	over, above, increased, excessive	hypertension	hy/per/TEN/sion
HYPO-	under, beneath, decreased	hypotension	hy/po/TEN/sion
HYSTER	uterus	hysterectomy	hys/er/ECT/o/my
-IASIS	condition of	psoriasis	psor/I/a/sis
ICTERO	jaudice	iceterus	IC/ter/us
ILEO	ileum (part of small intestine	ileitis	il/e/I/tis
ILIO	ilium (bone)	iliosacrum	il/i/o/SA/crum
INTER-	between	intercellular	inter/CELL/u/lar
INTRA-	within	intramuscular	in/tra/MUS/cu/lar
-ITIS	inflammation of	appendicitis	ap/pen/di/CI/tis
LAPARO	abdomen	laparotomy	la/par/OT/o/my
-LEPSY	seizure, convulse	narcolepsy	NAR/co/lep/sy
LEUKO	white	leukorrhea	leu/kor/RHE/a
LIPO	fat	lipoma	lip/O/ma
LITH	stone, calculus	lithotomy	lith/OT/o/my
-LYSIS	loosen, dissolve	hemolysis	hem/OL/y/sis
MACRO-	large, long	macrocyte	MAC/ro/cyte
MAL-	bad, poor, disordered	maladjusted	mal/ad/JUST/ed
-MANIA	insanity	kleptomania	klep/to/MAN/ia
MAST	breast	mastectomy	mas/TEC/to/my
MEGA-	large	acromegaly	ac/ro/MEG/a/ly
MEN	month	menstruation	men/stru/A/tion
MESO-	middle	mesentery	MES/en/ter/y
-METER	measure	thermometer	ther/MOM/e/ter
METRO	uterus	metrorrhagia	met/ror/RHA/gia
MICRO-	small	microscope	MIC/ro/scope
MONO-	single, one	monocyte	MON/o/cyte

Glossary of Word Elements (cont.)

Word Element	Refers to or Means		Example
MUCO	mucous membrane	mucocutaneous	mu/co/cu/TA/ne/ous
MYELO	spinal cord, bone marrow	myelomeningocele	my/el/o/men/IN/go/cel e
MYO	muscle	myopathy	my/OP/a/thy
NARCO	sleep	narcotic	nar/COT/ic
NASO	nose	nasopharynx	nas/o/PHA/rynx
NECRO	death	necropsy	NEC/rop/sy
NEO-	new	neoplasm	NE/o/plasm
NEPHRO	kidney	nephritis	ne/PHRI/tis
NEURO	nerve	neuralgia	neu/RAL/gi/a
NON-	no, not	nontoxic	non/TOX/ic
OCULO	eye	oculist	O/cu/list
-OLOGY	study of	bacteriology	bac/ter/i/OL/o/gy
-OMA	tumor	carcinoma	car/ci/NO/ma
OOPHOR	ovary	oophorectomy	o/opho/REC/to/my
OPHTHALMO	eye	ophthalmoscope	oph/THAL/mo/scope
-OPIA	vision	diplopia	dip/LO/pi/a
ORCHI	testicle	orchipexy	ORCH/i/pex/y
-ORRHAPHY	to repair a defect	herniorrhaphy	her/ni/OR/raphy/y
ORTHO-	straight	orthopedics	orth/o/PED/ics
-OSCOPY	look into, see	esophagoscopy	e/soph/a/GOS/co/py
OSIS	condition of	neurosis	neu/RO/sis
OSTEO	bone	osteoporosis	os/te/o/por/O/sis
-OSTOMY	surgical opening	colostomy	col/OST/o/my
OTO	ear	otolith	OT/o/lith
-OTOMY	incision, surgical cutting	gastrotomy	gas/TROT/o/my
PARA-	alongside of	paraplegia	par/a/PLE/gi/a
PATH	disease	pathology	pa/THOL/o/gy
PED (Latin)	foot	pedicure	PED/i/cure
PED (Greek)	child	pediatrics	pe/di/AT/rics
-PENIA	too few	leukopenia	leu/ko/PEN/i/a
PERI-	around, covering	pericarditis	pe/ri/car/DI/tis
-PEXY	to sew up in position	nephropexy	NEPH/ro/pex/y
PHARYNGO	throat	pharyngoplasty	pha/RYN/go/plas/ty
PHLEBO	vein	phlebitis	phle/BI/tis
-PHOBIA	fear, dread	photophobia	pho/to/PHO/bi/a
-PLASTY	operative revision	rhinoplasty	RHI/no/plas/ty

Glossary of Word Elements (cont.)

Word Element	Refers to or means	Example	
PLEGIA	paralysis	quadriplegia	qua/dri/PLE/gi/a
-PNEA	breathing	orthopnea	or/thop/NE/a
PNEUMO	air, lungs	pneumonia	pneu/MO/ni/a
POLY-	much, many	polyuria	po/ly/U/ri/a
POST	after	postpartum	post/PAR/tum
PRE-	before	preoperative	pre/OP/er/a/tive
PROCTO	rectum	proctoscopy	proc/TOS/co/py
-PTOSIS	falling	nephroptosis	neph/rop/TO/sis
PYELO	pelvis of kidney	pyelonephritis	py/el/o/neph/RI/tis
PYO	pus	empyema	em/py/E/ma
PYRO	heat, temperature	pyrexia	py/REX/i/a
RENAL	kidney	suprarenal	su/pra/RE/nal
RETRO-	behind, backward	retrosternal	ret/ro/STER/nal
-RHAGE	hemorrhage, flow	hemorrhage	HEM/or/rhage
-RHEA	flow	diarrhea	di/ar/RHE/a
RHINO	nose	rhinopathy	rhi/NOP/a/thy
SALPINGO	oviduct	salpingectomy	sal/pin/GEC/to/my
SEMI-	half	semicircular	sem/i/CIR/cu/lar
SEPTIC	poison, infection	septicemia	sep/ti/CEM/i/a
STOMATO	mouth	stomatitis	sto/ma/TI/tis
SUB-	under	subacute	sub/a/CUTE
SUPER	above	suprapubic	su/pra/PU/bic
-THERAPY	treatment	hydrotherapy	hy/dro/THER/a/py
-THERMY	heat	diathermy	DI/a/therm/y
THORACO	chest	thoractomy	thor/a/COT/o/my
THROMBO	clot	thrombosis	throm/BO/sis
THYRO	thyroid gland	thyroxine	thy/ROX/ine
TRANS-	across	transfusion	trans/FU/sion
-URIA, -URIC	condition of, presence in urine	glycosuria	gly/co/SUR/i/a
URO	urine	uremia	u/RE/mi/a
UNI	one	unicellular	u/ni/CELL/u/lar
VASO	blood vessel	vasoconstriction	vas/o/con/STRIC/tion

KEY IDEAS: FORMULATING MEDICAL TERMS

Many ordinary English terms referring to parts of the body systems and functions are followed by Latin and Greek root elements in parentheses. These roots should not be seen as synonyms for English equivalents. Rather, they should be understood as referring to the English terms coming before them. Careful study will increase your familiarity with Latin and Greek roots and the English words that come from them.

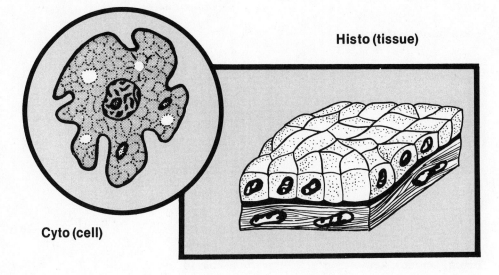

Histo (tissue)

Cyto (cell)

Definitions of Latin and Greek Root Words

Word Element	Refers to
Integumentary system (skin)	
dermo, dermato	skin
muco	mucous membrane
Musculoskeletal system	
myo	muscle
myocardio	heart muscle
myocolpo	vaginal muscle
myometro	uterine muscle
osteo	bone
chondro	cartilage
fibro	connective tissue
arthro	joint
costo	rib

Definitions of Latin and Greek Root Words (cont.)

Word Element	Refers to
cranio	skull
ilio	hipbone, ileum
sacro	tailbone, sacrum
myelo	bone marrow

Respiratory system

aero	air
naso, rhino	nose
pharyngo	throat
tracheo	windpipe
thoraco	chest
broncho	bronchus
pneumo	lung

Circulatory system

cardio	heart
hema, hemato, hemo	blood
vaso	blood vessel
arterio	artery
phlebo	vein
lympho	lymphatic system
angio	blood and lymphatic vessels
erythro	red
leuko	white
cyano	blue

Digestive system

stomato	mouth
denti	teeth
glosso	tongue
pharyngo	pharynx, throat
esophago	esophagus, food pipe
gastro	stomach
entero	small intestine
hepa, hepato	liver
cholecysto	gallbladder
chole	bile, gall
lipo	fat

Definitions of Latin and Greek Root Words (cont.)

Word Element	Refers to
choledocho	common bile duct
ileo	ileum
colo	large intestine
append	appendix
procto	rectum
ano	anus
laparo	abdomen

Nervous system

encephalo	brain
myelo	spinal cord
neuro	nerve
oculo, ophthalmo	eye
oto	ear

Endocrine system

adeno	gland
cephalo	head
thyro	thyroid
glyco, gluco	sugar
prostato	prostate

Urinary system

nephro, renal	kidney
pyelo	kidney pelvis
hydro	water
uro	urine
uretero	ureter
cysto	urinary bladder

Reproductive system

andro	man
gyne	woman
orchi, orchido	testicles
oophor	ovary
hyster, metro	uterus, womb
salpingo	oviduct
colpo	vagina
mast	breasts

KEY IDEAS: DISEASES AND DIAGNOSES

Throughout your hospital work you will run into medical terms that describe and define different diseases. You will be trying to figure out what these terms mean. To do this you will need to know the meanings of the roots

GYNE / *WOMAN*

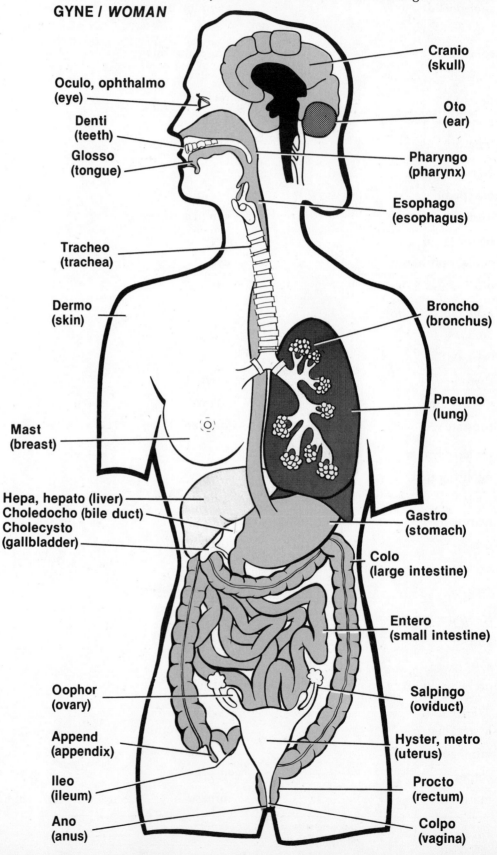

Cranio
(skull)

Oculo, ophthalmo
(eye)

Oto
(ear)

Denti
(teeth)

Glosso
(tongue)

Pharyngo
(pharynx)

Esophago
(esophagus)

Tracheo
(trachea)

Dermo
(skin)

Broncho
(bronchus)

Pneumo
(lung)

Mast
(breast)

Hepa, hepato (liver)
Choledocho (bile duct)
Cholecysto
(gallbladder)

Gastro
(stomach)

Colo
(large intestine)

Entero
(small intestine)

Oophor
(ovary)

Salpingo
(oviduct)

Append
(appendix)

Hyster, metro
(uterus)

Ileo
(ileum)

Procto
(rectum)

Ano
(anus)

Colpo
(vagina)

given in the earlier pages of this section. You will also need to know the suffixes that follow these roots to form words in the medical vocabulary. Understanding prefixes and their meanings will help you to be even better at defining these terms.

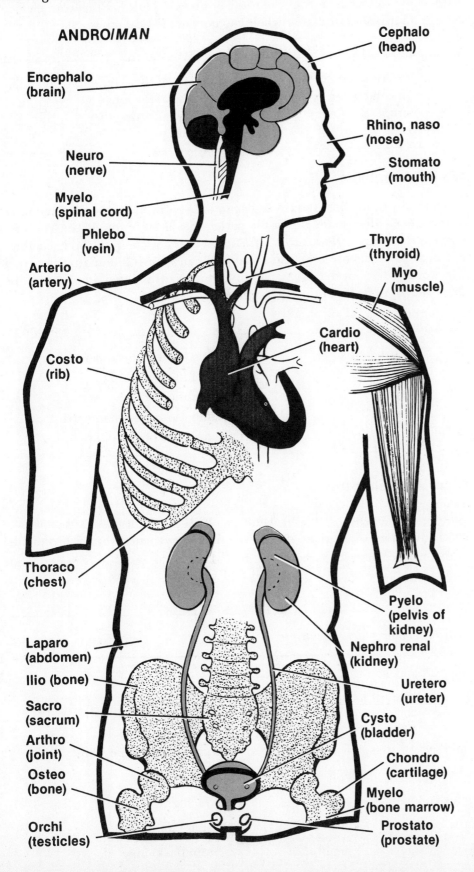

ANDRO/*MAN*

Encephalo
(brain)

Neuro
(nerve)

Myelo
(spinal cord)

Phlebo
(vein)

Arterio
(artery)

Costo
(rib)

Thoraco
(chest)

Laparo
(abdomen)

Ilio (bone)

Sacro
(sacrum)

Arthro
(joint)

Osteo
(bone)

Orchi
(testicles)

Cephalo
(head)

Rhino, naso
(nose)

Stomato
(mouth)

Thyro
(thyroid)

Myo
(muscle)

Cardio
(heart)

Pyelo
(pelvis of
kidney)

Nephro renal
(kidney)

Uretero
(ureter)

Cysto
(bladder)

Chondro
(cartilage)

Myelo
(bone marrow)

Prostato
(prostate)

Word Element: *Path*

When the word element *path* is found in a medical term, it always means *disease*. Examine the word *pathology*. The suffix *ology* means *the study of; pathology*, therefore, means the *study of disease*. Now use the word element *path* as a suffix to formulate a whole category of medical terms.

arterio*pathy*	any disease of the arteries
pneumono*pathy*	any disease of the lungs
uro*pathy*	any disease affecting the urinary tract

Word Element: *Itis*

The study of medical terminology can aid you in understanding the name of the specific disease for which the patient has been hospitalized. The word element *itis* means *inflammation of*. Almost every organ in the body is subject to infection by disease organisms that will cause an inflammatory reaction. The word to describe a diagnosis of this nature is formulated simply by adding the suffix *itis* to word for the body organ so affected.

appendic*itis*	inflammation of the appendix
dermat*itis*	inflammation of the skin
hepat*itis*	inflammation of liver tissue
rhin*itis*	inflammation of nasal mucosa
stomat*itis*	inflammation of the mouth

Other Word Elements

Many terms concerned with a disease, its many symptoms, the tools and procedures used to diagnose it, and the diagnoses themselves are formulated in the manner described above. Study and learn the terms in common usage listed below.

Word Element	*Example*	*Definition*
algia	neur*algia*	*pain* along the nerves
centesis	thora*centesis*	*puncture* of chest wall to remove fluids
emia	ur*emia*	urinary wastes in the *blood*
febr	*afebr*ile	absence of *fever*
genic	pyo*genic*	*producing* pus
iasis	cholelith*iasis*	gallstone *condition*
lith	nephro*lith*	*stone* in the kidney

Word Element	Example	Definition
oma	lip*oma*	fatty *tumor*
oscopy	an*oscopy*	*visualization* of the anus
osis	nephr*osis*	disease *condition* of the kidney
plegia	hemi*plegia*	*paralysis* of one-half of the body
pnea	a*pnea*	absence of *breathing*
pyo	*pyo*derma	skin disease caused by *pus*-forming bacteria
therapy	hydro*therapy*	water used in *treatment* of disease
uria	poly*uria*	excessive *urine* production and urination

KEY IDEAS: SURGICAL PROCEDURES

When you are working on a surgical floor, you will encounter another large group of medical terms. These describe surgical procedures. You will need to have some idea of the type of surgery done on a patient. For this you must learn the word elements used in the names for surgical procedures.

Word Element: *Ectomy*

The suffix *ectomy* means *surgical removal*. When used in combination with any word element denoting an organ or other body part, the term formed means that the organ or body part has been removed.

gastr*ectomy*	surgical removal of the stomach
thyroid*ectomy*	surgical removal of the thyroid gland
col*ectomy*	surgical removal of the large intestine

In many cases, an organ may be removed only partially. To indicate this procedure, other words are used to modify the medical term, for example:

subtotal thyroidectomy   *partial* cystectomy

Other modifying words may precede the medical term. This identifies the surgery performed even more accurately.

left salpingoophor*ectomy*	removal of the left ovary and oviduct
vaginal hyster*ectomy*	removal of uterus through the vagina
transurethral prostat*ectomy*	*removal of the prostate through the urethra*
total abdominal hyster*ectomy*	removal of the entire uterus through abdomen

Other Word Elements

Word Element	Example	Definition
orrhaphy	herni*orrhaphy*	*surgical repair* of a hernia
ostomy	ureter*ostomy*	*formation of an opening* for ureteral drainage
otomy	colp*otomy*	*surgical incision* into the vagina
pexy	cysto*pexy*	*fixation of bladder* to the abdominal wall
plasty	rhino*plasty*	*plastic surgery* of the nose

KEY IDEAS: MEDICAL SPECIALTIES

Name	Physician's Title	Description
Allergy	Allergist	A subspecialty of internal medicine dealing with diagnosis and treatment of body reactions resulting from unusual sensitivity to foods, pollens, dust, medicines, or other substances
Anesthesiology	Anesthesiologist	Administration of various forms of anesthesia in operations or diagnosis to cause loss of feeling or sensation
Cardiovascular diseases; Cardiology	Cardiologist	A subspecialty of internal medicine involving the diagnosis and treatment of disease of the heart and blood vessels
Dermatology	Dermatologist	Diagnosis and treatment of diseases of the skin
Gastroenterology	Gastroenterologist	A subspecialty of internal medicine concerned with diagnosis and treatment of disorders of the digestive tract
General practice	General practitioner	The diagnosis and treatment of disease by medical and surgical methods, without limitation to organ systems or body regions, and without restriction as to age of patients

Medical Specialties (Cont.)

Name	Physician's Title	Description
General surgery	Surgeon	The diagnosis and treatment of disease by surgical means, without limitation to special organ systems or body regions
Gynecology	Gynecologist	Diagnosis and treatment of diseases of the female reproductive organs
Internal medicine	Internist	The diagnosis and nonsurgical treatment of illnesses of adults
Neurological surgery	Neurosurgeon	Diagnosis and surgical treatment of brain, spinal cord, and nerve disorders
Neurology	Neurologist	Diagnosis and treatment of diseases of the brain, spinal cord, and nerves
Obstetrics	Obstetrician	The care of women during pregnancy, childbirth, and the interval immediately following
Ophthalmology	Ophthalmologist	Diagnosis and treatment of diseases of the eye, including prescribing glasses
Orthopedics	Orthopedist	Diagnosis and treatment of disorders and diseases of the muscular and skeletal systems
Otolaryngology	Otolaryngologist	Diagnosis and treatment of diseases of the ear, nose, and throat
Pathology	Pathologist	Study and interpretation of changes in organs, tissues, cells, and alterations in body chemistry to aid in diagnosing disease and determining treatment
Pediatrics	Pediatrician	Prevention, diagnosis, and treatment of children's diseases
Physical medicine and rehabilitation	Physiatrist	Diagnosis of disease or injury in the various systems and areas of the body and treatment by means of physi-

Medical Specialties (Cont.)

Name	Physician Title	Description
		cal procedures as well as treatment and restoration of the convalescent and physically handicapped patient
Plastic surgery	Plastic surgeon	Corrective or reparative surgery to restore deformed or mutilated parts of the body
Psychiatry	Psychiatrist	Diagnosis and treatment of mental disorders
Radiology	Radiologist	Use of radiant energy including x rays, radium, cobalt 60, etc., in the diagnosis of disease
Therapeutic radiology	Radiologist	The use of radiant energy, including x rays, radium, and other radioactive substances in the treatment of diseases
Thoracic surgery	Thoracic surgeon	Operative treatment of the lungs, heart, or the large blood vessels within the chest cavity
Urology	Urologist	Diagnosis and treatment of diseases or disorders of the kidneys, bladder, ureters, and urethra and of the male reproductive organs

Section 2: Continuing to Learn

OBJECTIVES: WHAT YOU WILL LEARN

When you have completed this section you should be able:

- To explain the function of the inservice education department or staff development department in your hospital
- To plan your career by using the career ladder

KEY IDEAS

Continue your education! To keep up with new developments in the medical field, all health care workers are expected to take refresher courses and study new medical developments that affect their employment all their working lives. As you continue to learn, your job will become more rewarding personally bend professionally. You and your employer, the health care institution, will be happy and grateful that you decided to be a nursing aide.

You can continue to learn while you are on the job. You can expand your knowledge of nursing care procedures. You can find better ways to do your work. You can learn more about other aspects of health care. All this can make you a more effective nursing aide. This means you will become more secure in your job.

Nursing inservice education departments, sometimes called staff development departments, in the hospital are designed mainly for continuing the educational process for all employees in the nursing department. These departments also orient new employees. They have classes and demonstrations of new equipment and techniques. There are refresher programs on procedures not often used. Staff development personnel constantly seek new methods for improving health care delivery for patients.

If you enjoy your work as a nursing aide, you may be interested in advancement where you are employed. Maybe you'd like to be a registered nurse or a licensed practical nurse. The *career ladder* shown here can give you a pattern to guide you in planning your advancement. The pattern can be changed to meet your own needs and goals. Skills, time, hard work, and careful planning are needed to climb to the top of the ladder.

Career Ladder

Attend graduate school for a master of science (MS) in nursing

↑

Work for one year as a registered professional nurse

↑

Attend a university to get a bachelor of science (BS) in nursing

↑

Work for one year as a registered nurse

↑

Become a registered nurse (RN) in an associate degree program

↑

Work for one year as a licensed practical nurse

↑

Become a licensed practical nurse (LPN)

↑

Work for one year as a nursing aide

↑

Become a nursing aide

If you don't have a high school diploma, that should be your first goal. Adult education programs given in the evening at local high schools offer basic education programs that lead to a high school equivalency diploma. Community colleges offer the prerequisite courses necessary to move up to a program for the licensed practical nurse or registered nurse level. They have counselors to advise you along the way. The director of nursing education in your hospital is the person to ask about planning your career ladder.

WHAT YOU HAVE LEARNED

You must have a good working knowledge of medical terminology and abbreviations. This includes the ability to spell, define, and pronounce these terms accurately. Then you can communicate effectively with the other members of your health care team. Remember: Learning medical terminology is similar to learning another language.

This chapter tells you how medical terminology is related to body parts and functions. This includes anatomy, the various body systems, diseases and diagnoses, and surgical procedures.

When you begin the study of medical terminology, you should understand that medical terms are combinations of words or word roots. The information in this chapter should help you to recognize word elements and their meanings. Time, thought, and practice are needed before you can become really expert in the language of medicine. When you have mastered the meanings of the prefixes, roots, and suffixes given in this chapter, you will be able to apply what you have learned to the medical terms you see and hear on the job. Your efforts will help you reach the goal of all health care workers—the delivery of better patient care.

If you find your work as a nursing aide enjoyable and rewarding, the career ladder can show you how to build a plan for advancement and further education.

You have started to climb the career ladder. You have taken the first step. You have succeeded in finishing this manual. Now you can be a success on the job. You are ready to be a truly productive and effective nursing aide.

Words To Remember

A

abdomen — the region of the body between the chest and the pelvis.

abdominal prep—the procedures for making the patient's abdomen ready for surgery. The preparation includes thorough cleansing of the skin and careful shaving of the body hair in the abdominal area.

ADL — an abbreviation for the activities of daily living.

admission — the administrative procedures followed when a person enters the hospital and becomes an inpatient. Admission covers the period from the time the patient enters the door of the hospital until he is settled in his room.

adrenal glands — two glands in the upper posterior part of the abdomen, near the kidneys.

afterpains — contractions of the uterus following childbirth.

alveoli — a microscopic sac made up of a single layer of squamous epithelial cells, which has a high content of oxygen that moves into the blood in the lung.

ambulatory — able to walk around.

amputation — the cutting off of a body part though accident or by surgery.

anal — pertaining to the anus.

anatomical position — a person standing facing you, feet together, palms forward, head up.

anatomy — the study of the structure of an organism— such as a plant, an animal, or a human being—and any of its parts.

anesthesia — loss of feeling or sensation in a part or all of the body. Local anesthesia is the loss of sensation in a part of the body. General anesthesia is complete loss of sensation in the entire body.

anesthetic — a drug used to produce loss of feeling in a person. An anesthetic can be given orally, rectally, by injection, or by inhalation. A person who has been given an anesthetic is anesthetized.

antagonistic action — action that happens when two sets of structures are doing exactly the opposite thing. An example is antagonistic action of the biceps and triceps. One relaxes while the other contracts.

anterior — located in the front. The opposite of posterior.

antibiotic — a drug used in medical treatment that prevents disease-causing microorganisms from multiplying.

anus — the posterior opening in the body through which feces is excreted.

aorta — the name for the major artery that carries blood away from the heart.

artery — a blood vessel that carries blood away from the heart.

asepsis — the condition of being free of disease-causing organisms.

aspirate — to remove material from a body cavity by using a tube. Aspirate also means to draw material such as saliva, mucus, or food particles into the lungs from the mouth.

atrium — one of the two smaller chambers of the heart. These chambers contract and push blood through the lungs where it picks up oxygen and returns to the ventricles.

auricles — the two upper chambers of the heart. They are side by side. Each is also known as an atrium (plural = atria).

autoclave — equipment used to sterilize instruments and other articles in the health care institution.

autonomic nervous system — the part of the nervous system that is made up of neurons that carry messages to and from the viscera, without our thinking about it.

axillary — the area under the arms; the armpits.

B

bacteria — sometimes called germs. A kind of microorganism. Many bacteria cause disease.

bassinet — a small crib made especially for newborn babies.

bed cradle — when in place over a body area such as a foot or arm, this equipment holds the bedclothes—sheets and blankets—away from the patient so that they do not touch that body part.

bedpan — a pan used by patients who are in bed so they can defecate or urinate.

bladder — a membranous sac that serves as the body's container for urine.

blood — the fluid that circulates through the heart, arteries, veins, and capillaries. It carries nourishment and oxygen to the tissues and takes away waste matter and carbon dioxide.

blood pressure — the force of the blood on the inner walls of the blood vessels as it flows through them.

body alignment — refers to the patient's position in bed.

body mechanics — special ways of standing and moving one's body to make the best use of strength and avoid fatigue.

brain — the main part of the central nervous system. It is the center of thought and controls coordination of the nerves and responses from the sense organs.

bronchial tubes — branches of the trachea that lead into the lungs.

bursa — a sac found within a joint capsule. It is filled with synovial fluid, which helps to buffer the movement of the bones against one another.

C

calories — units for measuring the energy produced when food is oxidized in the body.

cannula — a word used to mean any of the kinds of tubes that can be inserted into one of the body cavities. A cannula may be used to draw fluids out or to give oxygen.

capillaries — the very small blood vessels that carry blood to all parts of the body and the skin. Capillaries are a link between the ends of the arteries and the beginning of the veins.

carbohydrate — one of the basic kinds of food elements used by the body.

cardiac — pertaining to the heart.

cartilage — a tough connective tissue that holds bones together.

catheter — a tube inserted in a body cavity, usually used to withdraw fluid.

catheterization — inserting a catheter into any of the body's openings or cavities.

cell — the basic unit of living matter.

centigrade — a measurement of temperature using a scale divided into 100 units or degrees. In this system, the freezing temperature of water is 0° centigrade, written 0°C. Water boils at 100°C.

central nervous system — the part of the nervous system made up of the brain and the spinal cord.

cerebral — pertaining to the cerebrum, a part of the brain.

cerebrospinal fluid — fluid secreted by cells in cavities within the cerebrum. It circulates through the membranes that cover and protect the brain and spinal cord.

cervix — the narrow outer end of the uterus.

channel — path.

check and balance — a safeguard for health in which the systems of the body have built-in mechanisms that keep their activity in a state of balance.

circulation — the continous movement of blood through the heart and blood vessels to all parts of the body.

circulatory system — the heart, blood vessels, blood, and all the organs that pump and carry blood and other fluids throughout the body.

clean — a term used in health care institutions to refer to an object or area that is uncontaminated by harmful microorganisms.

clitoris — part of the external female genitals. It is located above the opening that leads from the bladder.

colon — the large bowel. It extends from the large intestine to the anus.

colostomy — a surgical procedure that provides the patient with an artificial opening, either temporary or permanent. The person's feces then can leave the body through this opening rather than through the rectum. The opening is usually made through the abdominal wall into a part of the large intestine.

coma — a state of deep unconsciousness often caused by disease, injury, or drugs.

communicable disease — a disease that is easily spread from one person to another.

complication — an unexpected condition, such as the development of another illness in a patient who is already sick.

compress — folded pieces of cloth or gauze used to apply pressure to part of the patient's body. The compress may also be used to supply moisture, heat, cold, or medications to a specific part of the body.

congenital — the term means born with, or from birth. It refers to a physical or mental characteristic present in a baby at birth.

congestion — unusually large amounts of blood or fluid in a body part. It means an abnormal condition exists.

connective tissue — tissue that connects and holds together cells of an organ. Also tissues between body structures, such as muscles and blood vessels.

continuous — uninterrupted, without a stop.

contract — get smaller.

contracture — when muscle tissue becomes drawn together, bunched up, or shortened because of spasm or paralysis, either permanently or temporarily.

convalescent — getting well or recovering after an illness or surgery.

coronary care unit — a special patient care unit where persons who have cardiac conditions receive intensive care; abbreviated CCU.

CSR — abbreviation for central supply room. This area may also be referred to as SPD (special purchasing department) or CSD (central supply department). This is a centralized area or place within the hospital used for storing supplies and equipment.

cyanosis — when the skin looks blue or has a gray color because there is not enough oxygen in the blood; often seen in the person's lips and nailbeds, and in the skin under the fingernails.

D

death rattle — a sound often made by a dying patient. It is caused by air passing through the mucus collected in his throat and bronchial tubes.

deceased — another word for dead.

decubitus ulcers — also called bed sores. These are areas of the skin that become broken and painful. They are caused by continuing pressure on the body part, and usually occur when a patient is kept in bed for a long time.

defecate — to have a bowel movement; to excrete waste matter from the bowels.

dehydration — a condition in which the body has less than the normal amount of fluid.

dentures — artificial teeth. Dentures may replace some or all of a person's teeth, and are described as being partial or complete, and upper or lower.

diabetes — a condition that develops when the body cannot change its sugar into energy. When this sugar collects in the blood, the patient needs a special diet and may have to be given insulin.

diagnosis — finding out what kind of disease or medical condition a patient has. A medical diagnosis is always made by a physician.

diagnostic examination — an examination that helps the physician make a diagnosis. The physician talks to the patient, examines him, and may order tests and x rays taken.

diagnostic testing — tests done to help the doctor in the diagnosis of a patient.

diaphragm — the muscular partition between the chest cavity and the abdominal cavity.

diarrhea — an abnormally frequent discharge of fluid fecal material from the bowel.

diastolic blood pressure — in taking a patient's blood pressure, one records the bottom number as the reading for the diastolic pressure.

digestive system — the group of body organs that carries out digestion. Digestion is the process in the body in which food is broken down mechanically and chemically, and is changed into forms that can enter the bloodstream and be used by the body.

dilates — gets bigger, expands.

dirty — a term used in the hospital to refer to an object or area as being contaminated by harmful microorganisms.

disability — loss of the ability to use a part or parts of the body in a normal way.

discharge — this word has two special meanings.
1. When a patient is ready to leave the hospital, the hospital's business office helps him with his arrangements and with the checking out procedure. This process is called discharge.
2. The term used for unusual material coming out from some part of the body. For example, after a patient has had surgery, there may be a discharge of some kind.

discoloration — change in color.

disinfection — the process of destroying most disease-causing organisms.

disposable equipment — equipment that is used one time only or for one patient only and then thrown away.

disposables — hospital supply and equipment items used once and then thrown away. There are many kinds; they range from tissues and napkins to syringes and surgeon's gloves.

DOA — abbreviation for dead on arrival.

doctor — *see* physician.

dorsal — refers to the back or to the back part of an organ; the posterior part.

drape — a covering used during an examination or an operation to cover the patient's body.

draping — covering a patient or parts of the patient's body with a sheet, blanket, bath blanket, or other material. Draping is usually done during physical examination of the patient, and during operations.

draw sheet — a small sheet made of plastic, rubber, or cotton. It is placed crosswise on the middle of the bed over the bottom sheet to help protect the bedding from a patient's discharges.

dry application — an application of warmth or cold in which no water touches the skin.

duodenum — the first part of the small intestine. Most digestion and most absorption of the end products of digestion occur in the duodenum.

E

edema — abnormal swelling of a part of the body caused by fluid collecting in that area. Usually the swelling is in the ankles, legs, hands, or abdomen.

ejaculate — also called semen. It is the fluid that carries the male sperm. It is ejaculated (expelled) when orgasm is reached.

emaciation — a wasting away of the flesh, caused by disease and sometimes by lack of food. An emaciated person is very thin.

embryo — the name for a new living human being during the first 8 weeks of its development in the uterus.

emergency department — an area in the hospital where patients are brought because they have suddenly become ill or have had an accident.

emesis basin — a pan used for catching material that a patient spits out or vomits.

endocrine gland — a ductless gland in the body which secretes hormones, a substance that affects the way some body systems do their work.

enema — a liquid injected into the rectum to wash out the contents of the rectum.

enzyme — a substance manufactured by living tissue that stimulates certain chemical changes in the body. For example, pancreatic enzymes cause complex food proteins to break down into simpler structures that can be absorbed by the intestines.

epithelium — the tissue cells composing the skin. Also the cells lining the passages of the hollow organs of the respiratory, digestive, and urinary systems.

esophagus — a muscular tube for the passage of food, which extends from the back of the throat (pharynx), down through the chest and diaphragm into the stomach.

evaporate — to pass off as vapor, as water evaporating into the air.

excreta — urine and feces; waste matter from the body.

excrete — to eliminate or expel waste matter from the body.

exhalation — the process of breathing out air in respiration.

expectoration — coughing up matter from the lungs, trachea, or bronchial tubes, and spitting it out.

extremities — the arms, legs, hands, and feet.

F

Fahrenheit — the name of a system for measuring temperature. In the Fahrenheit system the temperature of water at boiling is 212°. At freezing, it is 32°. These temperatures are usually written 212°F and 32°F.

fallopian tubes — the uterine tubes, one on either side of the uterus. These tubes are the passageways, also called the oviducts, through which the egg travels from the ovary to the uterus.

fanfold — a method of arranging bed linens so that the covers and spread are folded back out of the way, but still are on the bed and within easy reach.

feces — solid waste material discharged from the body through the rectum and anus. Other names for feces are stool, excreta, excrement, BM, bowel movement, and fecal matter.

fertile period — a period of 4 to 6 days at the time of ovulation when sperm may cause conception because a mature ovum is in the oviduct. This period varies in each woman at some time in her life.

fertilization — when a sperm cell and an egg cell meet, the two cells join, and the sperm cell is absorbed into the egg cell. This is also called "conception."

fetus — the name for the infant developing in the mother's body after the first 2 months.

fever — the term for a person's condition when his body temperature is above normal.

flatus — intestinal gas.

flex — to bend, as one's elbow.

➤ **fluid balance** — the same amount of fluid that is taken in by the body is given out by the body.

fluid intake — the fluid taken into the body, from whatever source.

fluid output — the fluid given out of the body, no matter how.

force fluids — extra fluids to be taken in by a patient according to his doctor's orders.

Fowler's position — the patient's position when the head of his bed is at a 45° angle.

fracture — a break in a bone.

friction — the rubbing of one surface against another. Friction between the patient's body and his bedclothes often produces bedsores.

G

gastrointestinal — the digestive system. Sometimes called "GI system," an abbreviation for gastro (stomach) and intestinal.

gatch handle — a handle used on manually operated hospital beds to raise or lower the backrest and kneerest.

gavage — feeding a patient by putting a tube into his stomach. Nasogastric gavage is putting the tube through the patient's nostril and then through the esophagus into his stomach.

generalized application — one in which warmth or coldness is applied to the entire body.

genital — refers to the external reproductive organs.

germicide — a chemical compound used to destroy bacteria.

gestation — the time from conception until the birth of a baby. The gestation period for a human baby is about 280 days. Another word for gestation is pregnancy.

GI — abbreviation for gastrointestinal.

gland — an organ that manufactures a chemical that will be used elsewhere in the body.

glans — the head of the penis.

graduate — a measuring cup marked along its side to show various amounts so the material placed in the cup can be measured accurately. The marks are called calibrations.

H

heart — a four-chambered, hollow, muscular organ that lies in the chest cavity, pointing slightly to the left. It is the pump that circulates the blood through the lungs and into all parts of the body.

hemorrhage — excessive bleeding.

hereditary — characteristics passed down from parent to child. An example is the color of your eyes. Some diseases apparently are hereditary. An example is diabetes.

homeostasis — stability of all body functions at normal levels.

hormone — a protein substance secreted by an endocrine gland directly into the blood.

hospital — a building where sick and injured people are given medical treatment and other kinds of care. A hospital is one kind of health care institution.

hypothalamus — a tiny structure at the base of the brain that has a lot of influence over all body activities, especially the activity of the pituitary gland.

I

incontinence — the inability to control one's bowels or bladder. An incontinent person can't stop himself from urinating or defecating.

incubator — a special crib used in the care of premature babies.

infection — a condition in body tissue in which germs or pathogens have multiplied and destroyed many cells.

inflammation — a reaction of the tissues to disease or injury. There is usually pain, heat, redness, and swelling of the body part.

inhalation — the process of breathing in air in respiration.

insensible fluid loss — fluid that is lost from the body without being noticed, such as in perspiration or air breathed out.

insulin — a hormone produced naturally in the body by the pancreas. Insulin helps the body change sugar into energy. Insulin can be produced artificially for use in the treatment of diabetes.

intensive care unit — an area in the health care institution for patients who need more intensive nursing care than ordinary patients.

intermittent — alternating; stopping and beginning again.

intracellular fluid — fluid within the cell.

intravenous — refers to the injection of fluids into a vein. Foods in liquid form and medications can be put into the patient's body in this way.

intravenous pole — also called IV pole or IV standard. A tall pole on rollers or casters used to hold the containers or tubes needed, for example, during a blood transfusion.

isolation gown — a special gown worn over a uniform when in the room of a patient with a communicable disease. The gown helps protect the uniform from being contaminated by harmful bacteria.

isolation procedures — special procedures used in caring for patients with communicable diseases to prevent the disease from spreading to other persons.

IV — abbreviation for intravenous, intravenous pole.

J

joint — a part of the body where two bones come together.

K

kidney — the organ lying in the upper posterior portion of the abdomen. It removes waste products and water from the bloodstream and excretes them as urine.

knee-chest position — a bent posture with the knees and chest touching the examining table. This position is sometimes used for examining the rectum. It is also used for women who have recently given birth, to get the uterus to fall forward into its normal position.

L

labia — lips of the vagina.

lactation — the body process of producing milk to feed a newborn baby.

lithotomy position — the patient lies on her back with her legs spread apart and her knees bent. This position is used for performing a pelvic (vaginal) examination.

liver — the body's largest gland, located in the abdominal cavity. The liver has many functions in the chemistry and metabolism of the body and is essential to life.

localized application — one in which warmth or coldness is applied to a specific area or small part of the body.

lubricant — a substance such as petroleum jelly, glycerine, or cold cream that is to make a surface smooth or moist.

lungs — the primary organs of breathing.

M

medical asepsis — special practices and procedures for cleanliness to decrease the chances for disease-causing bacteria to live and spread.

membrane — a thin layer of tissue. An example is the mucous membrane, as in the lining of the nose and throat.

meninges — the three membranes that protect the brain and spinal cord.

meniscus — a disc of cartilage found between two bones at a joint that acts to reduce wear and tear on the ends of the bones. The menisci found in the complicated knee joint are an example.

menstruation — the regular, usually monthly, bleeding from the uterus that occurs when a female of childbearing age is not pregnant.

metabolism — the total of all the physical and chemical changes that take place in living organisms and cells.

metric system — a system of measurement based on the decimal system. Units are 10s, 100s, 1000s, and so forth.

microorganism — a living thing so small it cannot be seen with the naked eye, but only through a microscope.

mitered corner — a special way to fold the bedding at the corners when making a hospital bed. The mitered corner keeps the bedding neat and stretched tightly so that wrinkles are avoided.

modified — changed.

moist application — an application of warmth or cold in which water touches the skin.

mucus — a sticky substance secreted by mucous membranes, mainly in the lungs, nose, and parts of the rectal and genital areas.

muscle — tissue composed of fibers with the ability to elongate and shorten, causing bones and joints to move. Voluntary muscles are in body parts such as the neck, arms, fingers, and legs. Involuntary muscles are in organs such as the heart and intestines.

muscle fiber — a cell in muscle tissue that may be smooth, striated, or indistinctly striated.

muscular system — the group of body organs that make it possible for the body and its parts to move.

N

nephron — the functional unit of the kidney that filters out those substances the body does not need, reabsorbing those it does need, and secreting those products that are harmful to the body. The result of this process is urine.

nerve impulse — a regular wave of negative electrical impulses that transmit information along the neuron from one part of the body to another.

nerves — bundles of neurons held together with connective tissue. They go to all parts of the body from the central nervous system, that is, from the brain and spinal cord.

nervous system — the group of body organs that control and regulate the activities of the body and the functioning of the other body systems.

neuron — a nerve, including the cell and the long fiber coming from the cell.

newborn — a baby in the first month of life.

nourishment — the process of taking food into the body to maintain life.

NPO — abbreviation for a Latin term, *nil per os*, which means nothing by mouth. A sign reading NPO is usually put at the head or foot of the patient's bed if he is not permitted to eat or drink anything by mouth.

nurse — a person educated and trained to care for sick people and to help physicians and surgeons. Nurses are licensed as registered nurses (RNs) and licensed practical nurses (LPNs).

nursing aide — a person who helps give nursing care to patients. Nursing aides usually work in hospitals or other health care institutions.

nutrients — food substances.

nutrition — the process by which the body takes in and uses food.

O

obese — very fat.

objective reporting — reporting exactly what you observe.

objective symptoms — symptoms that can be observed and reported exactly as they are seen.

omit — leave out.

ophthalmoscope — an instrument the doctor uses to look inside a patient's eye.

OR — abbreviation for operating room.

oral — anything to do with the mouth. Examples are eating and speaking.

oral hygiene — cleanliness of the mouth.

organ — a part of the body made of several types of tissue grouped together to perform a certain function. Examples are the heart, stomach, and lungs.

organism — a living thing.

orthopedics — the medical specialty that covers the treatment of broken bones, deformities, or diseases that attack the bones, joints, and muscles.

otoscope — an instrument the doctor uses to look at the inside of a patient's ear.

ovary — one of a pair of organs in the female that produce mature eggs (ova) as well as producing the primary sex hormones of the female, estrogen and progesterone.

ovulation — the period of time in which the ovum is pushed out from the surface of the ovary and usually picked up by the oviduct. This usually occurs 14 days before the onset of the next menstrual period.

ovum — the egg in the female. After fertilization, it develops into a new member of the same species.

oxidation — in the human body, this happens when food is combined with oxygen to create energy.

oxygen — a colorless, odorless gas making up about one-fifth of the volume of the air. It is essential for human life. Abbreviated as O_2.

oxygen tent — equipment used in the health care institution to provide large amounts of extra oxygen for a patient.

P

pancreas — a large gland, 6 to 8 inches long, that secretes enzymes into the intestines for digestion of foods. It also manufactures insulin, which is secreted into the bloodstream.

paralysis — loss of the ability to move a part or all of the body.

paraplegia — paralysis of the legs and lower part of the body.

parenteral — refers to a method of bringing substances into the body by some way other than the mouth and intestines. An example is intravenous feeding.

pathogens — disease-causing microorganisms.

patient care unit — an area of the hospital set aside for patients who have similar conditions or illnesses. For example, "3 West" might be the area where surgical patients are cared for.

patient lift — a mechanical device like a swinging seat used for lifting a patient into and out of such equipment as the hospital bed, bathtub, or wheelchair.

patient unit — the space for one patient including the hospital bed, bedside table, chair, and other equipment.

pediatrics — the medical specialty that has to do with the development and care of infants and children and with the treatment of their diseases.

percussion hammer — an instrument used by the doctor to test a patient's reflexes by tapping the body at certain places.

perineum — the body area between the thighs. It includes the area of the anus and the external genital organs.

peristalsis — movement of the intestines that pushes the food along to the next part of the digestive system.

phagocytosis — a process in which a cell engulfs and destroys a foreign protein, such as a germ.

physician — a doctor. A person who is licensed to practice medicine.

physiology — the study of the functions of body tissues and organs.

pituitary gland — sometimes called the master gland. It is attached to the base of the brain and directs the flow of all hormones in the body.

placenta — the oval, spongy structure in the uterus through which the unborn baby receives its nourishment. Sometimes called afterbirth. The umbilical cord is attached to the placenta. The placenta is discharged from the mother's body soon after childbirth.

plasma — the liquid portion of blood, or blood from which the red and white cells and platelets have been removed.

pleural cavity — the chest cavity containing the lungs. The *pleura* is the membrane lining the chest cavity and covering the lungs.

posterior — located in the back or toward the rear.

postmortem — after death.

postoperative — after surgery.

postoperative bed — a standard hospital bed made up in a special way for a patient who is coming back to his unit after an operation. Sometimes called recovery bed, stretcher bed, or operating room bed.

postpartum — following childbirth.

premature birth — birth of a baby before the normal period of gestation (pregnancy) is over.

preoperative — before surgery.

prepuce — the foreskin of the penis. The foreskin is often removed in an operation called a circumcision.

prone — lying on one's stomach.

prostate — a male gland behind the outlet of the urinary bladder.

prosthesis — an artificial body part. There are prostheses (plural) for legs, arms, hands, feet, breasts, eyes, and teeth.

psychiatric patient — a patient who is being treated for a mental illness.

pulmonary — refers to the lungs.

pulse — the rhythmic expansion and contraction of the arteries caused by the beating of the heart. The expansion and contraction show how fast, how regular, and with what force the heart is beating.

Q

quadriplegia — paralysis of both the upper and lower parts of the body.

R

radial pulse — this is the pulse felt at a person's wrist at the radial artery.

rectal irrigation — washing out the rectum by injecting a stream of water; giving an enema.

rectum — the lower 8 to 10 inches of the colon. The anus is the body opening from the rectum.

recumbent position — lying down or reclining.

rehabilitation — the processes by which people who have been disabled by injury or sickness are helped to recover as much as possible of their original abilities for the activities of daily living.

reproductive system — the group of body organs that makes possible the creation of new human life.

respiration — the body process of breathing; inhaling and exhaling air.

respiratory system — the group of body organs that carry on the body function of respiration. The system brings oxygen into the body and eliminates carbon dioxide.

restrict fluids — fluids that are limited to certain amounts.

reticuloendothelial system — the body system primarily responsible for our resistance to disease. The tissue is made up of cells from various systems, all of which are capable of either producing antibodies or the process of phagocytosis.

reverse isolation — procedures used to prevent harmful organisms from coming into contact with the patient. *See* isolation procedure.

rigor mortis — stiffening of a person's body and limbs shortly after death.

S

saliva — the secretion of the salivary glands into the mouth. Saliva moistens food and helps in swallowing. It also contains an enzyme (chemical) that helps digest starches.

scrotal prep — the procedures for making the genital area of a male patient ready for surgery. The preparation includes thoroughly cleansing the skin and carefully shaving hair in the area.

scrotum — a pouch below the penis that contains the testicles.

secrete — to produce a special substance and expel it. The salivary glands secrete saliva. The pancreas secretes insulin.

self-demand feeding — a schedule for feeding a baby when he cries or makes signs that he is hungry. It is not a strict, regular schedule. Also called self-regulatory feeding.

seminal vesicles — small glands in the male near the prostate and urethra where semen is stored before it is discharged.

sense organs — these organs make it possible for us to be aware of the outside world and ourselves through the senses of sight, hearing, smell, taste, and touch.

septicemia — a severe infection in the blood. Usually called blood poisoning.

shock — a state of collapse resulting from reduced blood volume and blood pressure, usually caused by severe injuries such as hemorrhage or burns on many parts of the body. Shock may also result from an emotional blow.

side lying — lying on one's side.

signs — objective evidence of disease. Signs can be observed by a trained person such as a doctor or nurse. Vital signs are special signals that doctors and nurses always look for. These are the patient's temperature, pulse, respiration, and blood pressure.

Sims' position — the patient lies on the left side with the right knee and thigh drawn up. This position permits a satisfactory rectal examination.

sitz bath — a bath in which the patient sits in a specially designed chair-tub or a regular bathtub with his hips and buttocks in water.

skeletal system — the bones and connections between them that provide the framework for the body.

skeleton — the bony support of the body.

solution — liquid containing dissolved substances.

specimen — a sample of material taken from the patient's body. Examples are urine specimens, feces specimens, and sputum specimens.

sperm — a tiny tadpole-like structure capable of causing conception, or the beginning of a baby, if it fuses with a mature egg or ovum.

sphincter — a ringlike muscle that controls the opening and closing of a body opening. An example is the anal sphincter.

sphygmomanometer — an apparatus for taking a patient's blood pressure.

spinal cord — one of the main organs of the nervous system. The spine is another name for the human backbone. The spinal cord is inside the spine. The spinal cord carries messages from the brain to other parts of the body and from parts of the body back to the brain.

spleen — an abdominal organ that manufactures blood cells during the life of the embryo.

splint — a thin piece of wood or other rigid material used to keep an injured part, such as a broken bone, in place.

spores — bacteria that have formed hard shells around themselves for protection. Spores can be destroyed only by sterilization.

sputum — waste material coughed up from the lungs or trachea.

staphylococcus — one type of infection found in health care institutions. Antibiotic drugs are used to fight staphylococcus infections.

sterilization — the process of destroying all microorganisms including spores.

stethoscope — an instrument that allows one to listen to various sounds in the patient's body, such as the heartbeat or breathing sounds.

stimulus — a change in the external or internal environment that is strong enough to set up a nervous impulse.

stoma — an artificially made opening connecting a body passage with the outside, such as in a tracheotomy or colostomy.

stomach — the part of the digestive tract between the esophagus (food pipe) and the duodenum. The stomach churns food and starts the process of digestion.

stroke — a sudden and severe attack such as apoplexy or paralysis. A paralytic stroke is a sudden attack of paralysis caused by injury to the brain or spinal cord. Strokes caused by damage to the blood vessels in the brain are sometimes called cerebrovascular accidents.

subjective reporting — giving your opinion about what you have observed.

suction — the action of, or capacity for, sucking up. This is accomplished by reducing the air pressure over part of the surface of a substance.

supine — lying on one's back.

suppository — a semisolid preparation (sometimes medicated) that is inserted into the vagina or the rectum.

surgical asepsis — when an area is made completely free of microorganisms. The area may be called surgically clean.

surgical procedure — the repair of an injury or a disease condition. In a surgical procedure, the surgeon usually makes an incision—that is, he cuts through the skin into the body.

symptom — evidence of a disease, disorder, or condition.

synovial fluid — a watery substance secreted by the epithelium that lines the joint capsule and fills the capsule to keep the ends of the bones in a healthy condition.

syringe — an instrument used for injecting liquids into body vessels and cavities or for drawing substances out of body tissues.

system — a group of organs acting together to carry out one or more body functions.

systolic blood pressure — the force with which blood is pumped when the heart muscle is contracting. When taking a patient's blood pressure, the top number is recorded.

T

taut — pulled or drawn tight. Not slack.

temperature — a measurement of the amount of heat in the body at a given time. The normal body temperature for an adult is 98.6°F (37°C).

tendons — tough cords of connective tissue that bind muscles to other body parts.

testes — a pair of reproductive organs in the male which lie in the scrotum hanging from the perineal area, dorsal to the penis.

testicles — another word for testes.

therapeutic — refers mainly to the treatment of disease. Something that helps heal.

thermometer — an instrument used for measuring body temperature.

thyroid — an endocrine gland, located in the front of the neck. It regulates body metabolism. This gland secretes a hormone known as thyroxine.

tissue — a group of cells of the same type.

tissue fluid — a watery environment around each cell that acts as a place of exchange for gases, food, and waste products between the cells and the blood.

tongue depressor — a flat blade-like instrument used to keep the patient's tongue flattened during an examination of the throat and mouth.

TPR — abbreviation for temperature, pulse, and respiration. Taking a patient's TPR is measuring these three vital signs.

trachea — an organ of the respiratory system. It is located in the throat area. The trachea is commonly called the windpipe.

tracheotomy — a surgical procedure to make an artificial opening in a person's neck connecting his trachea with the outside. This operation may be necessary when the person's trachea above the opening is blocked and he can't breathe.

traction device — equipment for pulling and stretching parts of the patient's body by using pulleys and weights. Traction is used to keep broken bones properly lined up while they are healing.

transfer — moving a hospital patient from one patient unit to another.

trapeze — a metal bar suspended over the bed. It is used by a patient to help him raise or move his body more easily.

traumatic — refers to damage to the body caused by injury, wound, or shock. Sometimes used to refer to mental disturbances caused by emotional shock.

Trendelenburg's position — the bed or operating table is tilted so the patient's head is about a foot below the level of the knees. This position is used to get more blood to the head and prevent shock. Also called the *shock position*.

tumor — a growth in or on the body. There are two kinds: 1) benign tumors, which grow slowly and can usually be removed by surgery; 2) malignant tumors, which grow wildly and are sometimes called "cancer." They often are a threat to a person's life, as well as to his health.

turning frames — reversible beds used in the care of patients with certain orthopedic conditions.

U

umbilical cord — a rather long, flexible, round organ that carries nourishment from the mother to the baby. It connects the umbilicus of the unborn baby in the mother's uterus to the placenta.

umbilicus — a small depression on the stomach that marks the place where the umbilical cord was originally attached to the fetus. Another name for the umbilicus is the navel.

ureters — tubes leading from the kidney to the bladder.

urethra — the tube leading from the urinary bladder to the outside of the body.

urinal — a portable pan given to male patients in bed so they can urinate without getting out of bed.

urinalysis — a laboratory test of the patient's urine done for diagnostic purposes.

urinary system — the group of organs that have the function of making urine and discharging it from the body.

urinate — to discharge urine from the body. Another word used for this function is void.

uterus — an expandable female reproductive organ in which the fetus grows and is nourished by membranes called the placenta until it is time for the baby to be born.

V

vagina — in the female, the birth canal leading from the vulva to the cervix of the uterus.

vaginal douche — a procedure by which a stream of water is sent into the patient's vaginal opening. The water may be plain or sterile and it may have medication in it.

vaginal prep — the procedures for making the genital area of a female patient ready for surgery. The preparation includes thoroughly cleansing the skin and carefully shaving the pubic hair.

varicose veins — an abnormal swelling of veins, especially veins in the legs.

vas deferens — the tube carrying sperm from the testicles to the glands where they are stored in preparation for ejaculation.

vein — a blood vessel that carries blood from parts of the body back to the heart.

ventricles — the lower two chambers of the heart. They are side by side.

villus — a tiny fingerlike projection in the lining of the small intestine into which the end products of digestion are absorbed and carried to the bloodstream and then to the individual cells.

virus — the microscopic living parasitic agent that can cause infectious disease.

viscera — refers to the organs within the main body cavity.

vital signs — temperature (T), pulse (P), respiration (R), and blood pressure (BP).

void — to urinate, pass water.

vomiting — throwing up; the contents of the stomach are cast up and out of the mouth.

vomitus — material vomited up; emesis.

W

well-balanced diet — a diet containing a variety of foods from each of the basic food groups.

Index

Page numbers followed by the letter **f** indicate illustrations; those followed by the letter **t** indicate tables.

Abbreviations, listed with meanings, 397–401t
  in medical terminology, 397
Abdominal binder, straight. *See* Straight abdominal binder
Abdominal cavity, organs of, 365
Abdominal prep, instructions for, 329, 329f
Accident prevention, 15f
Accuracy, need for, 10
Acetest, testing urine for acetone, 202
Acute illness, 18
Admission checklist, sample, 266
Admitting the patient
  procedure for, 263–266
  procedure for weighing and measuring, 267
  sample admission checklist, 266
  welcome, 263, 264f
Afternoon patient care, schedule of, 124
Air or rubber rings, 68
Alcohol sponge bath (moist cold application)
  procedure for, 319–321, 320f
  reasons for, 318–319
Alertness, need for, 32f
Alternating pressure mattress, 68
Anatomy, 358
Anesthesia, 336–337
  and chest complications in patient, 337
Anesthesiologist, 337
Anesthetics
  effects of, 337
  types of, 336
Anesthetist, 337
Anterior side of body, 364
Antiembolism elastic stockings, applying, 341–342
Apical pulse, 252
  procedure for taking, 252
Apical pulse deficit, 252
  procedure for measuring, 253
Appendicitis, 386
Appendix, 385–386
Aquamatic K-pad (dry heat application)
  procedure for, 298f, 313–314, 314f
Arteries, 381
Artificial eye, 227–229
  procedure for care of, 228–229
Asepsis, 191. *See also* Medical asepsis
  in specimen collection, 191
Aseptic, 43
Aspiration, of food, 382
Autoclave, in medical asepsis, 45, 46f
Autonomic nervous system, involuntary organ activity, 374–375
Axillary temperature, 233
  procedure for taking, 244–245, 248

Back prep, 331, 331f
Back rub, 141
  procedure for, 142–143, 142f, 143f
Bacteria. *See also* Microorganisms
  conditions for growth, 42f
  as microorganisms, 41
Bathing the patient, 130
  rules to follow, 130–131
  types of baths, 130
Bath thermometer, 133f
Battery-operated thermometers. *See* Thermometers, types of
Bed board, 68
Bed cradle, 68
Bedmaking, 71. *See also* specific procedures for bedmaking
  rules to follow, 72–73

tightened sheets, 72f
Bedpan
  procedure for giving, 152–155, 151f, 153f, 154f
  use of, 151, 151f, 152f
Bedsores. *See* Decubitus ulcers
Between-meal nourishments
  offering, 174–175, 175f
  procedure for serving, 174–175, 175f
Binders, 68, 341
  reasons for, 341
  rules to follow, 341
  types of, 341–345
Bladder drainage catheter, 226, 227f
Blood pressure, instruments for measuring, 256–258, 257f, 258f. *See also* Taking blood pressure
Blood pressure cuff. *See* Sphygmomanometer
Blue Code, for dying patient, 352
BM. *See* Feces, in specimen collection
Body cavities, 365, 366f
Body fluids, removed by suction, 287
Body mechanics
  importance of, 95
  rules for, 95–97, 96f, 97f
Body parts, 364–365, 365f
Body systems, 394–395t
Bones. *See also* Skeletal system
  functions of, 368–369
  and ligaments, 362f
  types of, 366, 367f
Bowel movement. *See* Feces, in specimen collection
Brachial pulse, listening to, 258
Brain, 371–375, 375f
Breast binder, 344, 344f
Bronchi, 382
Bursitis, 370

Calibrated graduate, in measuring fluids, 181–182, 181f, 182f
Capillaries, 381
Cartilage, in musculoskeletal system, 369
Catheters
  in measuring urinary output, 187. *See also* Daily catheter care
  and urine containers, 187f
Cells, 358–359, 358f, 361
Celsius. *See* Centigrade
Centigrade (Celsius) temperature, converting to Fahrenheit, 238f.
Centigrade (Celsius) thermometer. *See* Thermometers, types of
Central supply room, 66
  disposable prep kit, 325
  in specimen collection, 193, 202
Cerebellum, in brain, 373
Cerebrum, in brain, 373
Changing the patient's gown, 143
  procedure for, 144–145, 144f, 145f
Chest complications in patient, following anesthesia, 337
Chest prep, for thoracic surgery, 328, 328f
Children, 20–21
  classified by age, 21
  and importance of the family to, 20
  observation of, 35–37
  as pediatric patients, 20, 27–28
  reasons for being in hospital, 20–21
  precautions in patient unit, 65
  safety for, 91, 91f
Chronic illness, 18
Circular turning frame, 70, 70f
Circulatory system, 381
  organs, 381–382, 383f
  root words for, 414t

Clean (uncontaminated), 51
Clean-catch urine specimen. *See* Midstream clean-catch urine specimen
Cleanliness, importance of, 39
Cleansing enema. *See also* Ready-to-use cleansing enema
  procedure for, 210–214, 210f, 211f, 213f, 214f
  purpose of, 209
  ready-to-use, 214
  solution for, 210, 212f
Clean (uncontaminated) utility room, 53
Clinistix, used in testing urine for sugar, 202, 204
Clinistix test, procedure for, 205–206
Clinitest, testing urine for sugar, 202
Clinitest tablets, used in testing urine for sugar, 202, 204
Clitoris, in female reproductive system, 390, 391f, 392f
Closed bed, procedure for making, 73–80, 73f–79f
Cold applications, 293–295
  checking, 299
  equipment, 294f, 295
  length of time, 299
  patient comfort, 299–300
  patient safety, 299
  principle of, 296f
  signs of cyanosis, 299, 300f
  temperature control, 296
Cold compress (moist cold application)
  procedure for, 302–304, 303f, 304f
Cold soak (moist cold application), procedure for, 304–305
Colon, 385
Colostomy, 222–223, 223f
  procedure for care of, 224–225
Combing the patient's hair, 148
  procedure, 148f, 149
Commercial unit cold pack (dry cold application), procedure for, 310–311, 310f
Commercial unit heat pack (moist warm application), procedure for, 311–312
Communicable conditions
  and precautions, 53–58
  and preventive measures, 51
  special hospital areas for, 53
  and use of face masks, 53–54
Communicable diseases, 51. *See also* Diseases
Communicating
  with patients and other people, 29–31
  qualities for, 30–31
Community agencies assisting patient after discharge, 4
Complete bed bath, procedure for, 131–137, 132f, 134f–136f
Connective tissue, 360f, 361f
Contaminated linen, double-bagging technique, 58f
Contamination
  by disease germs, 51f
  in patient unit, 51
Cool wet pack (moist cold application), procedure, 314–315
Coronary care unit, 22
Coronary thrombosis, 382
Counting respirations, 253–255
  procedure, 255
Courtesy, importance of, 24
Cranial cavity, 365
Crisis intervention center, 21
Cross infection, 45
Cyanosis, signs of
  in cold applications, 299, 300f
  in shock, 394
Cystitis, 388

Daily catheter care, 226
  procedure for, 226–227
Daily patient care schedule, 123–124
Decubitus ulcers, 158, 158f
  causes, 158–159
  prevention of, 160, 160f
  in the incontinent patient, 161
  treatment of, 159
Deep-breathing exercises
  in postoperative nursing care, 337–338
  procedure for helping the patient, 337–338
Dentures, procedure for cleaning, 126–128, 127f
Dependability, meaning of, 10
Diabetes mellitus
  and related terms, 379
  signs and symptoms of, 378
Diabetic coma, signs and symptoms of, 380
Diabetic patients
  diagnostic tests on urine, 202
  testing urine for sugar and acetone, 202
Diaphragm, 365
Diastolic blood pressure, 256
Diets for patients, 166t. *See also* Therapeutic diets
Digestive system
  function of, 384
  organs of, 384–386, 386f
  root words, 414–415t
Dirty (contaminated), 51
Dirty utility room (contaminated), 53
Discharge planning. *See* Patient discharge planning
Discharging the patient, 271–272, 271f–273f
  procedure for, 272–273, 271f–273f
  using a wheelchair, 273f
Diseases. *See also* Communicable diseases
  caused by microorganisms, 40f, 41
  and diagnoses, word elements for, 416–419
  and importance of medical asepsis, 45–46
  types of, classified by cause, 18t
Disinfection, 44
  as a method of killing microorganisms, 44
Disposable equipment
  from central supply room, 66
  compared with standard equipment, 66, 66f
  in health care institutions, 66
Disposable prep kit, 327f
Disposable sitz bath (moist warm application), procedure for, 315–317, 316f
Dorsal cavity of the body, 365
Dorsal lithotomy position, 281, 281f
Dorsal recumbent position, 282, 282f
Double T binder, 343
Draping the patient for physical examination, 279f–283f
Drinking water, passing. *See* Passing drinking water
Dry applications, 297–298, 298f. *See also* specific types of
  types of, 297
Duodenum, 384
Dying patient
  caring for, 347–352
  emotional needs of, 347
  and family members, 348
  general instructions for, 347–349
  mouth care for, 351
  observations, 351
  postmortem care of, 352–356
  routine personal care, 349–350
  rules to follow, 349–351

signs of approaching death, 351–352
spiritual support for, 350
unconscious, 348
visitors of, 349

Ear, anatomy of, 378f
Edema, 178
Elastic bandages, 343, 345f
procedure for applying, 345–346
Elastic stockings, purpose of, 341, 345f
Electricity, misuses of, 93f
Emergency department, 22
Emergency patients, 22–23
Emotional control, 24, 24f
Endocrine glands, secreting hormones, 376, 379f
Endocrine system, root words for, 415t
Enemas. See also Cleansing enema; Specific types of enemas
preoperative preparations, 330–331, 331f
Enteric precautions, 54f
Epidermis, 394
Epithelial tissue, types of, 360f, 361f
Equipment, large, used in patient care, 60–70, 67f, 69f
Ethical behavior, code for, 12
Evening patient care, schedule for, 124
Excretory system, 387–388
Eye, anatomy of, 377f

Face mask. See also Mask techinque.
for communicable conditions, 53–54, 55f
Fahrenheit temperature, converting to centigrade, 238f
Fahrenheit thermometer. See Thermometers, types of
Family teaching, responsibility of professional nurse, 4
Feces, in specimen collection, 190
Feeding the helpless patient
preparations for, 170–171
procedure for, 171–174, 171f–173f
Female pelvic organs, 391f
Female reproductive organs, external, 392f
Fermentation, caused by microbes, 41
Fertilization and cell division, 388–390, 391f
Fire emergency procedures, 94f
Fire safety and prevention, rules for, 91–92, 91f, 92f
Fluid balance, in patient's body, 177–179, 178f
Fluid imbalance, in patient's body, 178, 178f
Fluid intake, 178. See also Measuring fluid intake
force fluids, 183–184
by mouth, 179–180, 180f
measuring, 179–181, 182–183, 181f
Fluid output, 178, 186
measuring, 186–187
Food service, therapeutic diets, 163, 165, 169f
Foot board, 68
Force fluids
measuring, 183–184, 184f
rules to follow, 184
Fowler's position, 282, 282f
Fresh fractional urine (FrU) specimen, procedure for collecting, 203–204
Frontal lobe, 373
Full diet. See Regular diet
Full-term babies, 20
Fungi, as microorganisms, 41

Gastrointestinal system. See Digestive system

Generalized warm and cold applications, 296, 297f
Geriatric patients, 22
Germs, See Microorganisms
Greek and Latin words, 413–415t

Handwashing, 47f–50f
in medical asepsis, 46–48
in prevention of disease and infection, 46
procedure for, 49–50
in specimen collection, 191
Harris flush (return-flow enema), 218–219
irrigation of rectum, 218–219
procedure for, 219–220
Head nurse, 2, 4
Health care institutions, 1
infection control in, 39–40
organization chart, 2f
and orientation for nursing aide, 1–2, 4–5
Health care team, nursing personnel, 2
Heart
anatomy, 380f
in circulatory system, 381–382
Heat cradle, 68
Heat lamp (dry warm application)
procedure for, 312–313, 312f
used as perineal lamp, 313
Helping a patient back into bed from a chair or wheelchair, procedure for, 115–116, 116f
Helping a patient into a chair or wheelchair, procedure for, 112–114, 113f, 114f
Helping the patient to stand, procedure for, 99–100, 99f, 100f
Hemispheres of the brain, 373
Hemorrhoids, 386
High blood pressure, 256
High Fowler's position. See Fowler's position
Horizontal recumbent position, 279, 279f
Hormones, 376
Hospital safety
general rules for, 89–94, 89f, 90f
side rails on bed, 90f
House diet. See Regular diet
Human rights of patients, 12
Hypertension. See High blood pressure
Hypotension. See Low blood pressure
Hypothalmus, and control of hormones, 377

I and O. See Intake and output
Ice bag, ice cap, ice collar (dry cold application), procedure for, 308–310, 309f, 310f
Incidents, 14
Incubators, for premature babies, 20
Infants, 21
observation of, 35–37
Infection
staphylococcus, 43
streptococcus, 43
Infection control
in health care institutions, 39–40
history of, 43–44
and medical asepsis, 44
Infections, communicable, 51
Inferior body areas (close to feet), 365
Insulin shock, signs and symptoms, 379–380
Intake and output
fluid balance, 177–179
recording on intake and output sheet, 179, 179f
recording postoperative patient's urine, 335
Integumentary system, 393, 393f
root words for, 413t
Intensive care unit, 22
Intestines, 385, 387f, 388f

Intravenous equipment, 284, 284f
and changing the patient's gown, 285
checking, 285f, 286f
observing and reporting, 286
rules to follow, 285–286
Intravenous poles, 67–68, 69f
Intravenous tubing, 284
Irregular pulse, reporting, 251
Irrigation of the rectum, 218–219
Isolation, 52, 52f
patient care in, 50–55
types of, 52f
Isolation gowns
and caring for patients in isolation, 55, 57
individual gown technique, 57, 57f
removing, procedure for, 58
types of, 55
Isolation technique, 50
"clean" and "dirty," 51, 53
for patient unit, 51
Isolation unit, 61
IV equipment. See Intravenous equipment

Joints (motion), 369–370

Ketostix, used in testing urine for acetone, 202
Ketostix reagent strip test, procedure for, 206–207, 207f
Kidneys, 387
Knee-chest position, 283, 283f

Labor and delivery rooms, 20
Labstix, used in testing urine for acetone and sugar, 202
Lamb's wool, 68
Larynx, 382
Latin words, 413–415
Leader. See Team leader
Left lateral position, 282, 282f
Left Sims' position, 283, 283f
Legal aspects of nursing care, 12–13
Licensed practical nurse (LPN), 4, 5f
as member of nursing care team, 4
qualifications, 5
Licensed vocational nurse (LVN), 5
Lifting patients, 97
procedures, 96f, 98–100, 98f–100f
Ligaments
and bones, 362f
in musculoskeletal system, 369
Lister, Joseph, in history of infection control, 43
Litter. See Stretcher
Liver, 385
Localized warm and cold applications, 296, 297f
Locking arms with the patient, procedure for, 98, 98f
Logrolling. See Rolling the patient
Low blood pressure, 256
Lungs, 382

Male reproductive organs, 392f
Malpractice, 13
Many-tailed binder. See Scultetus binder
Mask technique, procedure for, 55
Measuring blood pressure. See Blood pressure; Taking blood pressure
Measuring fluid intake. See also Fluid intake
importance of, 179–181
intake and output sheet, 182t
intravenous fluids, 182
preparations and steps for, 182–183
procedure for, 183
procedure for determining amounts, 183

recording, 182
Measuring fluid output, procedure for, 186–187
Measuring fluids
in calibrated containers, 181f, 182f
in cubic centimeters, 180–181
rules to follow, 181–182
Measuring urinary output
catheter drainage, 187
procedure for, 186
Medical asepsis, 45, 191
in infection control, 44
purposes of, 45–46
reasons for, 45–46
rules to follow, 46–48
Medical specialties, 420–422t
and physicians' titles, 420–422t
Medical-surgical patients, 18
Medical terminology, guide to pronunciation, 401–402, 402t
Medical terms, 413
in diseases and diagnoses, 416–419
and Latin and Greek root words, 413–415t
prefixes for, 401
similarity between, 405–406
suffixes for, 401
word elements, 401–416
for diseases and diagnoses, 416–419
Menstrual cycle, 390f
Menstruation, 389
Mental illness, 22
Menu card, 170f
Microbes. See Microorganisms
Microorganisms, 39f
and cause of disease, 41
entering the body, 41f
everywhere, 44f
harmful, 41, 43
helpful, 41
nature of, 41, 43
types of, 40f, 41
ways of spreading, 45
Microscope, 39f
Midstream clean-catch urine specimen, procedure for collecting, 193–195
Modified diet. See Therapeutic diets
Moist applications, 297–298, 298f
types of, 297
Morning patient care, schedule, 124
Mouth, organs of, 385f
Moving the helpless patient
to and from bed to stretcher, procedure for, 119–122, 121f
up in bed, procedure for, 101–102, 101f
to side of bed, procedure for, 106–107, 106f
into a wheelchair, procedure for, 113f, 114–115
Moving the mattress to the head of the bed with patient's help, procedure for, 103–104, 104f
Moving patient to head of bed with his help, procedure for, 102f, 103
Muscles, coordination of, 370f
Muscle tissue, 359f, 362, 363f, 364f
involuntary, 363–364
voluntary, 362–363
Muscular system, 371
Musculoskeletal system, root words for, 413–414t
Myocardial infarction, 382

Nasal cannulas, 288, 288f
Nasal catheter, 288, 288f
Nasogastric tubes, 286–287, 287f
rules to follow, 286
Negligence, 12–13
Neonates. See Newborn babies
Nerve tissue, types of, 359f
Nervous system, 371, 372f
root words, 415t
Neuron, 371, 373f